Intellectual Disability and Ill Health

A Review of the Evidence

Edited by

Jean O'Hara
Kings College London

Jane McCarthy
Kings College London

Nick Bouras
Kings College London

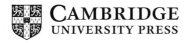

CAMBRIDGE
UNIVERSITY PRESS

CAMBRIDGE UNIVERSITY PRESS
Cambridge, New York, Melbourne, Madrid, Cape Town, Singapore,
São Paulo, Delhi, Dubai, Tokyo

Cambridge University Press
The Edinburgh Building, Cambridge CB2 8RU, UK

Published in the United States of America by
Cambridge University Press, New York

www.cambridge.org
Information on this title: www.cambridge.org/9780521728898

First published 2010

Printed in the United Kingdom at the University Press, Cambridge

*A catalogue record for this publication is available from the
British Library*

ISBN 978-0-521-72889-8 Paperback

Additional resources for this publication at
www.cambridge.org/9780521728898

362
2
OHA

Intellectual Disability and Ill Health

Contents

Contributors

Alaa Al-Sheikh MRCPsych
Locum Consultant Psychiatrist in Learning Disabilities, South London and Maudsley NHS Foundation Trust, Croydon, Surrey, UK.

Simon Bonell BSc (Hons.), MBBS, MRCPsych
Specialist Registrar, Psychiatry of Learning Disabilities, Oxleas Mental Health Trust, Greenwich CTLD, London, UK.

Nick Bouras MD, PhD, FRCPsych
Professor Emeritus, Institute of Psychiatry, King's College London David Goldberg Centre, Denmark Hill, London, UK.

Merlin G. Butler MD, PLD, FFACMG
Professor of Psychiatry, Behavioral Sciences and Pediatrics, ABMG Certified Clinical Geneticist and Clinical Cytogeneticist, Departments of Psychiatry and Behavioral Sciences and Pediatrics, University of Kansas Medical Center, Kansas City, Kansas, USA.

Basil Cardoza MBBS, DPM, MRCPsych
Consultant Psychiatrist Learning Disability Directorate, Abertawe Bro Morgannwg University NHS Trust, Caerau, Cardiff, UK.

Wai-Him Cheung
Kwai Chung Hospital, Kwai Chung, Hong Kong, China.

Robert W. Davis PhD, MBBS, FRACGP, Dip (Obst) RACOG, GDEB
Associate Professor Director, The Centre for Developmental Disability Health, Victoria School of Primary Health Care, Monash University Notting Hill, Victoria, Australia.

Shoumitro Deb MBBS, FRCPsych, MD
Clinical Professor of Neuropsychiatry and Intellectual Disability, Department of Psychiatry, University of Birmingham, National Centre for Mental Health, Birmingham, UK.

Neil A. Douglas MBBS, MSc, MRCGP, DCH, DCCH
General Practitioner and Honorary Clinical Lecturer, Barts and The London Hospital Medical College, Isle of Dogs, London, UK.

Maeve Eogan MD, MRCPI, MRCOG
Consultant Obstetrician and Gynaecologist, Rotunda Hospital, Dublin 1, Ireland.

Stefano Fedele DDS, PhD
Clinical Lecturer, UCL Eastman Dental Institute, London, UK.

William I. Fraser MD, FRCPsych, DPM
Professor, Welsh Centre for Learning Disabilities, Cardiff University Cardiff, UK.

John A. Grant MB, BCh, FRCS(C), FACS
Professor, Departments of Neurosurgery, History and Philosophy of Medicine, University of Kansas Medical Center, Kansas City, Kansas, USA.

Jessica A. Hellings MD
Associate Professor of Psychiatry, Department of Psychiatry and Behavioral Sciences, University of Kansas Medical Center, Kansas City, Kansas, USA.

Muthukumar Kannabiran MBBS, DPM, MRCPsych
Specialist Registrar, Mental Health in Learning Disability, South London and Maudsley NHS Foundation Trust, York Clinic, Guy's Hospital, London, UK.

Mike Kerr MBCHB, MRCGP, MRCPsych, MPhil, MSc
Professor of Learning Disabilities, Welsh Centre for Learning Disabilities, Cardiff University, Cardiff, UK.

Henry Kwok FRCPsych (UK), FHKAMP (Psychiatry), FHKCPsych (Hong Kong, China)
Psychiatric Unit for Learning Disabilities, Kwai Chung Hospital, Kwai Chung, Hong Kong, China.

Stefano Lassi MD
Psychiatrist, ODA Diacceto, Diacceto (Fi), Italy.

Lynette Lee FAFRM (RACP), FRACMA
Associate Professor, Staff Specialist, Rehabilitation Medicine and Disability Health Centre for Education and Research on Ageing, Concord Hospital, Concord, Australia.

Jane McCarthy MB, ChB, MRCGP, FRCPsych, MD
Consultant Psychiatrist and Visiting Research Associate Estia Centre, Institute of Psychiatry, King's College London York Clinic, Guy's Hospital, London, UK.

Seth A. Mensah MB ChB MSc DPM MRCPsych
Neuropsychiatrist, Welsh Neuropsychiatry Service, Cardiff and Vale NHS Trust Whitchurch Hospital, Cardiff, UK.

Joav Merrick MD, MMedSci, DMSc
Professor of Pediatrics, Child Health and Human Development Office of the Medical Director, Division for Mental Retardation, Ministry of Social Affairs, Jerusalem, Israel.

Mohammed Morad MD
Senior Lecturer and Medical Director, Clalit Health Services Shatal Clinic, Rehov Similanski, Beer Sheva, Israel.

Jean O'Hara MBBS, FRCPsych
Consultant Psychiatrist, Clinical Director and Visiting Research Associate Estia Centre, Institute of Psychiatry, Kings College London York Clinic, Guy's Hospital, London, UK.

Vishwa Radhakrishnan MD, MRCPsych
Specialist Registrar, Mental Health in Learning Disability, Maudsley and South East London rotational training scheme, Bassetts Resource Centre, Bromley, UK.

Stephen Reudrich MD
Associate Professor of Psychiatry, Department of Psychiatry, MetroHealth Medical Center, Cleveland Ohio, USA.

Norman Sartorius, MD, PhD, FRCPsych
Professor, President of the International Association for the Promotion of Mental Health Programmes.

Crispian Scully CB, MD, PhD, MDS, MRCS, BSc
Professor, Dean and Director of Studies and Research, UCL Eastman Dental Institute, London, UK.

Muhunthan Thillai BA, MBBS, MRCP
Wellcome Trust Research Training Fellow and Specialist Registrar in Respiratory Medicine, Tuberculosis Research Unit, Department of Respiratory Medicine, National Heart and Lung Institute, Wright-Fleming Institute of Infection and Immunity, Imperial College London, Norfolk Place, London, UK.

Jennifer Torr MBBS, MMed(Psychiatry), FRANZCP, Member FPOA GCHE
Director of Mental Health, Centre for Developmental Disability Health, Monash University Building One, Omnico Business Centre, 270 Ferntree Gully Rd, Notting Hill, Victoria, Australia.

Mary Wingfield MD, FRCOG
Consultant Obstetrician and
Gynaecologist, National Maternity
Hospital, Dublin 2, Ireland.

J. Margaret Woodhouse BSc, PhD
Senior Lecturer and Optometrist, School of
Optometry and Vision Sciences, Cardiff
University, Cardiff, UK.

Foreword

It is a great pleasure to see this volume in print not only because of the excellent quality of the contributions included in the volume and its comprehensive coverage of the subject, but also because this book is a further important contribution to the resolution of the problems arising because of co-morbidity between mental and physical disorders – one of the most serious problems in the field of health today.

The first book in the series that was initiated by the Association for the Improvement of Mental Health programmes dealt with schizophrenia and medical illness[1] and three further volumes are to appear after the volume that is presented here. These will deal with problems of co-morbidity in people with dementia, those with depression and those with problems related to the abuse of alcohol and drugs. It is possible that other volumes will follow: for the time being we have decided to concentrate on the most prevalent problems related to mental health and functioning.

Intellectual disability certainly belongs to that group of disorders. The estimates of prevalence and incidence of intellectual disability (under its various names) show it to be frequent in all countries and particularly in those that are poor and in the process of industrial development. What makes the problem even more important for public health is that the consequences of cognitive deficit of any type are becoming more and more a concern because of the constant growth of complexity of the world that surrounds us and that few of the numerous measures that could be taken (even in very poor countries) to prevent the occurrence of intellectual disability are used.

Those three characteristics – high frequency with potentially grave consequences, tendency of growth of the problem and the availability of effective measures of its prevention – should give intellectual disability a much higher priority for public health action. Unfortunately in most countries of the world this is not the case at present.

Problems related to intellectual disability are further complicated by the fact that people who have it are also at a higher risk for various forms of ill health. The reasons for this are many and range from genetic predisposition and neglect in childhood to discrimination in health services and self-neglect in later years. Two important components of the problem are that health authorities are often not aware of the frequency of co-morbidity between intellectual disability and ill health and that the current organisation of health services – with the significant distance between mental and physical illness services – does not provide comprehensive care to people with more than one health problem.

Care for people with intellectual disability requires – even more than care for people with mental health problems – a willing and intensive alliance between the health sector and other social sectors such as education and social welfare. The creation of such an alliance should be complemented by reforms of health services that will ensure that people who come forward to seek help get comprehensive care rather than partial responses to their problems. It is my hope that this volume – and the others in this series – will contribute to raising awareness of all concerned about the need for such alliances and reforms of health services. The realisation of this hope would not only improve the quality of life of people with intellectual disability, it would also be a most desirable reward to the many who have contributed their excellent chapters to this volume.

Professor Norman Sartorius MD, PhD, FRCPsych
President,
International Association for the Promotion of Mental Health Programmes

---

[1] Leucht, S. Burkard, T., Henderson, J. H. and Maj, M. (2007). *Physical illness and schizophrenia*. A Review of the Evidence. Cambridge: Cambridge University Press.

Preface

The key aim of this book is to provide a comprehensive and systematic review of the evidence base on the ill health of people with intellectual disability.

We have invited authors from around the world to contribute to the book to reflect the growing awareness of the health needs of people with intellectual disability across many countries.

The term intellectual disability as used in this book is the terminology used by the American Association on Intellectual and Developmental Disabilities, the European Association of Mental Health in Intellectual Disability, the International Association for the Scientific Study of Intellectual Disability and the World Psychiatric Association. Intellectual disability is defined as significant intellectual impairment, that is intelligence quotient (IQ) score below 70, with significant impairment of adaptive functioning, and is a disorder of early life occurring in the critical developmental period before adulthood. The terms intellectual disability, mental retardation, learning disability, developmental disability and moderate to severe learning difficulties are interchangeable. The International Classification of Diseases (ICD-10)[1] is the diagnostic classification system most often used worldwide followed by the Diagnostic and Statistical Manual of Mental Disorders (DSM-IV).[2] Both these classification systems use the term 'mental retardation' to refer to intellectual disability. Diagnostic systems have now been specifically developed for use with people with intellectual disability which are discussed in the relevant chapters of the book. The book has attempted to keep within the diagnostic categories of ICD-10.

People with intellectual disability are a heterogeneous group and so their health outcomes vary considerably with the severity of the impairment of their functioning, the aetiology of their intellectual disability, their risk for ill-health problems and environmental factors including access to health care. The book has therefore been divided into three sections with the first section looking at health needs and the causes of intellectual disability. This is in order to summarise the public health needs to policy makers, health authorities and service managers, so highlighting the critical importance of preventative health measures for this population. The focus is not only primary prevention but secondary and tertiary prevention of ill health which is covered in the review of the evidence base in the second and third sections in this book.

The second section of the book covers the major diseases and organ systems so giving a useful summary of the evidence on physical ill-health problems seen in people with intellectual disability. This section will be particularly useful to healthcare practitioners in primary care services and physicians in hospital- and clinic-based practice.

The third section covers mental illness and neurological and developmental disorders and contains the chapters with the largest evidence base available, partially due to higher prevalence of these disorders in people with intellectual disability. This section will be very useful for psychiatrists, neurologists, paediatricians and primary care physicians.

There is variation across the chapters in terms of length and focus, which is mainly a reflection of the evidence base available on specific disorders. Also we have allowed overlap, for example the ill health found in people with Down syndrome cuts across the chapters on infectious diseases, immune disorders, respiratory diseases and neurodegenerative disorders. Infectious diseases have a dedicated chapter but are also important in the chapters on aetiology of intellectual disability, gastrointestinal diseases and are a leading cause of mortality in respiratory diseases.

The book starts with a chapter by Jean O'Hara which gives an in-depth overview of the healthcare issues for people with intellectual disability, specifically the inequalities they experience and why it is essential to present the evidence base in a way that can be used by clinicians in their daily practice to influence not only the care they provide but the wider public health agenda for people with intellectual disability. This book is one of the first to attempt this task and is part of a series initiated by the International Association for the Promotion of Mental Health Programmes.

Finally, we would like to thank all our contributors and Lisa Underwood for her assistance in helping us with the final editing process.

Jean O'Hara, Jane McCarthy and Nick Bouras

---

[1] World Health Organization (1992). *The ICD-10 Classification of Mental and Behavioural Disorders.* Geneva: World Health Organization.
[2] American Psychiatric Association (1994). *Diagnostic and Statistical Manual of Mental Disorders: Fourth Edition.* Washington DC: American Psychiatric Association.

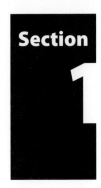

Section 1

Health care and aetiology

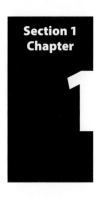

**Section 1
Chapter**

1

Health care and aetiology

Health care and intellectual disability

Jean O'Hara

Introduction

Although the presence of intellectual disability (ID) per se is not usually regarded as a health problem, the biopsychosocial implications of cognitive impairment contribute to the vulnerability of people with ID in any healthcare system (Wallace and Beange, 2008). The evidence for differences in health determinants, morbidity and mortality profiles and in the ability to access quality health care as compared to the general population is well established. This disparity cannot be explained by social deprivation or biological variations alone (Mencap, 2007; Stoddart *et al.*, 2005). People with ID are more likely to have significant health needs that may go unrecognised and untreated because of communication difficulties, diagnostic overshadowing, discrimination or indifference (Cumella and Martin, 2004; Disability Rights Commission, 2006; Health Care Commission, 2007; Michael, 2008). There is concern that public health measures aimed at reducing mortality in the general population will not address the main healthcare issues for people with ID and indeed may preferentially widen the inequality that already exists (Cooper *et al.*, 2004; NHS Health Scotland, 2004). Therefore, understanding the specific health needs of people with ID, including the impact of gender (O'Hara J, 2008a), ethnicity (McCarthy *et al.*, 2008) and physical and mental co-morbidities and how they determine care pathways is urgently needed.

Health indicators are being developed across nations in the hope of improving knowledge about people with ID worldwide (Scholte, 2008; Walsh, 2008; Walsh *et al.*, 2003). This chapter gives an overview of the main issues concerning health care in people with ID over the last decade.

Method

A search was made from a merged access to EMBASE, MEDLINE, PsycINFO and CINAHL (1967–2008), to find publications on the association between intellectual disabilities and physical illness or health care. The MeSH terms used were 'intellectual disability/disabilities', 'mental retardation', 'learning disability/disabilities', 'developmental disability/disabilities', 'healthcare' and 'physical illness'. The first search was made in May 2008 and updated in November 2008. All abstracts found in English were read. There was no restriction on age. Main ID journals published in the past year were hand searched, complemented by reference lists, good practice guidelines and government publications.

Intellectual Disability and Ill Health: A Review of the Evidence, ed. Jean O'Hara, Jane McCarthy and Nick Bouras. Published by Cambridge University Press. © Cambridge University Press 2010.

Table 1.1. Search results for health care and intellectual disabilities

MeSH headings: intellectual disability/disabilities, mental retardation, learning disability, developmental disability, healthcare, physical illness	Number of references	
	Before screen	After screen
Hand-searched journals, good practice guidance (2008)	–	34
Total number of references	482	106

Results

A total of 482 abstracts were found from the electronic searches. All were considered and grouped into themes for discussion. Following an evidence-based screen, 72 articles were read and an additional 34 articles were included through a hand search of journals and good practice guidance (see Table 1.1).

Discussion

The published evidence base available, predominantly from the last decade, is categorised into the following areas, acknowledging a degree of overlap:

a. Healthcare utilisation and inequalities
b. Service standards and quality issues
c. Competencies and identifying needs/support needs
d. User-led approaches and healthcare decision-making
e. Issues of transition
f. Service organisation and commissioning.

Healthcare utilisation and inequalities

Studies have suggested that mortality rates are higher for all age groups of people with ID compared to the general population. Specific risk factors influencing life expectancy include lower IQ, immobility, epilepsy, poor nutrition and low levels of verbal communication (Chaney and Eyman, 2000; Hollins *et al.*, 1998). The majority of adults with ID have a constellation of negative health determinants, including minimal education, low income, unemployment and poorly developed social networks, which are risk factors in their own right for poorer health outcome. The presence of cognitive impairment often means that people with ID have little capacity to overcome this (Wallace and Beange, 2008). Recognition of health needs requires regular assessment and reassessment (Kerr *et al.*, 2003; Lennox *et al.*, 2001) as well as initiatives to help increase health literacy in people with ID. Dodd and Brunker (1999) describe teaching body awareness and communication aids to help people with ID communicate with primary care teams, as well as facilitating an understanding of going to the doctor. The Books Beyond Words series (Hollins) has also helped bridge this gap for a range of health and life experience issues affecting people with ID.

Kerr *et al.*. (2003) reported that satisfactory health care can best be achieved by facilitated access to specialist services, monitoring and regular reassessments with reports clearly explained to carers. A cluster randomised controlled trial in Australia on annual health screening of 453 adults with ID using CHAP (Comprehensive Health Assessment Programme) found increased health promotion, disease prevention, detection of new disease and enhanced interaction between the adult with ID, their carer and their primary care physician (Lennox *et al.*, 2007). The authors suggest that the CHAP process alleviated barriers to health care and facilitated contact with primary care physicians who were then prompted to address known potential unmet health needs. It was also likely that CHAP assisted the transfer of information over time in services often characterised by high staff turnover. Cooper *et al.* (2006) demonstrated sustained benefits in health outcomes one year after a health screening intervention, with increased levels of met health need and increased levels of met new health needs compared to a control group. In the United States, Levy *et al.* (2006) call for a re-examination of healthcare needs of people with ID in community settings, with particular emphasis on integration of healthcare and psychiatric services. Lin *et al.*'s (2005) work on healthcare utilisation of people with ID and psychiatric disorders in Taiwan found that such patients were likely to be in poorer physical health and consume more healthcare resources (inpatients, outpatients and emergency care) than those without psychiatric disorders. Given they were also likely to be taking more medication it is suggested that healthcare systems should develop appropriate healthcare status monitoring and easily accessible mental health services.

Continuing evidence suggests that the prevalence of mental ill health in adults with ID is around 40% using assessment measures specifically aimed at this population (Cooper *et al.*, 2007; Mukherjee, 2007) (please refer to Chapter 16 on Mental illness), whilst children with severe developmental disorders and co-morbid behavioural disorders have significantly higher levels of special healthcare needs (McCarthy and Boyd, 2002). Kennedy *et al.* (2007) found no difference in the number or types of prescription medications the children received compared to children with severe developmental disorders without behavioural problems. They conclude that special healthcare needs may contribute to the occurrence and/or intensity of behavioural disorders in children and may require interdisciplinary care coordination.

However, in some countries the initial recognition of ID and its psychological, socio-economic impact on the individual and family is rare (Lazcano-Ponce *et al.*, 2008) and for many this is accompanied by discrimination, catastrophic costs often not covered by the State, lack of universal access to health care and lack of appropriate educational programmes and social services (Salud Publica de Mexico, 2008). Recent mapping of ID resources in all member states of the World Health Organization (WHO) concluded that there is no country in which a major policy and programme effort is not required (Lecomte and Mercier, 2008; WHO, 2007). Even in countries which have a relatively high standard of living, people with ID are very often denied the opportunity to enjoy the full range of economic, social and cultural rights. Both the WHO atlas-ID (WHO, 2007) and the right to health in international human rights law stress the importance of the underlying determinants of health by looking to the wider socio-economic, political and legal factors including public information and education.

Service standards and quality issues

The inequalities in health care experienced by people with ID have been well established (O'Hara J, 2008a, 2008b), however, recent investigations have highlighted disturbing evidence of discrimination and neglect in our hospitals and communities, with avoidable deaths and missed diagnoses (Health Care Commission, 2006, 2007; Mencap, 2007; Michael, 2008; Wallace and Beange, 2008). Collaborative projects around the world have tried to reach consensual agreement on basic health care (Scholte, 2008) as well as evidence-based health indicators for this population (Walsh *et al.*, 2005). The Pomona group agreed 18 indicators in

4 domains: demographics, health status, determinants and health systems. Pomona Phase II aims to test these indicator sets against a sample of 80 people with ID in each of the participating 17 European countries (www.pomonaproject.org).

In promoting access to health care three important principles underpin best practice and apply to all healthcare staff in contact with people with ID:

- The health needs of people with ID are greater and more complex and often present differently from those of the general population
- People with ID are more likely to have impaired communication and therefore require special consideration
- People with ID have the right to access health services and these should be provided within the current legislative framework.

The European manifesto on basic standards of health care for people with ID is the guiding document in the Netherlands and has been translated into several languages (Scholte, 2008). Its recommendations have now been adopted by the International Association for the Scientific Study of Intellectual Disabilities (IASSID). The five basic standards are:

1. Accessibility of mainstream health service with primary care playing a central role. This means adequate support in communication when needed; no barriers to using mainstream services and the provision of accessible health information and health promotion.
2. Health professionals in mainstream services will have competencies in ID (attitudinal and communication skills being seen as important as clinical skills).
3. Professionals specialised in the specific health needs of people with ID are available as back up to mainstream health services to advise, treat and take over (a part of) the medical care for people with ID if needed.
4. A multidisciplinary approach to specific health assessments and/or treatments if needed.
5. A proactive approach with a right to national screening programmes, implementation of health monitoring programmes and the right to aetiological investigations.

These standards are similar to those endorsed by government strategies in the UK (e.g. Department of Health, 2001; Northern Ireland, 2005; Scottish Executive, 2000; Welsh Assembly, 2004) and are now part of a monitoring process by external regulatory bodies. Basic checks on minimum standards will always be necessary (Campbell, 2008; Caton et al., 2007; O'Hara, 2006), but service excellence requires not only audit but research-driven evaluation (Clegg, 2008). Beadle-Brown et al.'s (2007) review of the process of deinstitutionalisation for ID services across the world cautions that whilst deinstitutionalisation continues to show that outcomes are better in the community than institutional care, there is more to this than just hospital closure. Quality of life includes choice, inclusion and self-identity as well as access to effective health care and treatment.

Competencies and support needs

People with ID are frequent users of general hospital services, often due to their complex and co-morbid health problems (Sowney et al., 2006), yet their length of stay for similar procedures is shorter than for those patients without ID (Morgan et al., 2000). Concerns about the basic competencies and level of training of all healthcare staff have been raised (Disability Rights Commission, 2006; Michael, 2008; Scholte, 2008) and some initiatives have been developed to address this (e.g. Hardy *et al.*, 2007; Hardy and Holt, 2007; Mencap, 2008; O'Hara and Sperlinger, 1997; RCGP 2006; van Schrojenstein Lantman-de Valk and Walsh, 2008) including raising awareness in support staff and family carers (Gratsa *et al.*, 2006; Hardy *et al.*, 2006; Holt and Bouras, 2004; Holt *et al.*, 2004).

Themes from focus groups with accident and emergency nursing staff in Northern Ireland reflected a lack of knowledge about the nature of ID. Staff felt fearful and vulnerable and tended to depend (or over-depend) on carers (Sowney and Barr, 2006), whilst social care staff identified attitudinal problems in some primary care staff (Jones *et al.*, 2008).

A survey in 2006 of six European countries (Finland, Germany, the Netherlands, Norway, Sweden and the UK) and Australia, Canada, Japan and the USA found that attention to the specific health aspects of ID in the total education programme for medical students varied from zero to 36 hours. In most countries there is no specific attention, just general information spread over psychiatry, paediatrics and genetics (Scholte, 2008). The education of doctors may prove to be the most important approach to improving health care for people with ID (Kerr, 2008).

Melville *et al.*'s (2006) pre- and post-intervention study addressing unmet training needs of primary care health professionals reported a statistically significant increase in knowledge and self-efficacy for the intervention group three months after the training event. Lin *et al.*'s (2008) investigation of primary care physicians' beliefs about their perceived role in providing health care to people with ID in Taiwan found they considered their role to be important but felt less satisfied with their ability to treat people with ID and that prior training experience in ID was statistically correlated with better satisfaction ($p < 0.05$). The whole support network plays an important part in recognising need and navigating access to appropriate services. Di Blasi *et al.*'s (2006) qualitative study of community pharmacists once again highlights the need for training and education.

Service provision has at times been subject to philosophical difference and a medical versus social model dichotomy. However, Lopez-Rangel *et al.* (2008) remind us that these need not be mutually exclusive. They emphasise a reciprocal cultural enrichment and cross-fertilisation of ideas and actions between medics and all other professionals and suggest that this is particularly true of the need for genetic diagnosis to optimise health care and function across the lifespan. Indeed, a comprehensive history focusing on health care during the pre-natal, perinatal and postnatal period; physical examination to focus on secondary abnormalities and congenital malformations and the need for neurological, behavioural phenotype, cytogenetics and metabolic evaluations are paramount (Katz and Lazcano-Ponce, 2008).

The interface between physical and mental health needs in people with ID is a common one (Kwok and Cheung, 2007). More recently, studies on substance misuse in people with ID have emphasised the importance of early identification and intervention before long-established patterns of use and associated related behaviours are reported (McCrystal *et al.*, 2007; Taggart *et al.*, 2006). Another focus of recent attention is the changing demographics of the population and the challenges this brings to services that were originally developed for younger adults focused on enabling individuals to lead full and productive lives (Ryan and McQuillan, 2005). Dementia is more prevalent in people with ID (Strydom *et al.*, 2007) and occurs at an earlier age than in the general population (Coppus *et al.*, 2006). Basic competencies in older adult services will be required in the future, or there is a danger of neglect (Fender *et al.*, 2007). Davies (2008) calls for knowledge and skills development to increase confidence in the workplace whilst Alexander *et al.* (2008) emphasise a preventative approach as the ageing process often affects the disabled person earlier.

Likewise, palliative care has been a recent issue to appear in the literature. Jacquemin (2005) investigated experiences of healthcare professionals faced with the death of residents with ID in a care home in Belgium. Tuffrey-Wijne's (2003) review reveals a lack of empirical data around the palliative care needs of people with ID. Potential problems highlighted included late presentation of illness and its implications, ethical issues around decision-making and consent to treatment. A small pilot study by Ng and Li (2003) explored the educational needs of qualified practitioners in ID settings in the South of England and showed major concerns around lack of skills, poor knowledge of psychosocial aspects of care and inconsistent policies. Issues of ID appear to override and obscure physical illness and palliative care needs. Services cannot afford to overlook this important issue any longer (NICE, 2008).

User-led approaches and decision-making

The ethical issues around decision-making and consent to treatment identified earlier have always challenged services. Recent developments in law and health-care policy on mental capacity and decision-making (e.g. Bamford Review, 2007; Keywood and Flynn, 2006; Mental Capacity Act, 2005; Scottish Parliament, 2000) tackle the concept of choice and best interests for vulnerable adults and the importance of creating time to engage and involve them in the decision-making process (Joyce, 2008).

Other initiatives have attempted to gain a better understanding from service users and carers on their experience when seeking primary health care (Jones et al., 2008). Emergent themes included access, communication and waiting around. These issues are not new and may reflect the lack of interest of services in general. Gibbs et al.'s (2008) focus group study of general hospital experiences also emphasise anxiety (often not understanding what the doctor said) and fear (of the unknown or needing to stay in hospital), issues of communication, practicalities of attending or being in hospital, behaviour problems (often caused by anxiety, long waits, the behaviour of others), perceived discrimination and negative comments. Patient safety issues have also been raised by people with ID (NSPA, 2004). Services in Scotland have begun formalising links between ID and hospital services to improve the quality of care and hospital experiences for people with ID (Scottish Executive, 2002). 'What people with disabilities want is an equal outcome – not an equal service' (Kerr, 2008).

Of particular note is the increasing interest in involving people with ID as active participants within the research process, allowing the adoption of research methods that enable and support them (e.g. Gilbert 2004; Lennox et al., 2005; Walmsley, 2004; Young and Chesson, 2007). Tuffrey-Wijne et al. (2008) also discuss the ethics and pitfalls of research into cancers, death and dying arguing that if conducted to the highest ethical standard, it will allow people with ID to be included and listened to when at their most vulnerable.

Transition issues

Healthcare transition is an essential part of healthcare provision. People with ID are particularly vulnerable to communication lapses between services/agencies during hospitalisation and subsequent discharge to home or another care facility – and these lapses can result in poor health outcomes (Brown and Censullo, 2008).

The need to plan for, and address, transition issues in general, especially for children with the most complex needs going into adult services, seems to be particularly problematic (Department of Health, 2008). Wallace and Beange (2008) outline the case for a tertiary model of health care for adults with ID, whilst respecting the principles of normalisation, to mirror the coordinated specialist paediatric services that often exist for children with ID under the age of 18.

There is an increasing awareness of the need to look at transition issues for adults as they age (Davies, 2008; Fender *et al.*, 2007). Further longitudinal studies are also necessary for better understanding of the ageing processes associated with particular syndromes (Schrander-Stumpel *et al.*, 2007).

Service organisation and commissioning issues

There has been controversy over the years about the value of a 'one-stop shop' model of health care, where adults with ID can access all their health needs from one location, rather than using generic healthcare systems. However, current philosophy favours a less institution-alised approach (Wallace and Beange, 2008). It has been suggested that such a model prevents mainstream services from acquiring the necessary skills for working with this population (Mir, 2007) and that traditional community ID teams are running parallel services and inadvertently sustaining this situation (Mencap, 2004). The most significant changes in healthcare delivery have occurred at the primary care level and health checks have been shown to make a real difference, but not enough is being done at a secondary care level (Kerr, 2008). There is little evidence in the literature regarding effective models of healthcare delivery. O'Hara D. (2008) concludes that the breadth of the problem for healthcare systems is not captured by focusing on the relatively small numbers of people with ID and concerns about their physical health care but rather by examining the costs associated with their care, including the healthcare delivery costs due to limited communicative and cognitive abilities.

From a cost-of-illness perspective, Polder *et al.* (2002) showed the cost of mental disorders are by far the largest in the Dutch healthcare system (25.8%), with the cost of ID and schizophrenia higher amongst men, and the cost of dementia and depression higher amongst women. However, demographic projections showed a less than average cost increase for ID and psychiatric disorders (0.2% and 0.4% respectively) compared to the costs of dementia and total health care (1.6% and 0.9% respectively). They caution that non-specific cost containment measures may endanger the quality of care for vulnerable people.

Hassiotis *et al.*'s (2008) investigation into the characteristics of a cohort of people with ID and severe behavioural problems in high-cost out-of-area accommodation from five London boroughs, found that 5% of the total service registered population accounted for 67% of the total expenditure. Spiller *et al.* (2007) also found that a small group of people with ID and mental health problems consumed a large proportion of service resources.

The need for better commissioning of health services for people with ID has recently been acknowledged (Department of Health, 2007a, 2007b; Emerson and Robertson, 2008; Mansell, 2007) at every level of health care. The knowledge and experience required of commissioners is a specialist area and across the world the literature reveals there is a lack of the most basic parameters upon which decisions to develop appropriate and integrated services are made. In some areas this includes basic prevalence rates and associated disabilities (Christianson *et al.*, 2002; O'Hara and Bouras, 2007; Salud Publica de Mexico, 2008).

The challenge for the future is to commission services based on the evidence. This means evidence from experiences of people with ID and their families, through to epidemiological data, health trends, inequalities and service gaps, to effective interventions and service models.

Conclusion

People with ID often do not have the capacity to overcome the constellation of negative health determinants that has been evidenced in the literature. It is incumbent on policy makers, commissioners and providers of health care to ensure that services are easily accessible, meaningful and effective in providing the same healthcare outcomes for people with ID as the general population. There is growing evidence that attitudinal change, education and training across the health economy are vital if this is to be a reality. Patient safety issues, human rights and capacity to determine their own health choices have recently been highlighted, as well as the need to include people with ID in the wider research agenda. The following chapters review the evidence base for a range of neuropsychiatric-related syndromes and organ system disorders as they affect people with ID.

References

Alexander, L. M., Bullock, K. and Maring, J. R. (2008). Challenges in the recognition of age-related conditions in older adults with developmental disabilities. *Top Geriatr Rehabil*, 24(1), 12–25.

Bamford Review of Mental Health and Learning Disability (2007). *A Comprehensive Legislative Framework: Consultation Report*. Belfast: Bamford Review. Available from: www.rmhldni.gov.uk.

Beadle-Brown, J., Mansell, J. and Kozma, A. (2007). Deinstitutionalization in intellectual disabilities. *Curr Opin Psychiatry*, 20(5), 437–42.

Brown, M. C. and Censullo, M. (2008). Supporting safe transitions from home to healthcare settings for individuals with intellectual disabilities. *Top Geriatr Rehabil*, 24(1), 74–82.

Campbell, M. (2008). The importance of good quality services for people with complex health needs. *Br J Learn Disabil*, 36(1), 32–7.

Caton, S., Starling, S., Burton, M., Azmi, S. and Chapman, M. (2007). Responsive services for people with learning disabilities from minority ethnic communities. *Br J Learn Disabil*, 35, 229–35.

Chaney, R. H. and Eyman, R. K. (2000). Patterns in mortality over 60 years among persons with mental retardation in a residential facility. *Ment Retard*, 38, 289–93.

Christianson, A. L., Zwane, M. E., Manga, P. et al. (2002). Children with intellectual disability in rural South Africa: prevalence and associated disability. *J Intellect Disabil Res*, 46(2), 179–86.

Clegg, J. (2008). Holding services to account. *J Intellect Disabil Res*, 52(7), 581–7.

Cooper, S.-A., Melville, C. and Morrison, J. (2004). People with intellectual disabilities: their health needs differ and need to be recognised and met. *BMJ*, 239, 414–15.

Cooper, S.-A., Morrison, J., Melville, C. et al. (2006). Improving the health of people with intellectual disabilities: outcomes of a health screening programme after one year. *J Intellect Disabil Res*, 50, 667–77.

Cooper, S.-A., Smiley, E., Morrison, J., Williamson, A. and Allan, L. (2007). Mental ill health in adults with intellectual disabilities: prevalence and associated factors. *Br J Psychiatry*, 190, 27–35.

Coppus, A., Evenhuis, H., Verberne, G.-J. et al. (2006). Dementia and mortality in persons with Down's syndrome. *J Intellect Disabil Res*, 50(10), 768–77.

Cumella, S. and Martin, D. (2004). Secondary healthcare and learning disability: results of consensus development conferences. *J Learn Disabil*, 8(1), 30–40.

Davies, N. (2008). Caring for older adults with learning disabilities. *Nurs Stand*, 22(24), 42–8.

Department of Health (2001). *Valuing People: A Strategy for Learning Disabilities for the 21st Century*. London: HMSO.

Department of Health (2007a). *Commissioning Specialist Adult Learning Disability Health Services: Good Practice Guidance*. Available from: www.dh.gov.uk/publications (last accessed 5 December 2008).

Department of Health (2007b). *Primary Care Service Framework: Management of Health for People with Learning Disabilities in Primary Care*. Available from: www.library.nhs.uk/learningdisabilities/ViewResource.aspx?resID=266202 (last accessed 5 December 2008).

Department of Health (2008). *Transition: Moving on Well. A Good Practice Guide for Health Professionals and their Partners on Transition Planning for Young People with Complex Health Needs or Disability*. London: Department of Health.

Di Blasi, A., Kendall, S. and Spark, M. J. (2006). Perspectives on the role of the community pharmacist in the provision of healthcare to people with intellectual disabilities: exploration of the barriers and solutions. *Int J Pharm Pract*, 14(4), 263–9.

Disability Rights Commission (2006). *Equal Treatment: Closing the Gap. A Formal Investigation into the Physical Health Inequalities Experienced by People with Learning Disabilities and/or Mental Health*

Problems. London: Disability Rights Commission.

Dodd, K. and Brunker, J. (1999). 'Feeling poorly': report of a pilot study aimed to increase the ability of people with learning disabilities to understand and communicate about physical illness. *Br J Learn Disabil*, 27(1), 10–15.

Emerson, E. and Robertson J. (2008). *Commissioning Person-centred, Cost-effective, Local Support for People with Learning Disabilities.* Adults' Services Knowledge Review 20, Social Care Institute for Excellence and Lancaster University. Available from: www.scie.org.uk.

Fender, A., Marsden, L. and Starr, J. M. (2007). Assessing the health of older adults with intellectual disabilities: a user-led approach. *J Intellect Disabil Res*, 11(3), 223–39.

Gibbs, S. M., Brown, M. J. and Muir, W. J. (2008). The experiences of adults with intellectual disabilities and their carers in general hospitals: a focus group study. *J Intellect Disabil Res*, 52(12), 1061–77.

Gilbert, T. (2004). Involving people with learning disabilities in research: issues and possibilities. *Health Soc Care Community*, 12, 298–308.

Gratsa, A., Spiller, J., Holt, G. *et al.* (2006). Developing a mental health guide for families and carers of people with intellectual disabilities. *J Appl Res Intellect Disabil*, 19, 223–4.

Hardy, S. and Holt, G. (2007). Autistic Spectrum Disorder: supporting people in primary care. *Prim Health Care*, 17(6), 31–3.

Hardy, S., Kramer, R., Holt, G., Woodward, P. and Chaplin, E. (2006). *Supporting Complex Needs. A Practical Guide for Support Staff Working with People with a Learning Disability who have Mental Health Needs.* London: Turning Point.

Hardy, S., Chaplin, E. and Woodward, P. (2007). *Mental Health Nursing of Adults with Learning Disabilities.* London: Royal College of Nursing.

Hassiotis, A., Parkes, C., Jones, L., Fitzgerald, B. and Romeo, R. (2008). Individual characteristics and service expenditure on challenging behaviour for adults with intellectual disabilities. *J Appl Res Intellect Disabil*, 21, 438–45.

Health Care Commission (2006). *Joint Investigation into the Provision of Services for People with Learning Disabilities at Cornwall Partnership NHS Trust.* London: Commission for Healthcare Audit and Inspection.

Health Care Commission (2007). *A Life Like No Other: A National Audit of Specialist Inpatient Healthcare Services for People with Learning Difficulties in England.* London: Commission for Health Care Audit and Inspection. Available from: www.healthcarecommission.org.uk.

Hollins, S. (ed.). Books Beyond Words series, Royal College of Psychiatrists, UK and Division of Mental Health, St George's, University of London. Available from: www.rcpsych.ac.uk/publications/booksbeyondwords/aboutbbw.aspx.

Hollins, S., Attard, M. T., von Fraunhofer, N., McGuigan, S. and Sedgwick, P. (1998). Mortality in people with learning disabilities: risks, causes and death certificate findings in London. *Dev Med Child Neurol*, 40, 50–6.

Holt, G. and Bouras, N. (2004). Training residential and day care staff on the mental health needs of people with intellectual disabilities. *J Intellect Disabil Res*, 48, 495.

Holt, G., Gratsa, A., Bouras, N. *et al.* (2004). *Guide to Mental Health for Families and Carers of People with Intellectual Disabilities.* London: Jessica Kingsley Publishers.

Jacquemin, D. (2005). Caring for people with learning difficulties. *Eur J Palliat Care*, 12(6), 249–50.

Jones, M. C., McLafferty, E., Walley, R., Toland, J and Melson, N. (2008). Inclusion in primary care for people with intellectual disabilities: gaining the perspective of service user and supporting social care staff. *J Intellect Disabil*, 12(2), 93–109.

Joyce, T. (2008). *Best Interests Guidance on Determining the Best Interests of Adults Who Lack Capacity to Make a Decision (or Decisions) for Themselves (England and*

Wales). London: British Psychological Society.

Katz, G. and Lazcano-Ponce, E. (2008). Intellectual disability: definition, etiological factors, classification, diagnosis, treatment and prognosis. *Salud Publica Mex*, 50(Suppl 2), S131–41.

Kennedy, C. H., Juarez, A. P., Becker, A. *et al.* (2007). Children with severe developmental disabilities and behavioral disorders have increased special healthcare needs. *Dev Med Child Neurol*, 49(12), 926–30.

Kerr, A. M., McCulloch, D., Oliver, K. *et al.* (2003). Medical needs for people with intellectual disability require regular reassessment, and the provision of client-and carer-held reports. *J Intellect Disabil Res*, 47(2), 134–45.

Kerr, M. (2008). Commentary on: 'On the need for a specialist service within the generic hospital setting' by Robyn A. Wallace and Helen Beange (2008). *J Intellect Dev Disabil*, 33(4), 365–6.

Keywood, K. and Flynn, M. (2006). Healthcare decision-making by adults with learning disabilities: ongoing agendas, future challenges. *Psychiatry*, 5(10), 360–2.

Kwok, H. and Cheung, P. W. (2007). Co-morbidity of psychiatric disorder and medical illness in people with intellectual disabilities. *Curr Opin Psychiatry*, 20(5), 443–9.

Lazcano-Ponce, E., Rangel-Eudave, G. and Katz, G. (2008). Intellectual disability and its effects on society. *Salud Publica Mex*, 50(Suppl 2), S119–20.

Lecomte, J. and Mercier, C. (2008). The WHO atlas on global resources for persons with intellectual disabilities: a right to health perspective. *Salud Publica Mex*, 50(Suppl 2), S160–6.

Lennox, N., Taylor, M., Rey-Conde, T. *et al.* (2005). Beating the barriers: recruitment of people with intellectual disabilities to participate in research. *J Intellect Disabil Res*, 49, 296–305.

Lennox, N., Bain, C., Rey-Conde T. *et al.* (2007). Effects of a comprehensive health assessment programme for Australian adults with intellectual disability: a cluster randomised control trial. *Int J Epidemiol*, 36, 139–46.

Lennox, N. G., Green, M., Diggens, J. and Ugoni, A. (2001). Audit and comprehensive health assessment programmes in the primary healthcare of adults with intellectual disability: a pilot study. *J Intellect Disabil Res*, 45(3), 226–32.

Levy, J. M., Botuck, S., Damiani, M. R. *et al.* (2006). Medical conditions and healthcare utilization among adults with intellectual disabilities living in group homes in New York City. *J Policy Pract Intellect Disabil*, 3(3), 195–202.

Lin, J., Hsu, S., Chou, Y. *et al.* (2008). Assessment of primary care physicians' beliefs relating to the care of people with intellectual disabilities: a Taiwan-based opportunity-guided approach. *Disabil Rehabil*, 30(9), 611–17.

Lin, J.-D., Yen, C. F., Li, C. W. and Wu, J. L. (2005). Health, healthcare utilization and psychiatric disorder in people with intellectual disability in Taiwan. *J Intellect Disabil Res*, 49(1), 86–94.

Lopez-Rangel, E., Mickelson, E. C. R. and Lewis, M. E. (2008). The value of a genetic diagnosis for individuals with intellectual disabilities: optimising healthcare and function across the lifespan. *Br J Dev Disabil*, 54, Part 2(107), 69–82.

Mansell, J. L. (2007). *Services for People with Learning Disabilities and Challenging Behaviours or Mental Health Needs*, revised edition. London: Department of Health. Available from: http://www.dh.gov.uk/en/ Publicationsandstatistics/Publications/ PublicationsPolicyAndGuidance/ DH_080129 (last accessed 5 December 2008).

McCarthy, J. and Boyd, J. (2002). Mental health services and young people with intellectual disability: is it time to do better?' *J Intellect Disabil Res*, 46, 250–6.

McCarthy, J., Mir, G. and Wright, S. (2008). People with learning disabilities and mental health problems: the impact of ethnicity. *Adv Ment Health Learn Disabil*, 2(2), 31–6.

McCrystal, P., Percy, A. and Higgins, K. (2007). Substance use behaviours of young people with a moderate learning disability: a longitudinal analysis. *Am J Drug Alcohol Abuse*, 33(1), 155–61.

Melville, C., Cooper, S.-A., Morrison, J. *et al.* (2006). The outcome of an intervention to reduce the barriers experienced by people with intellectual disabilities accessing primary health care services. *J Intellect Disabil Res*, 50, 11–17.

Mencap (2004). *Treat Me Right! Better Healthcare for People with a Learning Disability*. London: Mencap.

Mencap (2007). *Death by Indifference: Following Up the 'Treat Me Right' Report*. London: Mencap. Available from: www.mencap. org.uk.

Mencap (2008). *Getting It Right: When Treating People with a Learning Disability*. London: Mencap. Available from: www.mencap.org.uk/gettingitright (last accessed 23 December 2008).

Mental Capacity Act (2005). London: HMSO. Available from: http://www.opsi.gov.uk/ACTS/acts2005/pdf/ukpga_20050009_en.pdf (last accessed 5 December 2008).

Michael, J. (2008). *Health care for all. Report of the Independent Inquiry Into Access to Healthcare for People with Learning Disabilities: A Review*. Available from: http://www.iahpld.org.uk/Healthcare_final.pdf (last accessed 5 December 2008).

Mir, G. (2007). Meeting 'Valuing People' health targets: recommendations from a research workshop. *Br J Learn Disabil*, 35, 75–83.

Morgan, C., Ahmed, Z. and Kerr, M. (2000) Health care provision for people with a learning disability: record-linkage study of epidemiology and factors contributing to hospital care uptake. *Br J Psychiatry*, 176, 37–40.

Mukherjee, R. A. S. (2007). Prevalence of clinically diagnosed mental ill-health in adults with intellectual disabilities is around 40%. *Evid Based Ment Health*, 10(3), 94.

Ng, J. and Li, S. (2003). A survey exploring the educational needs of care practitioners in learning disability (LD) settings in relation to death, dying and people with learning disabilities. *Eur J Cancer Care*, 12(1), 12–19.

NHS Health Scotland (2004). *The Health Needs Assessment Report: People with Learning Disabilities in Scotland*. Glasgow: NHS Health Scotland.

NICE (2008). *Identifying and Supporting People Most at Risk of Dying Prematurely*. London: National Institute for Health and Clinical Excellence. Available from: www.nice.org.uk/PH15.

Northern Ireland (2005). *Review of Mental Health and Learning Disability (NI) 2005: Equal Lives – Review of Policy and Services for People with a Learning Disability in Northern Ireland*. Belfast. Available from: http://www.rmhldni.gov.uk/equallivesreport.pdf (last accessed 6 December 2008).

NSPA (2004). *Understanding the Patient Safety Issues for People with Learning Disabilities*. London: National Patient Safety Agency. Available from: www.npsa.nhs.uk.

O'Hara, D. (2008). Invited commentary on Wallace and Beange (2008): 'On the need for a specialist service within the generic hospital setting'. *J Intellect Dev Disabil*, 33(4), 362–4.

O'Hara, J. (2006). Standards and quality measures for services for people with intellectual disabilities. *Curr Opin Psychiatry*, 19(5), 497–501.

O'Hara, J. (2008a). Why should I care about gender? *Adv Ment Health Learn Disabil*, 2(2), 9–18.

O'Hara, J. (2008b). Attending to the health needs of people with intellectual disability: quality standards. *Salud Publica Mex*, 50 (Suppl 2), S154–9.

O'Hara, J. and Bouras, N. (2007). Intellectual disabilities across cultures. In *Textbook of Cultural Psychiatry*, ed. D. Bhugra and K. Bhui. Cambridge: Cambridge University Press, pp. 461–70.

O'Hara, J. and Sperlinger, A. (eds.) (1997). *Adults with Learning Disabilities: A Practical Approach for Health Professionals*. Chichester: J. Wiley and Sons.

Polder, J. J., Meerding, W. J., Bonneux, L. and van der Maas, P. J. (2002). Healthcare costs of intellectual disability in the Netherlands: a cost-of-illness perspective. *J Intellect Disabil Res*, 46(2), 168–78.

RCGP (2006). *Care of People with Learning Disabilities*. Royal College of General Practitioners Curriculum Statement 14. London: RCGP.

Ryan, K. R. and McQuillan, R. (2005). Palliative care for disadvantaged groups: people with intellectual disabilities. *Prog Palliat Care*, 13(2), 70–4.

Salud Publica de Mexico (2008). Intellectual disability, 50(Suppl 2). Available from: www.insp.mx/salud.

Scholte, F. A. (2008). European Manifesto: basic standards of healthcare for people with intellectual disabilities. *Salud Publica Mex*, 50(Suppl 2), pp. S273–6. Available from: www.insp.mx/salud.

Schrander-Stumpel, C. T., Sinnema, A., Van Den Hout, L. *et al.* (2007). Healthcare transition in persons with intellectual disabilities: general issues, the Maastricht model, and Prader-Willi syndrome. *Am J Med Genet C Semin Med Genet*, 145C(3), 241–7.

Scottish Executive (2000). *The Same as You? A Review of Services for People with Learning Disabilities*. Edinburgh: The Stationery Office. Available from: http://www.scotland.gov.uk/ldsr/docs/tsay-00.asp (last accessed 6 December 2008).

Scottish Executive (2002). *Promoting Health, Supporting Inclusion: The National Review of the Contribution of all Nurses and Midwives to the Care and Support of People with Learning Disabilities*. Edinburgh: The Stationery Office.

Scottish Parliament (2000). *Adults with Incapacity (Scotland) Act*. Edinburgh: Stationery Office. Available from: www.opsi.gov.uk.

Sowney, M. and Barr, O. G. (2006). Caring for adults with intellectual disabilities: perceived challenges for nurses in accident and emergency units. *J Advanced Nurs*, 55(1), 36–45.

Sowney, M., Brown, M. and Barr, O. (2006). Caring for people with learning disabilities in emergency care. *Emerg Nurse*, 14, 23–30.

Spiller, M., Costello, H., Bokszanska, A. *et al.* (2007). Service consumption of a specialist mental health service for people with intellectual disabilities. *J Appl Res Intellect Disabil*, 20, 430–8.

Stoddart, S. D. R., Griffiths, E. C. and Lilford, R. J. (2005). *A Confidential Inquiry into Excess Mortality in People with Learning Disability: Scoping Report to the National Patient Safety Agency*. London: NSPA.

Strydom, A., Livingston, G. and Hassiotis, A. (2007). Prevalence of dementia in intellectual disability using different diagnostic criteria. *Br J Psychiatry*, 191, 150–7.

Taggart, L., McLaughlin, D., Quinn, B. and Milligan, V. (2006). An exploration of substance misuse in people with intellectual disabilities. *J Intellect Disabil Res*, 50(8), 588–97.

Tuffrey-Wijne, I. (2003). The palliative care needs of people with intellectual disabilities: a literature review. *Palliat Med*, 17(1), 55–62.

Tuffrey-Wijne I., Bernal, J. and Hollins, S. (2008). Doing research on people with learning disabilities, cancer and dying: ethics, possibilities and pitfalls. *Br J Learn Disabil*, 36, 185–90.

van Schrojenstein Lantman-deValk, H. M. J. and Walsh, P. N. (2008). Managing health problems in people with intellectual disabilities. *BMJ*, 337:a2507 doi:10.1136/bmj.a2507

Wallace, R. A. and Beange, H. (2008). On the need for a specialist service within the generic hospital setting for the adult patient with intellectual disability and physical health problems. *J Intellect Dev Disabil*, 33(4), 354–61.

Walmsley, J. (2004). Involving users with learning difficulties in health improvement: lessons from inclusive learning disability research. *Nurs Inq* 11, 54–64.

Walsh, P. N. (2008). Health indicators in intellectual disability. *Curr Opin Psychiatry*, 21(5), 474–8.

Walsh, P. N., Kerr, M. and van Schrojenstein Lantman-de Valk, H. M. J. (2003). Health indicators for people with intellectual disabilities: a European perspective. *Eur J Public Health*, 13(Suppl 3), 47–50.

Walsh, P. N., Linehan, C., Kerr, M. P. *et al.* (2005). Brief research report developing a set of health indicators for people with intellectual disabilities: Pomona project. *J Policy Pract Intellect Disabil*, 2(3 & 4), 260–3.

Welsh Assembly (2004). *Learning Disability Strategy Section 7 Guidance on Service Principles and Service Responses*. Welsh Assembly Government. Available from http://www.ldiag.org.uk/information/sp-response-guide-e.pdf (last accessed 6 December 2008).

World Health Organization (WHO) (2007). *Atlas: Global Resources for Persons with Intellectual Disabilities*. Geneva, Switzerland: World Health Organization.

Young, A. F. and Chesson, R. A. (2007). Determining research questions on health risks by people with learning disabilities, carers and care-workers. *Br J Learn Disabil*, 36, 22–31.

2

Congenital causes

Jessica A. Hellings, Merlin G. Butler and John A. Grant

Introduction

Research during the past ten years in the fields of genetics, molecular biology and neuroimaging has given new insights into the congenital causes of intellectual disabilities (ID), as well as improved interventions and prevention. Functional brain imaging has allowed differences in brain function to be studied and comparisons made with cognitive and behavioural functioning. Genetic technology has advanced rapidly; gene microarrays allow simultaneous searching of the whole genome for functional and structural gene changes. Sharing of electronic gene databases promises even more rapid progress. At the same time, strategies for studying causes of other common conditions such as autistic spectrum disorders (ASD) have highlighted complexities in pinpointing genetic and environmental causes, since ASD is most likely heterogeneous and polygenic. This is also complicated by the scientific findings that regulatory genes and interaction with environmental factors influence the expression of candidate genes for ASD.

Furthermore, research has produced an appreciation of the critical role of brain structure (e.g. astroglia) in central nervous system (CNS) function, particularly with synaptogenesis. For example, the brains of individuals with ASD and those with Down syndrome (DS) are known to have abnormal neuronal dendritic spines. Neurotrophic factors including brain-derived neurotrophic factor (BDNF) have also been characterised and their role in neurotoxicity is being elucidated. Additionally, stress due to child abuse may alter maturing brain structure and function in the presence of predisposing gene variants. This research is being extended to fetal stress and outcomes. In terms of the broader population, prevention of congenital causes of ID remains an ultimate goal. Malnutrition, lack of obstetric and medical care and infectious diseases remain at the forefront of problems in developing countries.

Method

We reviewed published studies of congenital causes of ID by online computer searches, from 1950 to 2008 (please refer to Table 2.1). PubMed searches were performed using the phrases: 'congenital causes of mental retardation', 'intellectual disabilities' and 'mental retardation'.

Results

For the 'congenital causes of mental retardation' search, 5633 published articles were found, 38 publications were from January to mid-September 2008. For the 'intellectual disabilities'

Intellectual Disability and Ill Health: A Review of the Evidence, ed. Jean O'Hara, Jane McCarthy and Nick Bouras. Published by Cambridge University Press. © Cambridge University Press 2010.

Table 2.1. PubMed online search (1950–2008)

Key words		
Congenital causes of mental retardation	**Intellectual disabilities**	**Mental retardation**
5633	1529	77 654

search there were 1529 references, far fewer than for mental retardation since this is a newer term. For 'mental retardation' there were 77 654 references listed from 1950 to 2008.

Discussion

The commonest cause of ID remains unknown; as molecular and neuroimaging techniques improve presumably this 'unknown' group will diminish. A significant proportion of causes are also polygenic. Known congenital causes can be divided into (1) single gene and chromosome syndromes, (2) inborn errors of metabolism, (3) fetal infections, (4) fetal alcohol syndrome and other toxin-related syndromes and (5) congenital structural CNS anomalies amenable to surgery.

Select congenital syndromes

Down syndrome

Down syndrome (DS) or Trisomy 21 is the commonest known cause of ID, affecting 1 in 700–1000 live births (Cohen, 2005). Down syndrome differs from other congenital syndromes in that routine antenatal testing is recommended in all pregnant women over 35 years of age. In the case of an individual with DS with a chromosome 21 translocation, as occurs in about 5% of people with DS, parental chromosome studies are indicated due to increased recurrence risk (up to100% if the mother or the father carries a balanced 21 chromosome translocation).

Up to 50% of infants with DS have congenital heart defects, which are mostly mild or surgically correctable. Of the 100 identified physical features of DS, facial features are most easily recognisable. These include a flat face with a large protruding tongue, upward slanting eyes, small ears and mouth, and epicanthic folds. Individuals have poor muscle tone and short stature and are prone to obesity and hypothyroidism as well as atlantoaxial instability of the neck (Cohen, 2005; Prasher, 1995). Eye conditions such as strabismus and refractive errors are common, as are crowded teeth, dry skin and eczema. There is a small but increased risk for leukaemia (0.6% of individuals) (Roizen, 1996). Ongoing weight management and dental care are vital. Coeliac disease screening is recommended from two years of age. Neck X-rays are obtained from age three to detect atlantoaxial instability (American Academy of Pediatrics, 1994).

Down syndrome is associated with moderate ID, with average IQ in the 50s (Connolly, 1978; Gibson, 1978). Neuropsychiatric findings include significantly reduced total brain volume and underdeveloped temporal lobes (Golden and Hyman, 1994), associated with impaired auditory short-term memory. Frontal lobe underdevelopment is linked to problems with verbal fluency and expressive language (see Wang (1996) for review).

Fragile X syndrome

Fragile X syndrome (FRAX) is the commonest inheritable cause of ID, also amenable to prevention by genetic counselling. Fragile X syndrome is routinely diagnosed with DNA testing. The identified incidence is 1/4000 males and 1/8000 females. About one-third of all X-linked ID is due to FRAX (Turner *et al.*, 1996).

Two forms of FRAX have been identified. The typical group is FRAX-A, associated with the full mutation of > 200 CGG nucleotide repeats on the X chromosome and loss of function of the *FMR1 gene* and protein (Jacquemont *et al.*, 2003). Adult males with the full mutation have a mean IQ of 41 (Jacquemont *et al.*, 2005). The syndrome comprises ID, autistic-like behavioural abnormalities, macro-orchidism and a long face, large mandible and large ears, and connective tissue defects. The FRAX-E form is less common, but associated with ID and results from > 200 CGG repeats of the *FMR2 gene*.

Normally, FMR-protein provides nuclear export of neuronal mRNA, which in turn influences protein synthesis in dendritic spines. The abnormal gene becomes methylated and inactivated, to varying degrees, for as yet unknown reasons. Abnormal dendritic spines are identified in brains of humans with FRAX and in *FMR1* knockout mice. Usually individuals have 6 to 60 CGG repeats, most commonly 30, which are unmethylated. The mechanism of anticipation (expansion of trinucleotide repeats during meiosis) results in FRAX, only if the premutation is transmitted by a female carrier (Willems *et al.*, 1992). Males with the full mutation are presumed to have only premutation sperm. Males and females with the premutation are mostly normal phenotypically, cognitively and behaviourally. Almost all males with the full mutation manifest FRAX clinically. Over half of females with the full mutation manifest FRAX symptoms; while in the remaining females the normal second X chromosome compensates for the abnormal *FMR1* gene.

Direct DNA methylation testing for the fragile X is performed using blood samples or following amniocentesis on fetal cells. The extent of *FMR1* gene inactivation thus identified helps predict the child's prognosis. Also, a minority of males with the full mutation have only partial methylation and an average or low-average IQ (Hagerman *et al.*, 1994; Merenstein *et al.*, 1996). Physical features of FRAX are often subtle or missed in children. Prior to puberty, non-specific features occur, including connective tissue laxity, flat feet and soft skin, strabismus and scoliosis. Some cases are identified at birth by DNA testing, particularly when there is a positive family history or a benign mitral valve systolic ejection click. The long face, prominent fleshy ears and macro-orchidism mostly manifest post-pubertally. Avoidant gaze is a robust finding in males with FRAX. Approximately 20% of children with FRAX have seizures, which are mostly well controlled (Hecht, 1991).

Much early work focused on autism and FRAX, searching for a genetic cause for autism. This was based on the common finding of autistic features in males with FRAX, including gaze avoidance, rocking and other stereotypies, hyperacusis, restricted interests and poor social interactions. While 15% to 60% are identified with ASD, most males with FRAX have some autistic-like behaviour, as do many females (Dykens and Volkmar, 1997). Caudate nucleus enlargement correlates inversely with IQ (Reiss *et al.*, 1995). Caudate abnormality impacts on executive functions, motor and affect regulation, response inhibition and flexibility. Most boys referred clinically with FRAX manifest inattention and hyperactivity (Bregman *et al.*, 1988; Hagerman, 1996). Girls with FRAX are more prone to inattention and impulsivity (Lachiewicz, 1992; Lachiewicz and Dawson, 1994). The smaller posterior cerebellar vermis in males with FRAX may relate to hyperactivity and impaired gating of tactile and sensory stimuli. Cohen in 1995 suggested hyperarousal of the autonomic nervous system which may account for the social anxiety, tactile defensiveness, shyness, perseveration and hand-biting problems.

Treatment studies are extremely limited. Initially, high-dose folic acid therapy was tried, but showed no difference from placebo for attentional problems in double-blind controlled trials (Fisch *et al.*, 1988; Froster-Iskenius *et al.*, 1986; Hagerman *et al.*, 1986; Strom *et al.*, 1992). A single case study reported a favourable response in a six-year-old boy with FRAX and behaviour problems to the tricyclic antidepressant, imipramine, although worsening occurred when methylphenidate was added (Hilton *et al.*, 1991). L-acetylcarnitine has reportedly reduced behaviour problems in boys with FRAX, at 50 mg dosed twice daily (Torrioli *et al.*, 1999). More recent studies using compounds that target specific neurochemical and synaptic abnormalities include ampakine (AMPA) compound X 516, which potentiates brain AMPA receptors (Berry-Kravis *et al.*, 2006). The antiglucocorticoid compound, mifepristone, was tried to 'reset' the hypothalamic–pituitary–adrenal axis, based on elevated cortisol levels observed in FRAX syndrome which are linked to hyperarousal and hyperactivity (Hessl *et al.*, 2002). Both studies were inconclusive. Social skills training and systematic exposure to social situations using escape extinction are also effective. Further research is needed to determine how *FMR1* gene methylation and protein deficiency act at brain level.

Prader-Willi syndrome

Findings from genetic studies of Prader-Willi syndrome (PWS) led to the novel concept of genomic imprinting regarding gene expression according to parent of origin, and thus changed the field of molecular genetics. Prader-Willi syndrome is characterised by extreme hyperphagia, hypogonadism, short stature, skin-picking, obsessive-compulsive behaviour and explosive outbursts. However, infants with PWS are floppy and suck poorly. Recent brain imaging studies support research suggesting the hyperphagia relates to lack of satiation (Holsen *et al.*, 2006).

Prader-Willi syndrome results most commonly from a paternal deletion of the 15q11-q13 chromosome region (in 75% of cases) (Bittel and Butler, 2005). Two types of the 15q11-q13 deletion are recognised; larger (Type I) and smaller (Type II). Individuals with these deletions are more prone to hypopigmentation, skin-picking, repetitive behaviours and explosive outbursts, compared to other genetic subtypes of PWS. Twenty-five per cent of individuals with PWS have no deletion but have two maternal chromosome 15s, thus called uniparental maternal disomy or UPD (Nicholls *et al.*, 1989). In these cases, the chromosome 15 pair appears normal in structure and number, but has an incorrect inheritance pattern (both 15s of maternal origin). Advanced maternal age may increase UPD risk. Interestingly, individuals with UPD are prone to psychosis (Vogels *et al.*, 2004).

One gene of particular interest and critical to the PWS phenotype, is *SNRPN* (Bittel and Butler, 2005; Khan and Wood, 1999). Fewer than 5% of individuals with PWS have neither UPD nor deletions subtypes, but have a defect of the imprinting centre which controls the activity of the imprinted genes within the 15q11-q13 region (Buiting *et al.*, 1995; Saitoh *et al.*, 1996). The PWS recurrence risk is less than 1%, but 50% in cases where the unaffected father carries a defect in the imprinting centre on his maternal chromosome 15, and passes the imprinting defect to his children.

Treatments for PWS include strict locking up of food, dietary control, treatment of sleep apnoea, monitoring for diabetes mellitus and orthopaedic follow-up for scoliosis. Growth hormone treatment increases stature, decreases fat mass and increases muscle, thereby also increasing metabolic rate. Selective 5-hydroxytryptamine (5-HT, serotonin) reuptake inhibitors (SSRIs) such as fluoxetine are effective for treating obsessive-compulsive and depressive disorders, as well as skin-picking (Benjamin and Buot-Smith, 1993; Dech and Budow, 1991; Hellings and Warnock, 1994; Warnock and Kestenbaum, 1992). Psychosis and/or mania, which are more common in the maternal disomy subgroup, respond to antipsychotics and mood stabilisers, although clinical trials are needed.

Angelman syndrome

Angelman syndrome (AS) involves the same chromosome region as PWS and also results from genomic imprinting (Williams, 2005). However, the defect is a maternal deletion of the 15q11-q13 region (in 75% of cases), paternal disomy 15 (3%), an imprinting centre defect (6%), or due to a fourth mechanism, notably a mutation of the causative UBE3A gene (15%). The latter gene encodes for ubiquitin protein ligase which regulates brain cell protein turnover. Damaging abnormal molecules accumulate and interfere with normal synaptic function. Interestingly, the maternal copy of the UBE3A gene is expressed only in the cerebellum and hippocampus. Individuals with only a mutation in the UBE3A gene, generally, do not develop the epilepsy characteristic of AS. Part of the PWS/AS critical region contains genes for subunits of the gamma-aminobutyric acid (GABA)-A receptors which are deleted in most individuals with PWS or AS and could contribute to epilepsy occurring in people with AS.

Velo-cardio-facial syndrome

Velo-cardio-facial syndrome (VCFS) or 22q11.2 deletion syndrome occurs in 1 in 5000 live births (Tezenas Du Montcel et al., 1996) and is associated with a high prevalence of birth defects and associated psychiatric disorders. Due to mild and variable phenotypic expression, VCFS is often missed clinically. Velo-cardio-facial syndrome is currently the commonest known genetic cause of schizophrenia. Midline structures developing from the rostral embryonic neural crest are abnormal in VCFS, notably (1) velopharyngeal insufficiency or cleft palate; (2) cardiac malformations: tetralogy of Fallot or a ventriculoseptal defect; (3) dysmorphic facies: a large nose, nasal tip and root, thin upper lip, narrow eyes, a long expressionless face, a long philtrum and small cupped ears. Other features include immunodeficiency, hypocalcaemia and borderline intelligence to mild ID. Autistic features or social deficits and inattention in childhood are common (Feinstein et al., 2002). Psychosis often begins in late adolescence, in 32% of cases (Gothelf and Martin, 2007). This may relate to several genes in the deletion region, however, the main aetiological hypothesis relates to catechol-o-methyl transferase (COMT) deficiency resulting in deficient breakdown of dopamine, noradrenaline and adrenaline neurotransmitters. Polymicrogyria of the cerebral cortex, likely due to ischaemic injury during neural crest brain development, is common in VCFS, most likely resulting from the cardiac abnormalities and hypoxaemia (Robin et al., 2006).

Velo-cardio-facial syndrome research has evolved rapidly, providing a model for studying gene–brain–behaviour relationships. Studying the gene–dosage effect may identify risk factors and markers for development of psychosis (Schaer and Eliez, 2007). Treatment studies are lacking in VCFS, apart from case reports of antipsychotic efficacy for the psychosis (Brewington et al., 2008; Gladston and Clarke, 2005).

Rett syndrome

Rett syndrome (RS) was originally believed to occur only in girls; however, some males with the syndrome are now identified. Estimated RS prevalence is 1/10 000 girls, thus RS represents one of the more frequent causes of severe ID in girls (Percy, 2002). A hallmark of RS is global deceleration of psychomotor development and subsequent loss of acquired cognitive and motor skills, after 6–18 months of apparently normal development. The deterioration progresses to severe dementia with loss of speech, autistic features, repetitive truncal rocking and ataxia and loss of purposeful use of the hands and the classical hand-wringing movements. Irregular breathing occurs, with hyperventilation and slowing of head growth. The reasons for this neurological deterioration and slowing head growth are unclear, however, studies have shown an altered expression of specific proteins in certain cerebral neurons and decreases in synaptic numbers. There is no apparent alteration in myelin, no consistent evidence of cell loss or atrophy, no ventriculomegaly and no obvious brain malformation. However, dendritic trees are significantly diminished in regions of the RS brain including the prefrontal and motor cortex (Bienvenu, 2005).

In 2001, the methyl CpG binding protein 2 (*MECP2*) gene responsible for RS was identified (Van den Veyver and Zoghbi, 2001). The *MECP2* gene is thought to repress transcription in methylated regions of DNA. It may act as a mechanistic bridge between DNA methylation and histone methylation. It is highly expressed in the brain, lung and spleen, and moderately expressed in the kidney and heart. The MECP2 protein may repress genes that are vital for neuronal development and may be detrimental to mature neurons. The MECP2 protein has also been implicated in imprinted gene regulation. Up to 95% of classical RS cases have *MECP2* gene alterations.

There is no cure for RS. Treatment requires a team approach and aims to slow disease progression, improve or maintain mobility and balance, promote hand use, reduce hand stereotypies and foster non-verbal communication and social interactions.

Inborn errors of metabolism

The major inborn errors of metabolism can be grouped into: (a) amino acids, (b) lipids, (c) carbohydrates and (d) miscellaneous.

a. *Disorders of amino acid metabolism* include phenylketonuria (PKU) which is the prototype of such disorders causing ID. Since the PKU gene was cloned in 1983 (Woo *et al.*, 1983), hundreds of mutations have been identified. Interestingly, the correlation between the metabolic phenotype and IQ is variable rather than direct. Phenylketonuria is a classical autosomal recessive metabolic disorder in which dietary intervention, by exclusion of phenylalanine, is effective in preventing ID. Therefore, it is routinely screened for at birth in all states in the USA.

   Other inborn errors of amino acid metabolism include maple syrup urine disease, mannosidosis, urea cycle disorders and mitochondrial abnormalities. Routine workup for all new cases of ID includes a urine test for elevated levels of organic acids. Population variations in incidence exist for several amino acid metabolic disorders, for example homocystinuria is five times more common in Ireland than in other countries.

b. *Disorders of lipid metabolism* include Tay-Sachs disease, Gaucher disease, metachromatic leukodystrophy and progressive leukoencephalopathy. Tay-Sachs and Gaucher diseases occur mostly in Jewish children of Eastern European descent. Both are autosomal recessive causes of cerebromacular degeneration, with tissue damage due to accumulation of gangliosides in the CNS and retina. Tay-Sachs disease usually causes death within two to four years; a chronic form of Gaucher disease exists with gradual onset before ten years old and mostly includes physical disabilities. Metachromatic leukodystrophy or sulphatide lipidosis may present first as a childhood disintegrative disorder. Metachromatic lipids accumulate in the CNS white matter, peripheral nerves and viscera causing mental and physical deterioration and hepatosplenomegaly. The pathogenic arylsulphatase deficiency results from an arylsulphatase A gene mutation on chromosome 22 (Gieselmann, 2003). Progressive leukoencephalopathies begin ambiguously, with irritability and hypersensitivity to stimuli. Progressive dementia and paralysis start by age two and prove fatal in about ten years. Laughing spells, spasticity, ataxia, cortical blindness and deafness occur early in the disease.

c. *Carbohydrate storage diseases* include classical galactossaemia, which is autosomal recessive, glycogen storage diseases, fructose intolerance and hypoglycaemias. The latter can be neonatal, leucine-sensitive or familial-type.

d. *Miscellaneous metabolic causes of ID* include hypothyroidism ('goitrous cretinism'), hyperparathyroidism and idiopathic hypocalcaemia due to vitamin D hypersensitivity. Congenital hypothyroidism can result not only from iodine deficiency, but also from maternal thyroid antibodies passed transplacentally to the fetus.

Other miscellaneous metabolic causes include Lesch-Nyhan syndrome, Wilson disease, familial non-haemolytic jaundice (Crigler-Najjar syndrome), pyridoxine dependency, and mucopolysaccharidoses Type I (Hurler syndrome) and Type II (Hunter syndrome). Lesch-Nyhan syndrome is X-linked recessive, therefore occurring in boys and is due to deficiency of the enzyme hypoxanthine-guanine phosphoribosyltransferase (HGPRT). This leads to an accumulation of uric acid and associated ID with severe self-biting of the fingers and lips. Allopurinol may improve the medical and behavioural problems (Robey *et al.*, 2003).

Fetal infections

Intrauterine infections constitute a group of preventable causes of ill health and congenital ID that are still extremely common in developing countries (please refer to Chapter 4 on Infectious diseases). Maternal infection during the first trimester results in the worst fetal outcomes including stillbirth, miscarriage, prematurity and the most severe neuropsychiatric and congenital manifestations if the fetus lives. The central pathogens are cytomegalovirus (CMV), *Toxoplasma gondii*, *Treponema pallidum*, rubella virus and human immunodeficiency virus (HIV). More recently, the zoonotic Ljungan virus (LV) has been found to be associated with hydrocephaly and anencephaly, amongst other CNS malformations in humans as well as intrauterine fetal death (Niklasson *et al.*, 2009).

Cytomegalovirus

Cytomegalovirus (CMV) is often asymptomatic in women, while transmission to the fetus occurs in 24–75% of the cases (Stoll and Kliegman, 2004). The virus may exist in a latent state and be reactivated during pregnancy, although the greatest risk to the fetus occurs with primary infection during pregnancy. Symptoms of CMV inclusion disease include hepatosplenomegaly, petechiae, jaundice, microcephaly, chorioretinitis and growth retardation. Most infants infected with CMV (90%), and fewer who are asymptomatic but were exposed (5–15%), will have ID, microcephaly, optic atrophy, chorioretinitis, hearing loss and speech abnormalities. A safe and effective vaccine is under development, while treatment with ganciclovir is being used for symptomatic congenital CMV.

Toxoplasmosis

Approximately 4000 cases of toxoplasmosis are identified in the USA each year (Montoya and Liesenfeld, 2004). Maternal infection by *Toxoplasma gondii* is amenable to prevention. Acute signs and symptoms include intracranial calcifications, dilated ventricles, hepatomegaly and placental thickening in utero. The classic toxoplasmosis triad postnatally includes cerebral calcifications, chorioretinitis and hydrocephalus. Intellectual disability, seizures, blindness, anaemia and low platelet count also can occur. Prenatal diagnosis is made by polymerase chain reaction (PCR) detection of DNA in the fluid. Prenatal treatment from the time of diagnosis until delivery is with spiramycin; combination treatment with pyrimethamine and sulphonamides is used during the first year of life (Bell, 2007).

Congenital syphilis

In Sub-Saharan Africa, the rate of syphilis during pregnancy is as high as 3000 per 100 000; in the USA the rate is 30 per 100 000 (Bell, 2007). The *Treponema pallidum* spirochete is transmitted to the fetus either transplacentally or from the mother's genital syphilitic lesions during birth. Prior to penicillin use, 60% of infants with syphilis were stillborn, died shortly after birth or had severe brain impairment (Golden *et al.*, 2003). Early maternal treatment with a single intramuscular injection of penicillin may prevent up to 98% of congenital syphilis cases, unless fetal damage has already occurred and is not reversible.

Congenital rubella syndrome

Under 20 infants are born in the USA each year with congenital rubella syndrome since vaccination programmes began (Atreya *et al.*, 2004; Danovaro-Holliday *et al.*, 2003). The syndrome includes cataracts, deafness and congenital heart disease. Unilateral or bilateral deafness (occurring in 80% of cases) may be the only diagnosable feature. Other symptoms may include microcephaly, ID and progressive encephalopathy. Laboratory diagnosis is made by detection of rubella-specific immunoglobulin M (IgM) in the serum, together with the above features.

Congenital human immunodeficiency virus

Although almost all infants born to women infected with HIV will be positive for the HIV antibody, only about 25% of the infants become actively infected, in the absence of treatment. In developing countries, and in undiagnosed mothers, transmission by breast-feeding is significant (Berk *et al.*, 2005; Newell *et al.*, 2004). Viral load, or copies of virus per millilitre of blood, is the strongest predictor of disease progression, notably 750 000 copies of the virus in rapid progressors, versus 300 000 in infected infants showing less rapid disease progression. In infants who become infected, the HIV retrovirus infects CD4 cells which are vital to cellular immunity, producing the acquired immunodeficiency syndrome (AIDS).

Congenital HIV causes significant brain injury and ID for multiple reasons. Antiretroviral drugs cross the blood–brain barrier poorly. Microglial cells have CD4 receptors and become a site of latent HIV infection. The HIV retrovirus damages neurons and glia directly, and indirectly by release of neurotoxins or by predisposing to opportunistic infections of the brain, including CMV encephalitis, toxoplasma encephalitis, cryptococcal meningitis, and progressive multifocal leukoencephalopathy.

Zoonotic Ljungan virus

The Ljungan virus (LV) has been identified recently as a cause of CNS malformations in laboratory mouse models, as well as intrauterine fetal death in humans. Niklasson *et al.* (2009) diagnosed LV infection in 9 out of 10 cases of elective abortions for hydrocephaly and 5 out of 9 with anencephaly versus 1 out of 18 controls with Trisomy 21. When 47 mouse neonates were exposed to LV all developed encephalitis with 8 manifesting hydrocephalus, versus zero out of 52 control mouse neonates.

Apart from the specific infections described above, other non-specific maternal infections and inflammation during pregnancy may injure the fetus and produce cerebral palsy by damaging developing brain white matter. The resulting periventricular leukomalacia is a significant cause of ID (Grether and Nelson, 1997).

Fetal alcohol syndrome and other toxin-related disorders

Fetal alcohol syndrome

The genetics of both alcoholism and fetal alcohol syndrome (FAS) still require elucidation (Adam and Hoyme, 2005). However, the adverse effects of alcohol on the developing fetus, in terms of phenotype, behaviour and neuro-cognitive outcomes, are well documented (Barr and Streissguth, 2001). Estimated prevalence of FAS in the USA has varied between 0.0/1000 children and 10.7/1000 children, depending upon the population studied and method used (Warren *et al.*, 2001). The FAS full diagnosis includes: (1) a confirmed history of excessive maternal alcohol intake during pregnancy, (2) pre- and postnatal growth retardation, (3) facial anomalies including a broad midface region, flattened philtrum, thin upper lip, thin palpebral fissures and mandibular hypoplasia and (4) CNS neurodevelopmental abnormities which include microcephaly, cerebellar hypoplasia, complete or partial agenesis of the corpus callosum, impaired hand–eye coordination and fine motor skills deficits.

As such individuals' environments usually suffer from poverty, instability, poor family functioning and deficient community supports, it is important not to attribute all problems to the FAS. Since the youngest child is not uncommonly the most severely affected in a family, it is important to also carefully screen the older siblings and obtain appropriate interventions. This includes evaluation for renal and cardiac defects and visual and hearing impairments, and developmental and educational assessments. Also, since FAS can be superimposed on or confused with other genetic and dysmorphic syndromes, the FAS diagnosis is one of exclusion. Women who drank several drinks prior to confirmation of their pregnancy but then abstain from alcohol use have a low FAS offspring risk. The most severely affected offspring are born to mothers that binge-drink during pregnancy to the point of intoxication or who drank steadily during pregnancy.

Other toxins or gene abnormalities can produce increased neuronal death in the cephalic premigratory and migratory neural crest, causing facial dysmorphology. Chick embryos receiving antibodies that block Sonic Hedgehog protein (Shh), which is greatest in the developing head region and is a signalling molecule that leads into a cascade of events causing activation and transcription of target genes, develop FAS-type craniofacial phenotypes and cranial neural crest cell death (Ahlgren *et al.*, 2002). It is postulated that alcohol may inhibit the Shh pathway in the developing fetus. However, alcohol probably disrupts brain growth on many levels, including astroglial development, cell–cell and cell–matrix signalling, retinoic acid abnormalities, and by triggering neuronal apoptosis through blockade of N-methyl-D-aspartate (NMDA) glutamate receptors and inactivation of GABA-A receptors (Ikonomidou *et al.*, 2000).

Heavy metals

The two most neurotoxic heavy metals are lead and mercury. Other neurotoxins include polychlorinated biphenyls (PCBs), dioxins, pesticides, herbicides and fungicides (please refer to Chapter 3 on Disorders of environmental origin).

Congenital structural CNS anomalies

Congenital CNS malformations occur in 1 in 1000 live births, and are best conceptualised by the stage of neural development at which deviation occurs. Central nervous system development, while extraordinarily complex, comprises neurulation and post-neurulation phases. During neurulation, the cell ribbon constituting the primitive neural plate folds over to form a vertical tube. The tube must close lengthwise as well as rostrally and caudally initially, for normal development to occur, at about eight weeks of pregnancy. Disruption of this process by genetic factors such as the *Dlx5* gene (Depew *et al.*, 1999) or environmental factors such as decreased serum folate result in open neural tube defects, including exencephaly (open brain) or spina bifida (open spinal cord). Anencephaly and myelomeningocoele result from incomplete closure. Normally the rostral neural tube reopens and expands on each side to form the cerebral hemispheres. A later failure of rostral tube reopening and positioning produces a posterior fossa 'Dandy-Walker' cyst. At least 60% of children with a diagnosed Dandy-Walker cyst are significantly intellectually delayed, although occasionally neither ID nor hydrocephalus are present.

Post-neurulation defects include encephalocoele (rostral neural tube extrusion through defective mesoderm), schizencephaly (loss of the entire tube wall thickness in one or more places) and holoprosencephaly (failure of rostral neural tube expansion into two cerebral hemispheres). Outcomes correlate directly with anatomical malformation size. Encephalocoele affects mostly occipital brain, due to a skull defect allowing protrusion, often of malformed brain tissue outside of the skull. There is associated hydrocephalus, ID, seizures and leg spasticity.

Other malformations, such as myelomeningocoele and associated hydrocephalus, originate in aberrations occurring throughout pregnancy. All such malformations often but not invariably result in ID. Anencephaly is the only congenital CNS malformation incompatible with life.

Like Dandy-Walker malformation, craniosynostosis is relatively common and can be isolated or familial, due to several recognised genetic syndromes (e.g. Apert). Cranial suture absence or premature closure can produce an unacceptable head shape, with increased risk for intracranial pressure elevations and resulting ID. Surgery for these conditions is not purely cosmetic, but facilitates normal brain development.

The neural tube wall comprises inner ependymal and outer pial layers. Astrocytes have foot processes in both layers, being transmantle. Where astrocyte cell bodies migrate to during this stage and how the tube folds and divides dictates the final brain shape. Irregularities in this process, such as migrational disorders (e.g. heterotopias) and cortical disorders (e.g. lissencephaly or smooth brain), are again associated with variable degrees of ID.

Hydrocephalus is present in 60% to 95% of children with neural tube defects; lesions lower down in the spinal cord are less likely to result in hydrocephalus (Tuli *et al.*, 2003). Massive hydrocephalus in utero is a poor prognostic indicator for intelligence. Up to 75% of children with a myelomeningocoele have average IQ (Barf *et al.*, 2004), although attention span, perception, organisational skills and motor skills are often impaired (Snow, 1994). The remaining 25% of children have ID that is mostly mild. Those with severe ID and myelomeningocoele often have had infections of the surgical shunt and brain, or severe prenatal hydrocephalus. (Please refer to Chapter 18 on Diseases of the nervous system.)

While occasionally an isolated birth defect, hydrocephalus most frequently results from intraventricular hemorrhage following premature birth (by definition an acquired form), or from myelomeningocoele. Studies of prenatal fetal surgery on myelomingocoele show promising results, notably decreased need for ventricular shunts, and less severe Chiari II malformations, but no improvement in leg or bladder function. Prenatal surgery is not currently standard practice (Bannister *et al.*, 2000), although multicentre trials are underway in the USA.

Migration defects of neocortical projection neurons are classified according to the stage in which radial migration is disrupted (Gleeson and Walsh, 2000). Mutations in the X-linked *filamin* gene produce ectopic neuron collections near brain ventricles (Gleeson and Walsh, 2000). Mutations in *DCX* and *LIS* genes disrupt migration and cortical lamination by altering microtubule function, producing various subtypes of lissencephaly (agyria or smooth brain). Associated clinical features include significant ID, intractable epilepsy and shortened lifespan. Gene mutations in the reelin pathway produce disorganisation of cortical layers, while mutations in *presenilin* lead to neuronal migration out of brain and into meninges, also producing lissencephaly (Epstein *et al.*, 2004). (Please refer to Chapter 18 on Diseases of the nervous system.)

Fortunately, prevalence of neural tube defects (NTDs) is decreasing worldwide due to maternal serum alphafetoprotein (AFP) testing and early prenatal diagnosis (Feldkamp *et al.*, 2002). About half of these pregnancies are electively terminated (Forrester and Merz, 2000). Currently, all pregnant women are advised to take a daily supplement of 400 µg of folic acid, based on 50% reduction of NTDs by this practice (Martinez De Villareal *et al.*, 2002). Guidelines recommend 4 mg of folic acid daily from around conception to early pregnancy for women who themselves have an NTD, or who have a child or first-degree relative with one. Clarification of these diagnoses prenatally is by maternal serum AFP measurement, high-resolution ultrasound and then amniocentesis for AFP level and acetylcholinesterase. Parents not choosing pregnancy termination are advised to have the child delivered by Caesarean section at a hospital with a neonatal intensive care and neurosurgical unit, to allow early surgical closure of the back lesion, which may reduce future paralysis.

Conclusion

Major advances have been made in the past ten years into identifying the molecular, genetic, surgical and neuropsychiatric aspects of congenital causes of ID. The largest and as yet unknown group of causes will hopefully be elucidated in the next decade. Development of brain and tissue banks, access to computer databases and more sophisticated brain imaging techniques, with collaboration among neuroscientists, will afford a better understanding of brain anatomy and function. Challenges to gene–protein and gene–brain studies include the complexity of gene modifiers and interactions and environmental influences that turn identified genes on or off. While genetic engineering is still in the future, studies of specific protein replacement may begin soon, as in Fragile X syndrome. Due to the diversity of causes, prevention of ID remains a significant but highly worthwhile challenge.

References

Adam, M. P. and Hoyme, H. E. (2005). Fetal alcohol syndrome. In *Genetics of Developmental Disabilities*, ed. M. G. Butler and F. J. Meaney. Boca Raton, FL: Taylor and Francis Group, pp. 665–91.

Ahlgren, S. C., Thakur, V. and Bronner-Fraser, M. (2002). Sonic hedgehog rescues cranial neural crest from cell death induced by ethanol exposure. *Proc Natl Acad Sci U S A*, 99(16), 10476–81.

American Academy of Pediatrics (1994). Health supervision for children with Down syndrome. *Pediatrics*, 93, 855–9.

Atreya, C. D., Mohan, K. V. and Kulkarni, S. (2004). Rubella virus and birth defects: molecular insights into the viral teratogenesis at the cellular level. *Birth Defects Res A Clin Mol Teratol*, 70(7), 431–7.

Bannister, C. M., Russell, S. A., Rimmer, S., Thorne, J. A. and Hellings, S. (2000). Can prognostic indicators be identified in a fetus with an encephalocele? *Eur J Pediatr Surg*, 10(Suppl 1), 20–3.

Barf, H. A., Verhoef, M., Post, M. W. *et al.* (2004). Educational career and predictors of type of education in young adults with spina bifida. *Int J Rehabil Res*, 27(1), 45–52.

Barr, H. M. and Streissguth, A. P. (2001). Identifying maternal self-reported alcohol use associated with fetal alcohol spectrum disorders. *Alcohol Clin Exp Res*, 25(2), 283–7.

Bell, M. J. (2007). Infections and the fetus. In *Children with Developmental Disabilities*, 6th edn, ed. M. L. Batshaw, L. Pellegrino and N. J. Roizen. Baltimore, MD: Paul Brookes Publishing Company, pp. 71–82.

Benjamin, E. and Buot-Smith, T. (1993). Naltrexone and fluoxetine in Prader-Willi syndrome. *J Am Acad Child Adolesc Psychiatry*, 32(4), 870–3.

Berk, D. R., Falkovitz-Halpern, M. S., Hill, D. W. *et al.* (2005). Temporal trends in early clinical manifestations of perinatal HIV infection in a population-based cohort. *JAMA*, 293(18), 2221–31.

Berry-Kravis, E., Krause, S. E., Block, S. S. *et al.* (2006). Effect of CX516, an AMPA-modulating compound, on cognition and behavior in fragile X syndrome: a controlled trial. *J Child Adolesc Psychopharmacol*, 16(5), 525–40.

Bienvenu, T. (2005). Rett syndrome. In *Genetics of Developmental Disabilities*, ed. M. G. Butler and F. J. Meaney. Boca Raton, FL: Taylor and Francis Group, pp. 477–519.

Bittel, D. C. and Butler, M. G. (2005). Prader-Willi syndrome: clinical genetics, cytogenetics and molecular biology. *Expert Rev Mol Med*, 7(14), 1–20.

Bregman, J. D., Leckman, J. F. and Ort, S. I. (1988). Fragile X syndrome: genetic predisposition to psychopathology. *J Autism Dev Disord*, 18(3), 343–54.

Brewington, R., Hellings, J. and Butler, M. G. (2008). Velocardiofacial syndrome-associated psychiatric illness and response to aripiprazole: A case study. *Am J Psychiatry*, 3, 1–4.

Buiting, K., Saitoh, S., Gross, S. *et al.* (1995). Inherited microdeletions in the Angelman and Prader-Willi syndromes define an imprinting centre on human chromosome 15. *Nat Genet*, 9(4), 395–400.

Cohen, I. L. (1995). A theoretical analysis of the role of hyperarousal in the learning and behavior of fragile X males. *Ment Retard Dev Disabil Res Rev*, 1, 286–97.

Cohen, W. I. (2005). Medical care of the child with Down syndrome. In *Genetics of Developmental Disabilities*, ed. M. G. Butler and F. J. Meaney. Boca Raton, FL: Taylor and Francis Group, pp. 223–45.

Connolly, J. A. (1978). Intelligence levels of Down's syndrome children. *Am J Ment Defic*, 83(2), 193–6.

Danovaro-Holliday, M. C., Gordon, E. R., Woernle, C. *et al.* (2003). Identifying risk factors for rubella susceptibility in a population at risk in the United States. *Am J Public Health*, 93(2), 289–91.

Dech, B. and Budow, L. (1991). The use of fluoxetine in an adolescent with Prader-Willi syndrome. *J Am Acad Child Adolesc Psychiatry*, 30(2), 298–302.

Depew, M. J., Liu, J. K., Long, J. E. *et al.* (1999). Dlx5 regulates regional development of the branchial arches and sensory capsules. *Development*, 126(17), 3831–46.

Dykens, E. M. and Volkmar, F. R. (1997). Medical conditions associated with autism. In *Handbook of Autism and Pervasive Developmental Disorders*, 2nd edn., ed. D. J. Cohen and F. R. Volkmar. New York: John Wiley and Sons, pp. 338–407.

Epstein, C. J., Erickson, R. P. and Wynshaw-Boris, A. (eds.). (2004). *Inborn Errors of Development*. New York: Oxford University Press.

Feinstein, D. L., Heneka, M. T., Gavrilyuk, V. *et al.* (2002). Noradrenergic regulation of inflammatory gene expression in brain. *Neurochem Int*, 41(5), 357–65.

Feldkamp, M., Friedrichs, M. and Carey, J. C. (2002). Decreasing prevalence of neural tube defects in Utah, 1985–2000. *Teratology*, 66(Suppl 1), S23–8.

Fisch, G. S., Cohen, I. L., Gross, A. C. *et al.* (1988). Folic acid treatment of fragile X males: a further study. *Am J Med Genet*, 30(1–2), 393–9.

Forrester, M. B. and Merz, R. D. (2000). Prenatal diagnosis and elective termination of neural tube defects in Hawaii, 1986–1997. *Fetal Diagn Ther*, 15(3), 146–51.

Froster-Iskenius, U., Bodeker, K., Oepen, T. *et al.* (1986). Folic acid treatment in males and females with fragile-(X)-syndrome. *Am J Med Genet*, 23(1–2), 273–89.

Gibson, D. (1978). *Down's Syndrome. The Psychology of Mongolism*. Cambridge: Cambridge University Press.

Gieselmann, V. (2003). Metachromatic leukodystrophy: recent research developments. *J Child Neurol*, 18(9), 591–4.

Gladston, S. and Clarke, D. J. (2005). Clozapine treatment of psychosis associated with velo-cardio-facial syndrome: benefits and risks. *J Intellect Disabil Res*, 49(7), 567–70.

Gleeson, J. G. and Walsh, C. A. (2000). Neuronal migration disorders: from genetic diseases to developmental mechanisms. *Trends Neurosci*, 23(8), 352–9.

Golden, J. A. and Hyman, B. T. (1994). Development of the superior temporal neocortex is anomalous in trisomy 21. *J Neuropathol Exp Neurol*, 53(5), 513–20.

Golden, M. R., Marra, C. M. and Holmes, K. K. (2003). Update on syphilis: resurgence of an old problem. *JAMA*, 290(11), 1510–14.

Gothelf, D. and Martin, A. (Eds.). (2007). Neuropsychiatric genetic syndromes. *Child Adolesc Psychiatr Clin N Am*, 16, 541–743.

Grether, J. K. and Nelson, K. B. (1997). Maternal infection and cerebral palsy in infants of normal birth weight. *JAMA*, 278(3), 207–11.

Hagerman, R. J. (1996). Fragile X syndrome. *Child Adolesc Psychiatr Clin N Am*, 5, 895–911.

Hagerman, R. J., Jackson, A. W., Levitas, A. *et al.* (1986). Oral folic acid versus placebo in the treatment of males with the fragile X syndrome. *Am J Med Genet*, 23(1–2), 241–62.

Hagerman, R. J., Hull, C. E., Safanda, J. F. *et al.* (1994). High functioning fragile X males: demonstration of an unmethylated fully expanded FMR-1 mutation associated with protein expression. *Am J Med Genet*, 51(4), 298–308.

Hecht, F. (1991). Seizure disorders in the fragile X chromosome syndrome. *Am J Med Genet*, 38(2–3), 509.

Hellings, J. A. and Warnock, J. K. (1994). Self-injurious behavior and serotonin in Prader-Willi syndrome. *Psychopharmacol Bull*, 30(2), 245–50.

Hessl, D., Glaser, B., Dyer-Friedman, J. *et al.* (2002). Cortisol and behavior in fragile X syndrome. *Psychoneuroendocrinology*, 27(7), 855–72.

Hilton, D. K., Martin, C. A., Heffron, W. M., Hall, B. D. and Johnson, G. L. (1991). Imipramine treatment of ADHD in a fragile X child. *J Am Acad Child Adolesc Psychiatry*, 30(5), 831–4.

Holsen, L. M., Zarcone, J. R., Brooks, W. M. *et al.* (2006). Neural mechanisms underlying hyperphagia in Prader-Willi syndrome. *Obesity (Silver Spring)*, 14(6), 1028–37.

Ikonomidou, C., Bittigau, P., Ishimaru, M. J. *et al.* (2000). Ethanol-induced apoptotic neurodegeneration and fetal alcohol syndrome. *Science*, 287(5455), 1056–60.

Jacquemont, S., Hagerman, R. J., Leehey, M. *et al.* (2003). Fragile X premutation tremor/ataxia syndrome: molecular, clinical and neuroimaging correlates. *Am J Hum Genet*, 72(4), 869–78.

Jacquemont, S., des Portes, V. and Hagerman, R. J. (2005). Fragile X and X-linked mental retardation. In *Genetics of Developmental Disabilities*, ed. M. G. Butler and F. J. Meaney. Boca Raton, FL: Taylor and Francis Group, pp. 247–78.

Khan, N. L. and Wood, N. W. (1999). Prader-Willi and Angelman syndromes: update on genetic mechanisms and diagnostic complexities. *Curr Opin Neurol*, 12(2), 149–54.

Lachiewicz, A. M. (1992). Abnormal behaviors of young girls with fragile X syndrome. *Am J Med Genet*, 43(1–2), 72–7.

Lachiewicz, A. M. and Dawson, D. V. (1994). Behavior problems of young girls with fragile X syndrome: factor scores on the Conners' Parent's Questionnaire. *Am J Med Genet*, 51(4), 364–9.

Martinez De Villareal, L., Perez, J. Z., Varquez, P. A *et al.* (2002). Decline of neural tube defects after a folic acid campaign in Nuevo Leon, MX. *Teratology*, 66(5), 249–56.

Merenstein, S. A., Sobesky, W. E., Taylor, A. K. *et al.* (1996). Molecular-clinical correlations in males with an expanded FMR1 mutation. *Am J Med Genet*, 64(2), 388–94.

Montoya, J. G. and Liesenfeld, O. (2004). Toxoplasmosis. *Lancet*, 363(9425), 1965–76.

Newell, M.-L., Hoosen, C., Cortina-Borja, M. *et al.* (2004). Mortality of infected and uninfected infants born to HIV-infected mothers in Africa; a pooled analysis. *Lancet*, 364, 1236–43.

Nicholls, R. D., Knoll, J. H., Butler, M. G., Karam, S. and Lalande, M. (1989). Genetic imprinting suggested by maternal heterodisomy in nondeletion Prader-Willi syndrome. *Nature*, 342(6247), 281–5.

Niklasson, B., Samsioe, A., Pappadogiannakis, N., Gustafsson, S. and Klitz, W. (2009). Zoonotic Ljungan virus associated with central nervous system malformations in terminated pregnancy. *Birth Defects Res A Clin Mol Teratol* [Epub ahead of print], DOI: 10.1002/bdra.20568.

Percy, A. K. (2002). Rett syndrome. Current status and new vistas. *Neurol Clin*, 20(4), 1125–41.

Prasher, V. P. (1995). Overweight and obesity amongst Down's syndrome adults. *J Intellect Disabil Res*, 39(5), 437–41.

Reiss, A. L., Abrams, M. T., Greenlaw, R., Freund, L. and Denckla, M. B. (1995). Neurodevelopmental effects of the FMR-1 full mutation in humans. *Nat Med*, 1(2), 159–67.

Robey, K. L., Reck, J. F., Giacomini, K. D., Barabas, G. and Eddey, G. E. (2003). Modes and patterns of self-mutilation in persons with Lesch-Nyhan disease. *Dev Med Child Neurol*, 45(3), 167–71.

Robin, N. H., Taylor, C. J., McDonald-McGinn, D. M. *et al.* (2006). Polymicrogyria and deletion 22q11.2 syndrome: window to the etiology of a common cortical malformation. *Am J Med Genet A*, 140(22), 2416–25.

Roizen, N. J. (1996). Down syndrome and associated medical disorders. *Ment Retard Dev Disabil Res Rev*, 2, 85–9.

Saitoh, S., Buiting, K., Rogan, P. K. *et al.* (1996). Minimal definition of the imprinting center and fixation of chromosome 15q11-q13 epigenotype by imprinting mutations. *Proc Natl Acad Sci U S A*, 93(15), 7811–15.

Schaer, M. and Eliez, S. (2007). From genes to brain: understanding brain development in neurogenetic disorders using neuroimaging techniques. *Child Adolesc Psychiatr Clin N Am*, 16(3), 557–79.

Snow, J. H. (1994). Memory functions for children with spina bifida: Assessment in rehabilitation and exceptionality. *Pediatrics*, 1, 20–7.

Stoll, B. J. and Kliegman, R. M. (2004). Nervous system disorders. In *Nelson Textbook of Pediatrics*, 17th edn., ed. R. E. Behrman,

R. M. Kliegman and H. G. Jenson. Philadelphia, PA: W. B. Saunders Co, pp. 561–9.

Strom, C. M., Brusca, R. M. and Pizzi, W. J. (1992). Double-blind, placebo-controlled crossover study of folinic acid (Leucovorin) for the treatment of fragile X syndrome. *Am J Med Genet*, 44(5), 676–82.

Tezenas Du Montcel, S., Mendizabai, H., Ayme, S., Levy, A. and Philip, N. (1996). Prevalence of 22q11 microdeletion. *J Med Genet*, 33(8), 719.

Torrioli, M. G., Vernacotola, S., Mariotti, P. *et al.* (1999). Double-blind, placebo-controlled study of L-acetylcarnitine for the treatment of hyperactive behavior in fragile X syndrome. *Am J Med Genet*, 87(4), 366–8.

Tuli, S., Drake, J. and Lamberti-Pasculli, M. (2003). Long-term outcome of hydrocephalus management in myelomeningoceles. *Childs Nerv Syst*, 19(5–6), 286–91.

Turner, G., Webb, T., Wake, S. and Robinson, H. (1996). Prevalence of fragile X syndrome. *Am J Med Genet*, 64(1), 196–7.

Van den Veyver, I. B. and Zoghbi, H. Y. (2001). Mutations in the gene encoding methyl-CpG-binding protein 2 cause Rett syndrome. *Brain Dev*, 23(Suppl 1), S147–51.

Vogels, A., De Hert, M., Descheemaeker, M. J. *et al.* (2004). Psychotic disorders in Prader-Willi syndrome. *Am J Med Genet A*, 127A(3), 238–43.

Wang, P. P. (1996). A neuropsychological profile of Down syndrome: cognitive and brain morphology. *Ment Retard Dev Disabil Res Rev*, 2102–8.

Warnock, J. K. and Kestenbaum, T. (1992). Pharmacologic treatment of severe skin-picking behaviors in Prader-Willi syndrome. Two case reports. *Arch Dermatol*, 128(12), 1623–5.

Warren, K. R., Calhoun, F. J., May, P. A. *et al.* (2001). Fetal alcohol syndrome: an international perspective. *Alcohol Clin Exp Res*, 25(5), Suppl 202S–6S.

Willems, P. J., Van Roy, B., De Boulle, K. *et al.* (1992). Segregation of the fragile X mutation from an affected male to his normal daughter. *Hum Mol Genet*, 1(7), 511–15.

Williams, C. A. (2005). Angelman syndrome. In *Genetics of Developmental Disabilities*, ed. M. G. Butler and F. J. Meaney. Boca Raton, FL: Taylor and Francis Group, pp. 319–35.

Woo, S. L., Lidsky, A. S., Guttler, F., Chandra, T. and Robson, K. J. (1983). Cloned human phenylalanine hydroxylase gene allows prenatal diagnosis and carrier detection of classical phenylketonuria. *Nature*, 306(5939), 151–5.

3

Disorders of environmental origin

Alaa Al-Sheikh

Introduction

Disorders of environmental origin in the general population, especially in children, have attracted significant research attention. This may be due to the detrimental effect that these disorders can have on large populations of vulnerable young people. In developed countries the biggest environmental concern is the presence of hazardous environmental agents, while in the developing world poverty and malnutrition are more worrying.

The burden and cost of disease attributed to selected environmental factors and injury among children and adolescents specifically can lead to long-term disability. This subject was reviewed by Valent *et al.* (2004). They examined published studies and reports from international agencies for calculation of risk-factor exposure for children in Europe. Mild intellectual disability (ID) resulting from lead exposure, for example, accounted for 4.4% of Disability-Adjusted Life Years (DALYs), defined as 'the sum of years of potential life lost due to premature mortality and the years of productive life lost due to disability' (WHO Website). Other factors found were non-specific to ID. This can provide a framework to assess the impact of disease on a population and to better allocate scarce health resources. Disorders of environmental origin in ID can be examined from two main perspectives, one causative and the other co-morbid to ID; although the two may overlap.

This chapter examines the evidence base for disorders of environmental origin according to the International Statistical Classification of Diseases and Related Health Problems (ICD-10) Chapters XIX and XX including selected subcategories (WHO, 1992). (Please refer to Box 3.1).

Method

A broad search strategy included a literature search in peer-reviewed journals from the following sources: MEDLINE (1950–2008), EMBASE, PsycINFO, Health Business Elite, CINAHL, British Nursing Index and Health Management Information. A similar search was made of the World Health Organization website. A selection of accessible textbooks on ID, child psychiatry and paediatrics were also hand searched.

The MeSH terms used were intellectual disabilities, learning disabilities, mental retardation, developmental disabilities, environmental disorders, environmental factors, external causes of morbidity and mortality. Subcategories such as injury and poisoning were also searched; the terms used are mentioned below in the relevant section. There was no restriction as to language. The first search was made in July 2008 and updated in September 2008.

Intellectual Disability and Ill Health: A Review of the Evidence, ed. Jean O'Hara, Jane McCarthy and Nick Bouras. Published by Cambridge University Press. © Cambridge University Press 2010.

Table 3.1. Summary of literature search

Search results including hand-search, relevant websites and text books	222
References included in this review	51

Box 3.1 ICD-10

International Statistical Classification of Diseases and Related Health Problems, 10th Revision, Version for 2007.

Chapter XIX

Injury, poisoning and certain other consequences of external causes (S00–T98), excluding birth and obstetric trauma

Includes the following subcategories (this is not a complete but a selective list of categories)

- Injuries to the head and other parts of the body
- Effects of foreign body entering through natural orifice
- Burns and corrosions
- Frostbite
- Poisoning by drugs, medicaments and biological substances
- Toxic effects of substances chiefly non medicinal as to source

Chapter XX

External causes of morbidity and mortality (V01–Y98)

Includes the following subcategories (this is not an exclusive list)

- Accidents including transport accidents
- Falls
- Accidental drowning and submersion
- Exposure to smoke, fire and flames
- Accidental poisoning by and exposure to noxious substances
- Intentional self-harm
- Assault

All abstracts found were read, and potentially relevant articles, chapters and documentation were inspected in more detail.

Exclusion criteria were birth trauma and environmental disorders during pregnancy. Self-injurious behaviour and intentional self-harm were also excluded as they are beyond the scope of this chapter. Evidence included high-quality population-based studies with a control group, population-based studies, systematic reviews, cohort and case control studies. Case reports, case series and review articles were also included due to the dearth of information in this area and the lack of high-quality large population studies specific to people with ID.

Results

The search found 222 relevant studies, articles, policy documentation and book chapters on the association between ID and disorders of environmental origin including searching subcategories. Summary of the results are included in Table 3.1.

Discussion

Intellectual disability has attracted some research attention with regard to environmental disorders, however, there is a dearth of high-quality evidence, with more emphasis on studies related to children and young people. There are a few large population or controlled inter-vention studies but the results are conflicting. In a population-based 35-year follow-up study causes-specific mortality of people with ID differed significantly from the general popula-tion, with reduced mortality from neoplasms and external causes (Patja *et al.*, 2001). On the other hand an Australian study found that the overall standardised mortality ratio (SMR) in people with ID was higher than that of the general population. External causes of mortality (see Box 3.1) were the second main cause of death after respiratory disease (Durvasula *et al.*, 2002).

Environmental causes

The causes of ID can be classified according to the timing of the damage to the brain into pre-natal (during pregnancy), perinatal (during labour) and postnatal (following birth) (Harris, 2005). Each of these stages can be further divided into hereditary and environmental. This section focuses on some of the environmental postnatal causes of ID. (Please refer to Box 3.2).

Box 3.2 Environmental causes of ID in the postnatal period

1. Infections: some childhood infections that can damage the brain such as encephalitis and meningitis.
2. Trauma and injury: accidental injury in children resulting from road traffic accidents or general domestic accidental injury. Non-accidental injury can be due to physical abuse of children.
3. Toxic agent and metal poisoning: this is an evolving area of research. Common agents which can cause ID are lead, mercury, copper, environmental pollutant, pesticides and polychlorinated biphenyls (PCBs).
4. Nutrition: protein-calorie malnutrition including Kwashiorkor and Marasmus can cause physical and intellectual disability.
5. Environmental, sensory and social deprivation: social exclusion, child abuse and neglect, chronic sensory deprivation can all affect child development and may lead to ID.

Adapted from Harris, 2005; Watson, 2005

Margai and Henry's (2003) American study of the potential association between exposure to pollutants and toxicants and incidence of ID found areas of high risk were strongly associ-ated with historically significant sources of lead toxicity and air pollution facilities. However, in some parts of the world, especially those affected by famine, malnutrition may lead to physical and mental developmental delay while severe sensory and social deprivation (as in the case of institutionalisation) are other recognised environmental causes of ID (Watson, 2005). However it is beyond the scope of the chapter to discuss this in further detail.

Injury and trauma

Injury and trauma are considered major causes of death and disability worldwide and place a significant burden on countries with limited resources. In general, people with ID are at high risk of injury. Injury prevalence was higher for children with ID compared to others without ID in a study by Slayter *et al.* (2006). However the prevention of unintentional injury to people with ID has not been addressed sufficiently. Injury prevention programmes are needed to protect the quality of life for people with ID and their families (Sherrard *et al.*, 2004). This section (please refer to Table 3.2) focuses on recent studies of injuries in people with ID, including two areas of particular importance.

Table 3.2. Studies related to specific injury in children and adults with ID

Injury type	Authors	Description and results of the study
Traumatic injury	Steinmann et al., 2007	This article looks at the recent growing experience in the field of rehabilitation after trauma of those with ID. It presumes that with increasing awareness of the benefits of comprehensive and early rehabilitation, all medical professionals who work in intensive care units will be referred more patients who had never before gained from this specialty
Concussion	Sim, 2006	Sports-related concussion in the high school athlete: an analysis of incidence rates, neuropsychological deficits, and recovery patterns. Participants included 420 male and female athletes (mean age = 15.69) who underwent baseline testing of neuropsychological functioning prior to their sports season. Participants with a history of ID or attention deficit hyperactivity disorder (ADHD) demonstrated significantly poorer baseline performance. The study concludes that history of premorbid symptoms of ADHD and ID must be assessed in order to accurately evaluate the impact of a concussive injury and monitor an athlete's recovery
General injury	Konarski and Tasse, 2005	Assessing risk of injury in people with ID living in an intermediate care facility. A brief instrument designed to assess risk of injury was applied retrospectively for 2 years and prospectively for 1 year. Results suggest that the percentage of people who experienced an injury significantly increased across the levels of increasing risk indicated by the instrument. This instrument promises a reliable and valid method for predicting injury risk level
Non-fatal injury in children	Xiang et al., 2005	Non-fatal injuries among US children with disabling conditions. Among 57 909 children aged 5–17 years who participated in the 2000–2002 National Health Interview Survey, 711 had ID. Higher percentage of children with disabilities reported non-fatal injuries (3.2% for ID); however after controlling for confounding factors children with ID did not have a statistically significantly higher injury risk
Fall	Bruckner and Herge, 2003	Assessing the risk of falls in people with ID and developmental disabilities. Eighteen community-based people with ID, aged 55+ with high risks for falls, were examined using a reliable screening tool under 3 conditions: free walking, walking with a rolling walker and walking with a personal assistant. Conclude that typical strategies (use of assisted devices and personal assistance) can decrease the patients walking speed. They conclude that people with ID have a high risk of falls and this can put them at risk of injury and higher healthcare costs
Head trauma	Hardman and Manoukian, 2002	Review article looking at the essential primary and secondary injuries attributable to traumatic brain injury (TBI). Motor vehicle crashes, falls, assaults, guns, sports and recreational activities are the major causes of TBI. Increased risk for accidents in people with ID was reported
General injury	Wang et al., 2002	Analysis of hospital use for injury among individuals with ID. In comparison with the general population, persons with ID had a lower proportion of accident and emergency department visits related to injury. Admissions to hospital were more likely to be due to falls rather than road traffic accidents. Persons with ID were more likely to be seen for poisoning
Injury in children	Gaebler-Spira and Thornton, 2002	Review article of injury in children with disabilities and their prevention. Little injury data exist. There is an urgent need to address injury prevention and to improve safety standards. The article suggests strategies to help prevent injuries in this group

Table 3.2. (*cont.*)

Injury type	Authors	Description and results of the study
Injury and falls in adults with ID	Hsieh *et al.*, 2001	Short report. Risk factors for injuries and falls among adults with ID. Identified risk factors for injuries including falls and non-fall-related injuries in 268 adults with ID. Eleven per cent of the sample reported to have injuries. Over 50% of injuries were caused by falls. Individuals who had a higher frequency of seizures, had more destructive behaviour and used antipsychotic drugs had the highest risk of injuries. A sub-analysis of fall-related injuries indicated that individuals who were > or = 70 years of age, ambulatory and had a higher frequency of seizures had the highest risk of injurious falls. Adaptive behaviour, destructive behaviour and physical health were positively related to non-fall-related injuries. Individuals with ID who have better health and greater adaptive behaviour may be more active and, therefore, at an increased risk of non-fall-related injuries
Injury in young people with ID	Sherrard *et al.*, 2001	Important cohort study of injury in young people with ID. Carer reports of medically attended injury to subjects were collected. Annual injury mortality and morbidity rates were 150/100 000 and 55.6/1000 persons; the rate for injury hospitalisations was twice that of the general population. Falls were more common and transport injury and intentional injury less common causes of morbidity compared with the general population. It is essential that injury prevention programmes be implemented and evaluated for their effectiveness in reducing the substantial additional burden of suffering, care and cost resulting from injury to young people with ID
Fracture	Lohiya *et al.*, 1999	American study of fracture epidemiology and control in a centre for residents with developmental disabilities. During 3 and a half years, 182 fractures occurred among 994 residents. The fracture rate was 1.7 times greater than the rate in the US population. Fracture rate was significantly greater in residents with epilepsy, but it was not affected by severity of ID. A fall contributed to 41 fracture cases (23%)
Shaken baby syndrome	lund *et al.*, 1998	Case series of shaken baby syndrome (Danish study). Many cases were fatal or led to severe disability including blindness, cerebral palsy, ID or epilepsy in about 60% of the children
General injury	Konarski *et al.*, 1994	Case study of the relationship between census reduction and injuries to residents in an intermediate care facility (ICF). Compared the frequency and severity of injuries of adults living in an ICF for one year before and one year after the number of residents in that facility was reduced from 28 to 19. The study group had severe or profound ID, few sensory deficits and limited communication skills; most had severe behaviour problems. Results suggest that reducing the number of residents was clearly related to lowering the number of injuries
Paediatric craniocerebral trauma	Maier-Hauff *et al.*, 1993	German study of paediatric craniocerebral trauma. Presents the standardised diagnostic procedures and therapeutic strategies for the management of traumatic brain damage in children. They conclude that optimised medical management and intensive rehabilitation may help to reduce the frequency of intellectual and physical disability following such injuries in children
Depressed skull fracture in childhood	Zbinden and Kaiser, 1989	Retrospective study of 35 children with depressed skull fractures. They found ID and/or post-traumatic epilepsy were the most important sequel. The most important causes were falls and road accidents

Table 3.3. Studies identified in poisoning and toxicity search

Toxins	Authors	Description and the results of the study
Lead	Grosse et al., 2002; Landrigan et al., 2002; Needleman, 1990	These studies examined the cost of childhood lead poisoning and preventions. Concluded that removing lead paint is cost-effective if it prevents even two-thirds of lead exposure for any single year's cohort of 2-year-olds
Lead	Pocock et al., 1994	Systematic review of environmental lead and children's intelligence. Measured cognitive impairment by IQ tests and is the best-studied effect of lead exposure in children. The strength of this association and its time course has been observed to be similar in multiple studies across several countries.
Lead	Ali, 2001	Literature review of aetiology, epidemiology and complications of pica in people with ID. Pica is a common problem in this population which can be a manifestation of a range of medical conditions and can lead to a variety of complications including lead and nicotine toxicity. Rates are low in community samples in contrast to institutionalised ones
Mercury	Goldman et al., 2001	Review article on mercury toxicity, treatment and prevention. Young children can be affected disproportionately by mercury exposure because brain development can be disturbed by the presence of mercury. There have been many measures taken in the USA to reduce exposure to mercury such as the collaboration between regulatory organisations, the pharmaceutical industry and the medical community to decrease or eliminate exposure to mercury from vaccines and other medical products
Mercury	Gilbert and Grant-Webster, 1995	Review article of neurobehavioural effects of developmental methylmercury exposure. Confirms previous findings that the fetus and infant are more sensitive to adverse effects of mercury
Iron	Robotham and Lietman, 1980	Review article on the effect of iron poisoning especially in children. Found that substantial iron ingestion can result in profound ID
Arsenic	Dakeishi et al., 2006	Reviewed the long-term consequences of arsenic poisoning during infancy due to contaminated milk powder. Part of an overview of inorganic arsenic poisoning outbreaks among Japanese infants. The surviving victims were reported to suffer from severe sequelae, such as ID, neurological diseases and other disabilities
Organophosphate pesticide	Eskenazi et al., 2007	Study of organophosphate pesticide exposure and neurodevelopment in young Mexican-American children. One of the first studies to look at the effect of both prenatal and postnatal organophosphate exposure on early neurodevelopment. Reports an adverse association with prenatal organophosphate pesticide exposure, as measured by one of the metabolites, with mental development and pervasive developmental problems at 24 months of age

Of particular note is Alden et al.'s (2002) retrospective study of burn injuries in people with early onset neurological impairments of ID, autism and others. The average total body surface area (TBSA) burned was 8.9% yet resulted in unexpectedly prolonged hospitalisations. The authors attributed this to the complicated discharge needs of these patients. Another case identified is a report of accidental burns in a seven-year-old girl with ID and the circumstances of the incident in relation to neglect and abuse in this vulnerable group of children (Johnson et al., 2000).

In a recent retrospective Japanese study of 35 children with airway foreign bodies, Watanabe *et al.* (2007) identified only three children with ID. This concurred with Das's (1998) earlier study which regarded ID as a minor aetiological factor for foreign bodies in ears and noses. Other studies identified in the search were either case reports or case series (including Haanstra *et al.*, 2007; Karcher *et al.*, 2006; Muller *et al.*, 1999; Noguchi *et al.*, 2000; Ohno *et al.*, 2004; Schulz *et al.*, 2006; Ucar *et al.*, 2008).

Poisoning and toxicity

People with ID may be more vulnerable to further injury from toxins compared to the general population as they may have less control over exposure to and escape from toxins. Examples of common toxins include: lead, pesticides and herbicides, cleaning products and mercury (please refer to Table 3.3).

Lead is a very potent neurotoxin. Effects of lead exposure include: ID, decreased growth, hyperactivity, impaired hearing, behavioural tendencies toward violence and even brain damage. Lead poisoning in American children has decreased dramatically since the 1970s, however, more work is needed in trying to minimise it and other chemicals' toxicity risk in children and young adults.

Accidents and drowning

Intellectual disability is associated with an increased incidence of accidents which in turn can lead to traumatic brain injury and further disability (Hardman and Manoukian, 2002).

In an epidemiological study of drowning in children and young people in New Mexico, over a six-year period, two of the major risk factors identified were epilepsy and ID (Asano *et al.*, 1991). The study investigated the relationship between serial cranial CT findings and prognoses in 11 children after near-drowning incidents. Computed tomography scans were performed within two weeks, at three weeks to one month, two to four months and more than five months after admission. After a few months more than half (six cases) had ID and enlargement of the third ventricle. In Molnar *et al.*'s (2000) retrospective review of 32 children after drowning incidents, they found little data on long-term functional outcome of survivors with disability. Approximately 85% of the 32 children achieved age-appropriate functioning in activities of daily living with less favourable outcomes in cognitive function, as most children showed residual ID.

Assaults and intentional self-harm

People with ID are vulnerable to assaults including sexual and physical abuse (McNally, 2000). Their level of disability and social functioning are important factors as demonstrated in a matched case-control study of 174 sexual assault cases (87 with and 87 without ID) (Li *et al.*, 2007). After multivariate analysis of sexual self-defence capacity in people with ID, the researchers concluded that the level of social functioning should be properly considered in the assessment of sexual self-defence capacity. Intentional self-harm and self-injurious behaviour are not discussed here as it is beyond the scope of this chapter.

Autistic spectrum disorder and disorders of environmental origin

In an American study into the causes of death in autism, more than 13 000 people with autism were followed up between 1983 and 1997 (Shavelle *et al.*, 2001). Elevated death rates were observed for several causes, including seizures and accidents such as suffocation and drowning.

A recent link between autism and the measles, mumps, and rubella (MMR) vaccine drew a great deal of attention but has not been validated by research. A study in the UK found no association between the vaccine and autism (Taylor *et al.*, 1999). A Cochrane review of the MMR vaccine in children by Demicheli *et al.* (2005) also concluded that exposure to the MMR vaccine was unlikely to be associated with autism. The CHARGE (Childhood Autism Risks from Genetics and Environment) project is an epidemiological investigation of genetic and environmental factors contributing to autism. The CHARGE project will address a wide spectrum of chemical and biological exposures, susceptibility factors and their interactions. It is a large case-control investigation of underlying environmental and genetic causes for autism and is still in its recruiting stage (Hertz-Picciotto *et al.*, 2006).

Conclusion

Disorders of environmental origin are well studied in the general population especially in children and young people, but not greatly researched in the field of ID. Though many of the environmental causes of ID are understood and preventable, proven methods of prevention are not being fully implemented especially in developing countries. Therefore regulating policies and raising public awareness are key; preventive environmental health policy should prioritise the brain, because it is the most vulnerable and valuable human asset (Williams, 1997).

Further research in this area especially for children needs to be backed up by strong national public health information. Prospective studies may be the best avenue to fully address several of these concerns (Goldman and Koduru, 2000). Specific attention to disorders of environmental origin as they relate to ID is required, and may prove to have major implications in preventing accidents, injury and further disability in this already vulnerable population.

References

Alden N. E., Rabbitts A., Rolls J. A., Bassey P. Q. and Yurt R. W. (2002). Burn injury in patients with early-onset neurological impairments. ABA Paper. *J Burn Care Rehabil*, 25(1), 107–11.

Ali, Z. (2001). Pica in people with intellectual disability: a literature review of aetiology, epidemiology and complications. *J Intellect Dev Disabil*, 26(3), 205–15.

Asano, J., Ieshima, A., Kisa, T. and Ohtani, K. (1991). [CT findings and prognoses of anoxic brain damage due to near-drowning in children.] *No to Hattatsu*, 23(3), 227–33.

Bruckner, J. and Herge, E. A. (2003). Assessing the risk of falls in elders with mental retardation and developmental disabilities. *Top Geriatr Rehabil*, 19(30), 206–11.

Dakeishi, M., Murata, K. and Grandjean, P. (2006). *Long-Term Consequences of Arsenic Poisoning During Infancy Due to Contaminated Milk Powder*. Environmental Health: A Global Access Science Source, 5/31., 476–069X

Das, S. K. (1998). Aetiological evaluation of foreign bodies in the ear and nose: a clinical study. *J Laryngol Otol*, 98(10), 989–91.

Demicheli, V., Jefferson, T., Rivetti, A. and Price, D. (2005). Vaccines for measles, mumps and rubella in children. *Cochrane Database Syst Rev*, Issue 4. Art. No.: CD004407. DOI: 10.1002/14651858.CD004407.pub2.

Durvasula, S. Beange, H. and Baker, W. (2002). Mortality of people with intellectual disability in northern Sydney. *J Intellect Dev Disabil*, 27(4), 255–64.

Eskenazi, B., Marks, A. R., Bradman, A. *et al.* (2007). Organophosphate pesticide exposure and neurodevelopment in young Mexican-American children. *Environ Health Perspect*, 115(5), 792–8.

Gaebler-Spira, D. and Thornton, L. S. (2002). Injury prevention for children with disabilities. *Phys Med Rehabil Clin N Am*, 13(4), 891–906.

Gilbert, S. G. and Grant-Webster, K. S. (1995). Neurobehavioral effects of developmental methylmercury exposure. *Environ Health Perspect*, 103(Suppl 6), 135–42.

Goldman, L. R. and Koduru, S. (2000). Chemicals in the environment and developmental toxicity to children: a public health and policy perspective. *Environ Health Perspect*, 108(Suppl 3), 443–8.

Goldman, L. R., Shannon, M. W. and the Committee on Environmental Health (2001). Technical Report: Mercury in the environment: implications for paediatricians. *Pediatrics*, 108(1), 197–205.

Grosse, S. D., Matte, T., Schwartz, J. and Jackson, R. J. (2002). Economic gains resulting from the reduction in children's blood lead in the United States. *Environ Health Perspect*, 110, 563–9.

Haanstra, H. B., Vastert, S. J., Vos, G. D. and Pelleboer, R. A. (2007). Two children with severe complications following incomplete removal of a percutaneous endoscopic gastrostomy (PEG) catheter. *Ned Tijdschr Geneesk*, 151(10), 607–10.

Hardman, J. M. and Manoukian, A. (2002). Pathology of head trauma. *Neuroimaging Clin N Am*, 12(2), 175–87.

Harris, J. C. (2005). *Intellectual Disability: Understanding its Development, Causes, Classification, Evaluation and Treatment.* New York: Oxford University Press US, pp. 166.

Hertz-Picciotto, I., Croen, L. A., Hansen, R. *et al.* (2006). The CHARGE study: an epidemiologic investigation of genetic and environmental factors contributing to autism. *Environ Health Perspect*, 114(7), 1119–25.

Hsieh, K., Heller, T. and Miller, A. B. (2001). Short report. Risk factors for injuries and falls among adults with developmental disabilities. *J Intellect Disabil Res*, 45(P 1), 76–82.

Johnson, C. F., Oral, R. and Gullberg, L. (2000). Diaper burn: accident, abuse, or neglect. *Pediatr Emerg Care*, 16(3), 173–5.

Karcher, J. C., von Buch, C., Waag, K. L. and Reinshagen, K. (2006). Gastrobronchial fistula after toothbrush ingestion. *J Pediatr Surg*, 41(10), 1768–70.

Konarski, E. A. and Tasse, M. (2005). Assessing risk of injury in people with mental retardation living in an intermediate care facility. *Am J Ment Retard*, 110(5), 333–8.

Konarski, E. A. Jr., Riddle, J. I. and Walker, M. (1994). Case study of the relation between census reduction and injuries to residents in an ICF/MR. *Ment Retard*, 32(2), 132–6.

Landrigan, P. J., Schecter, C. B., Lipton, J. M., Fahs, M. C. and Schwartz, J. (2002). Environmental pollutants and disease in American children: estimates of morbidity, mortality, and costs for lead poisoning, asthma, cancer, and developmental disabilities. *Environ Health Perspect*, 110, 721–8.

Li, B.-H., Wang, B. and Hu, J. M. (2007). Multivariant analysis of sexual self-defense capacity in patients with mental retardation. *Chin J Evid Based Med*, 7(2), 108–11.

Lohiya, G. S, Crinella, F. M., Tan-Figueroa, L., Caires, S. and Lohiya, S (1999). Fracture epidemiology and control in a developmental center. *West J Med*, 170(4), 203–9.

Lund, A. M., Sandgren, G. and Knudsen, F. U. (1998). Shaken baby syndrome. *Ugeskr Laeg*, 160(46), 6632–7.

Maier-Hauff, K. Gatzounis, G. and Borschel, M. (1993). Pediatric craniocerebral trauma. Special characteristics, therapy and prognosis. *Unfallchirurg*, 96(11), 604–8.

Margai, F. and Henry, N. (2003). A community-based assessment of learning disabilities using environmental and contextual risk factors. *Soc Sci Med*, 56(5), 1073–85.

McNally, S. (2000). Learning disability nursing. Caring for people with a learning disability who are victims of crime. *Br J Nurs*, 9(8), 493–6.

Molnar, G. E., Brezner, A., Aguilar, C. and Haining, R. (2000). Rehabilitation and outcome of children following near drowning. *Phys Med Rehabil*, 14(2), 301–9.

Muller, R., Schmidt, M., Muller, K.-M. and Breuer, H.-W. M. (1999). Aspiration pneumonia caused by vertebra of a dove in a 39-year old patient with Down syndrome. *Pneumologie*, 53(7), 360–3.

Needleman, H. L. (1990). The future challenge of lead toxicity. *Environ Health Perspect*, 89, 85–9.

Noguchi, I., Sasao, M., Takano, K., Sekita, S. and Amemiya, Y. (2000). Three cases of dental foreign bodies in airways. *J Jpn Dent Soc Anesthesiol*, 28(2), 237–42.

Ohno, S., Miura, M. and Ichimaru, K. (2004). Two cases of denture foreign body in the esophagus in the aged with mental disorder. *Pract Otorhinolaryngol (Basel)*, 97(11), 983–6.

Patja, K., Mölsä, P. and Iivanainen, M. (2001). Cause-specific mortality of people with intellectual disability in a population-based, 35-year follow-up study. *J Intellect Disabil Res*, 45(P 1), 30–40.

Pocock, S. J., Smith, M. and Baghurst, P. (1994). Environmental lead and children's intelligence: a systematic review of the epidemiological evidence. *BMJ*, 309, 1189–97.

Robotham, J. L. and Lietman, P. S. (1980). Acute iron poisoning. A review. *Am J Dis Child*, 134(9), 875–9.

Schulz, M., Wild, L., Konig, C., Kiess, W. and Siekmeyer, W. (2006). An esophagobronchial fistula caused by an unusual foreign body in the esophagus leading to mediastinitis with fatal outcome. *Klin Paediatr*, 218(2), 85–7.

Shavelle, R. M., Strauss, D. J. and Pickett, J. (2001). Causes of death in autism. *J Autism Dev Disord*, 31(6), 569–76.

Sherrard, J., Tonge, B. J. and Ozanne-Smith, J. (2001). Injury in young people with intellectual disability: descriptive epidemiology. *Inj Prev*, 7(1), 56–61.

Sherrard, J., Ozanne-Smith, J. and Staines, C. (2004). Prevention of unintentional injury to people with intellectual disability: a review of the evidence. *J Intellect Disabil Res*, 48(P 7), 639–45.

Sim, A. H. (2006). *Sports-Related Concussion in the High School Athlete: An Analysis of Incidence Rates, Neuropsychological Deficits, and Recovery Patterns.* 01 January

2006, /(0–71)ETD collection for University of Nebraska – Lincoln. Paper AAI3218334. http://digitalcommons.unl.edu/dissertations/AAI3218334.

Slayter, E. M, Garnick, D. W., Kubisiak, J. M. *et al.* (2006). Injury prevalence among children and adolescents with mental retardation. *Ment Retard*, 44(3), 212–23.

Steinmann, M., Hadad, N., Shemesh, F., Goldin, D. and Ohry, A. (2007). The rehabilitation of patients with intellectual disability who sustained traumatic injury. *Harefuah*, 146(1), 7–10, 80.

Taylor, B., Miller, E., Farrington, C. P. *et al.* (1999). Autism and measles, mumps, and rubella vaccine: no epidemiological evidence for a causal association. *Lancet*, 353, 2026–9.

Ucar, D., Paker, N. and Bugdayci, D. (2008). Intravaginal foreign body in a girl with spastic diplegic cerebral palsy: Case report. *Turkiye Klinikleri J Med Sci*, 28(2), 243–5.

Valent, F., Little, D., Bertollini, R. *et al.* (2004). Burden of disease attributable to selected environmental factors and injury among children and adolescents in Europe. *Lancet*, 363(9426), 2032–9.

Wang, D., McDermott, S. and Sease, T. (2002). Analysis of hospital use for injury among individuals with ID. *Inj Control Saf Promot*, 9(2), 107–11.

Watanabe, K., Kagawa, K., Kinouchi, K. *et al.* (2007). [Perioperative management of airway foreign bodies in 35 pediatric patients.] *Masui*, 56(9), 1065–70.

Watson, D. (2005). Causes and manifestation of learning disability. In *Learning disability*, 4th edn., ed. B. Gates. Edinburgh: Churchill Livingstone, pp. 21–39.

World Health Orgnization (WHO) (1992). International Statistical Classification of Disease and Related Health Problems, 10th revision. Geneva: World Health Organization.

World Health Organization (WHO) Website www.who.int/mental_health/management/depression/daly/en/ (last accessed December 2008).

Williams, C. (1997). *Terminus Brain: The Environmental Threats to Human Intelligence*. Cassell: London and the summary from the St George's, University of London (SGUL) website @ www.intellectualdisability.info (last accessed August 2008).

Xiang, H., Stallones, L., Chen, G., Hostetler, S. G. and Kelleher, K. (2005). Nonfatal injuries among US children with disabling conditions. *Am J Public Health*, 95(11), 1970–5.

Zbinden, B. and Kaiser, G. (1989). Specific aspects of depressed skull fractures in childhood. *Z Kinderchir*, 44(1), 3–7.

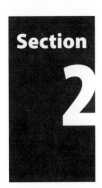

Section 2

Systems disorders

Infectious diseases

Neil A. Douglas

Introduction

Although accounting for a small proportion of the aetiological causes of intellectual disability (ID), infectious diseases are important because of the potential for primary prevention by treatment, vaccination or public health measures. People with ID can be vulnerable to infection through behavioural factors related to their level of disability, due to living in institutional settings and through the depressed immunity that is characteristic of syndromes such as Down syndrome. If ID is complicated by communication difficulties then infection may present atypically and diagnosis and treatment may be delayed. This is particularly true in respiratory infection and endocarditis, both of which contribute significantly to the morbidity and mortality associated with ID.

In primary care, consultation rates for infectious diseases are significantly higher for people with ID than for a matched control population, with the highest rates seen for fungal skin infections and respiratory infection (Straetmans *et al.*, 2007). This chapter will discuss recent reviews and research with particular emphasis on common infectious diseases which have special relevance in ID. The review will highlight areas of concern where gaps in knowledge indicate opportunities for further research.

Method

A search (1998 to last update December 2008) was made to find literature on the association between intellectual disabilities and infection. A broad search strategy included MEDLINE, AMED, BNI, EMBASE, HMIC, PsycINFO, CINAHL and Health Business Elite databases. The MeSH terms used were 'mental handicap', 'mental retardation', 'mental retardation/ aetiology', 'learning disability', 'intellectual disability' and 'infection'.

The initial search was supplemented by PubMed searches for studies on the association of particular infectious diseases including hepatitis, *Helicobacter pylori*, HIV, cytomegalovirus, tuberculosis and toxoplasmosis with intellectual disability. The focus was on studies and reviews that represent recent advances or opinions on common current issues. Some earlier studies of particular relevance were included.

All abstracts found were read and grouped into broad categories. Potentially relevant studies were inspected in more detail.

Intellectual Disability and Ill Health: A Review of the Evidence, ed. Jean O'Hara, Jane McCarthy and Nick Bouras. Published by Cambridge University Press. © Cambridge University Press 2010.

Table 4.1. Search results for infection

	Number of references
Mental retardation/aetiology and infection	106
Infection and mental retardation	364
Infection and learning disability	121
Infection and mental handicap	48
Infection and intellectual disability	71

Table 4.2. Search results for particular infectious diseases

	Mental retardation	Mental handicap	Learning disability	Intellectual disability
Hepatitis	497	16	18	5
Helicobacter	14	0	2	8
HIV	113	5	151	4
CMV	160	1	9	2
Toxoplasmosis	147	1	5	2
TB	98	6	7	2

CMV, cytomegalovirus; HIV, human immunodeficiency virus; TB, tuberculosis.

Results

The number of references for the initial search was 710. PubMed searches yielded an additional 1273 references (see Tables 4.1 and 4.2).

Exclusion criteria were articles published before 1980 and references that did not have an abstract or an abstract in English. Evidence included reviews, meta-analyses, trials, case-control studies, surveys, guidelines and opinion pieces.

Discussion

Infection as an aetiological factor

A recent review of aetiological factors identified infection as a cause in a relatively small percentage of cases of ID (Bhate and Wilkinson, 2006). The expression of the disease and subsequent disability is dependent on several factors and in particular the time point during nervous system development at which the infection occurs (Meyer *et al.*, 2006). It is important to note that the cause may be multifactorial with infection complicating factors such as genetic susceptibility, poor nutritional status, low socio-economic status and low levels of maternal education (Durkin, 2002). This is particularly salient in the developing world where for example helminth infections which are associated with poor cognitive performance in children (Ezeamama *et al.*, 2005; Jardim-Botelho *et al.*, 2008; Stephenson, 2001) can interact with other vulnerability factors.

A review in the USA looking at data from 1950 to 2000 researched the impact of specific medical interventions to reduce the prevalence of ID (Brosco *et al.*, 2006). Infections studied included congenital syphilis, measles, *Haemophilus influenzae* type b, meningitis and congenital rubella. The review concluded that despite preventing thousands of cases of ID by screening and immunisation the overall effect on the prevalence of ID was relatively small. Despite this, efforts have continued to find primary preventive measures for infectious diseases that continue to burden individuals, families and society. Immunisation can be extremely effective as in the case of the rubella vaccine programme which was introduced in the USA in 1969 and has reduced the incidence of congenital rubella syndrome (sensori-neural deafness, cataracts, heart abnormalities and ID) by 99% (Centers for Disease Control and Prevention, 2005).

Immunisation as a preventive measure may have a more significant role in developing countries where resources and facilities to identify and treat infection are limited. This is illustrated by a case series from Paraguay that describes the sequelae of *Haemophilus influenzae* type b infection in children (Basualdo and Arbo, 2004). In this study 39% (28/72) of the sample developed severe adverse outcomes such as bilateral hearing loss, hydrocephalus and ID. Further research in the Gambia demonstrated that 25% and 50% of the survivors of *Haemophilus influenzae* type b and *Streptococcus pneumoniae* meningitis respectively had major disability including ID as sequelae to infection (Goetghebuer *et al.*, 2000). The potential benefits from cost-effective vaccination programmes are therefore considerable. However, proven methods of prevention are often not implemented in developing countries and further epidemiological studies are needed to raise awareness and set priorities for interventions (Durkin, 2002). One study in South Africa exploring ID and secondary epilepsy identified reducing meningitis, tuberculosis and neurocysterosis as key elements in such a preventive campaign (Leary *et al.*, 1999).

In contrast one can observe the furore surrounding the MMR (measles, mumps and rubella) vaccine in the UK. A published case series suggested a role for the vaccine in the aetiology of autism (Wakefield *et al.*, 1998). This generated public and parental anxiety and despite much evidence refuting a causative link with autism (Hornig *et al.*, 2008; Kaye *et al.*, 2001; Taylor *et al.*, 2002) immunisation rates fell (Owens, 2002). Herd immunity dropped with a subsequent increase in the prevalence of measles and mumps. Ironically this increased the risk of children developing ID as a consequence of these infections (Mayor, 2003).

However, recent research on the aetiological role of infection in ID has concentrated on cytomegalovirus (CMV) and to a lesser degree toxoplasmosis. (Please refer to Chapter 2 on Congenital causes.)

Cytomegalovirus

Cytomegalovirus is a herpes type virus and is the most common cause of congenital infection in humans, affecting 0.5–3% of all newborns worldwide (Damato and Winnen, 2002). It is the leading infectious cause of deafness and ID in children. Primary maternal infection occurs in 1–4% of pregnant women and presents a 40% risk of intrauterine transmission. Infection in the first trimester is most likely to have sequelae and 11% of live-born infants are symptomatic (Kenneson and Cannon, 2007). Symptomatic infection in the neonate with neurological signs including microcephaly presents a poor prognostic indicator (Noyola *et al.*, 2001). Congenital infection without neurological deficit generally has a good developmental outcome (Noyola *et al.*, 2001).

Maternal infection may be asymptomatic and there has been debate about the accuracy and use of diagnostic serological testing (Revello and Gerna, 2004). Although some countries have introduced antenatal screening this remains controversial. However, recent advances using polymerase chain reaction (PCR) techniques to detect DNA on blood used for the

Guthrie test (originally introduced to detect neonatal hypothyroidism and phenylketonuria) have opened the possibility of early diagnosis and treatment of infected neonates. Hearing loss may be prevented by antiviral chemotherapy but it is not known if treatment prevents ID (Schleiss, 2008).

Although the deployment of a vaccine is still some way off, studies have been undertaken in healthy adult subjects and this holds the prospect of being the most effective preventive measure (Wloch *et al.*, 2008). Relatively low numbers are infected by an index case so it has been suggested that a moderately effective vaccine with modest coverage rates may make a significant difference (Colugnati *et al.*, 2007). In the meantime reduction of viral transmission by good hygiene and hand washing has been suggested (Cannon and Davis, 2005). Racial, ethnic and low income disparities in the prevalence of CMV infection in the USA (Colugnati *et al.*, 2007) suggest that there may be wide geographical variations in the impact of CMV and this warrants further research.

Toxoplasmosis

Toxoplasmosis is a parasitic zoonosis caused by ingestion of cysts present in undercooked meat and cat litter. In the USA, up to 85% of women of child-bearing age are susceptible to infection (Jones *et al.*, 2003). Co-infection with human immunodeficiency virus (HIV) causes toxoplasmosis infection to be more severe (Simpore *et al.*, 2006). The infection is asymptomatic but screening and treatment are relatively expensive (Thiebaut *et al.*, 2007). It is not known if antenatal treatment reduces transmission and a recent systematic review concluded that evaluation of treatment and screening programmes is needed (Peyron *et al.*, 1999). Other authors argue that treatment of the infection in the fetus and infant during the first year of life significantly improves clinical outcome (Montoya and Remington, 2008). At present there is no recommendation to introduce screening and preventive measures include educational programmes to increase awareness in women around the issues of food and animal hygiene (Ogunmodede *et al.*, 2005).

Human immunodeficiency virus

Children with perinatally acquired symptomatic HIV have been shown to have an increase in non-verbal ID associated with white matter disturbance in the brain caused by the infection (Harris, 1999). Children with more severe HIV-1 disease and immune problems have more developmental delay than children with milder symptomatology and treatment with antiretrovirals may not improve this (Foster *et al.*, 2006). As HIV becomes a chronic disease due to more sophisticated retroviral drug regimes in the developed world we may see a cohort of HIV infected children with ID surviving into adulthood (McIntosh, 2005).

Research however focuses on the risk of acquiring HIV. Children with ID are at similar or greater risk of contracting sexually transmitted infections as other youth but risk behaviours are not well understood (Mandell *et al.*, 2008). Paradoxically, it is felt that people with ID are particularly at risk exactly because they are not perceived to be at risk by other people (Clark and O'Toole, 2007). Studies in men have suggested that low levels of knowledge and passivity may make negotiation of safer sexual practices including condom use more difficult despite work on behavioural education (Thompson, 1994). This is supported by research in adolescents and young adults where poor decision-making and low confidence around safe sexual practice are areas for concern (Dawood *et al.*, 2006; McGillivray, 1999). Attitudes and awareness by staff caring for individuals with ID on issues of sexuality are felt to be important in addressing this problem (MacDonald *et al.*, 1999).

Existing literature does not however inform specifically about the incidence or preva-lence of HIV infection in people with ID or on issues of treatment and outcome. Two studies suggest a low seroprevalence in institutionalised settings (Pincus *et al.*, 1990. Lohiya, 1993). However, it is interesting to note that individuals with ID were least likely to report having been tested for HIV (Neri *et al.*, 2007). Specific programmes designed to accommodate indi-vidual needs are required (Scotti *et al.*, 1996).

Helicobacter pylori

The bacteria *Helicobacter pylori* (*H. pylori*) is one of the most common human infections and has been associated with peptic ulcer and increased risk of developing gastric cancer and gastric lymphoma. Eradication of the infection by combination antibiotic regimes used with proton pump inhibitors has shown to be of benefit in these conditions (Fuccio *et al.*, 2008). (Please refer to Chapter 8 on Digestive system diseases.)

Worldwide the prevalence varies from 20% in Scandinavia to 80% in Japan and South America but it is estimated that about half the world's population carries this organism. Par-ticularly high prevalence has been noted in adults and children with ID (Morad *et al.*, 2002). Studies have also related high rates of gastric malignancy and severe dyspeptic symptoms in adults with ID to infection with *H. pylori* (Duff *et al.*, 2001). Risk factors associated with high rates of infection are living in an institution for longer than five years, more severe disabil-ity, maladaptive behaviour and contact with others who have excess oral secretions or faecal incontinence (Clarke *et al.*, 2008; Wallace *et al.*, 2002). Infection of carers is also a recognised occupational risk (De Schryver *et al.*, 2008; Wallace *et al.*, 2003b).

Difficulties in diagnosis have been highlighted. The presentation of typical dyspepsia may be rare in those with communication difficulties. Confirmation of diagnosis and eradication by using the urea breath test, which requires an ability to understand and cooperate with the testing technique, presents a further problem (Wallace *et al.*, 2003a). Although stool antigen testing provides an acceptable alternative it is less accurate than the breath test (Manes *et al.*, 2005).

Treatment side effects due to the antibiotics appear higher in the ID population, with lower eradication rates (Wallace *et al.*, 2004a). Subsequent recurrence rates are higher than for the general population (7% vs. under 1%) and although screening has not been rec-ommended it is suggested that adults are retested 3–5 years after treatment (Wallace *et al.*, 2004b).

Down syndrome

Increased susceptibility to infection has been described in several syndromes including monosomy 14 (McConnell *et al.*, 2004) and Prader-Willi syndrome (Butler *et al.*, 2002). However, most of the literature focuses on Down syndrome (DS) and its association with deficiencies in the immune system (please refer to Chapter 5 on Immune system diseases).

Studies of cohorts with DS (trisomy 21 chromosome) have shown that there is an increased relative risk of dying in childhood (Baird and Sadovnick, 1988). Congenital heart disease and respiratory infections are the most common causes of this excess mortality (Bell *et al.*, 1989). Acute respiratory infection is a common cause for hospitalisation in children with DS and there is increased morbidity in this group due to an increased incidence of acute lung injury and respiratory distress syndrome (Brujin *et al.*, 2007) (please refer to Chapter 7 on Respiratory diseases).

There are several haematological disorders associated with DS that may account for these observations (Choi, 2008; Nespoli *et al.*, 1993). These include dysplasia of the thymus, abnormal antibody formation and disrupted cytokine production. Chromosome 21 carries the gene encoding interferon receptor and in trisomy 21 lymphocytes are more sensitive to interferon than normal cells (WHO Scientific Group, 1995). More recent research suggests that early senescence of the immune system and ineffective lymphocyte activation may underline the immune defects noted (Prada *et al.*, 2005). Acute leukaemia is more common and the prognosis of children with DS with this condition is worse due to the increased susceptibility to infection (Levitt *et al.*, 1990).

Early onset and enhanced deterioration of periodontal disease have also been noted (Cichon *et al.*, 1998) and it has been suggested that this is due to deficiencies in the phagocyte system and impaired cell-mediated immunity (Morgan, 2007). Congenital heart disease is also common in DS and therefore the treatment of dental disease complicated by bacteraemia presents a risk of endocarditis for those individuals with structural heart disease. To prevent this prophylactic antibiotics are recommended for dental procedures but the evidence for this is from consensus statements or expert opinion rather than trials (Dennis and Elliman, 2007; Pueschel *et al.*, 1995).

Prevalence of hepatitis B surface antigen (HBsAg) is higher in DS (Vellinga *et al.*, 1999; Wallace, 2007) and long-term carriage of HBsAg is more likely in hepatitis B infection in DS (Hawkes *et al.*, 1980). This appears to be the case in both residential and non-residential settings compared to other people with ID (van Schrojenstein Lantman-de Valk *et al.*, 1996). However, it is suggested that the high rates of chronic carriage are not due to a deficient humoral response and small studies have suggested a normal response to vaccination (Hawkes *et al.*, 1980.) although other authors suggest that this response may decline significantly with age (Heijtink *et al.*, 1984). In contrast, hepatitis A may be less prevalent in DS but there is no explanation for this (Renner *et al.*, 1985).

Efforts to prevent diseases resulting from these problems are hampered by the fact that measures such as immunisation require a functioning immune system. The antibody response to pneumococcal vaccine has been shown to be lower in adults with DS (Nurmi *et al.*, 1982). Despite this some authorities recommend vaccination for *Streptococcus pneumoniae* and *Haemophilus influenzae* but again the level of evidence is from expert consensus rather than clinical trials (Dennis and Elliman, accessed 2008). Some support for this recommendation comes from a study indicating that some subclasses of immunoglobulin are significantly reduced in children with DS, increasing the susceptibility to infections with encapsulated bacteria like *Haemophilus influenzae* type b (Anneren *et al.*, 1992).

Infection in hospitals and institutions

In many developed countries there has been a move away from large institutions and hospitals into the community. However, many opportunities exist for exposure to infectious disease in school, day-care facilities or respite settings. People with ID, particularly with severe disability, are resident for a significant proportion of their lives in institutional settings. Non-tubercular respiratory infection was the commonest cause of death in one survey (Puri *et al.*, 1995).

Residents with immune problems such as occur in DS or with multiple disabilities are particularly vulnerable to infections transmitted by close contact, respiratory droplets and the faecal-oral route. Impaired neutrophil function in residents was thought to be responsible for the pathogenesis of recurrent furunculosis caused by methicillin resistant *Staphylococcus aureus* (MRSA) in one setting (Gilad *et al.*, 2006). In another setting abnormal behaviour by residents was thought to be responsible for an outbreak of amoebiasis (Ono *et al.*, 1999). In developing countries this vulnerability may be exacerbated by poor nutritional status (Monteno *et al.*, 2000) and infection with intestinal parasites.

This difference is illustrated by two studies examining the prevalence of intestinal parasitic infection. In an institutionalised Thai population the prevalence was 57.6% as opposed to a non-institutionalised prevalence of 7.5% (Sirivichayakul *et al.*, 2003). *Trichuris* and *entamoeba* were the most common infecting parasites. In Italy the prevalence in one institution was 23% (75% of which were protozoal infections, 20% helminths) (Gatti *et al.*, 2000). Although different parasites are endemic in the two regions the relatively low prevalence in Italy was explained as a reflection of relatively good facilities, sanitary conditions, adequate staffing and control in susceptible subjects in this institution. High rates of infection in endemic areas have led to calls for active surveillance and mass screening for amoebiasis in institutional settings (Su *et al.*, 2007).

Further evidence of increased vulnerability in residential settings is provided by two studies of chicken pox outbreaks. One in a home setting for children demonstrated higher than expected complication rates (Enright *et al.*, 2006) and another highlighted the high risk of infection for institutionalised adults (Noorda and Hoebe, 2004). As a result post-exposure prophylaxis has been suggested for children in these circumstances and further research in sero-prevalence of protective antibodies and the use of prophylaxis or vaccination for adults has been proposed.

Methods to prevent nosocomial transmission of respiratory infection have been promoted by two studies describing outbreaks of pertussis (whooping cough) (Karino *et al.*, 2001; Steketee *et al.*, 1988) and SARS (severe acute respiratory distress syndrome) (Wong *et al.*, 2005) in hospital settings in populations with severe ID. For pertussis, prophylaxis and early treatment with a macrolide antibiotic is recommended. However, there are risks in inducing toxicity reactions with other drugs such as carbamazepine in using this approach. With SARS, grouping of cases within isolation areas and intensive infection control training for staff is the management strategy recommended.

Outbreaks of tuberculosis have potentially high mortality which is felt to be secondary to the degree of disability and co-morbid conditions (Abramovic *et al.*, 1990). Isolation by transferring patients to a general hospital (Huang *et al.*, 2007) and chemoprophylaxis (Wiggins *et al.*, 1989) have been suggested as methods of control and management. However, other authors have pointed out the difficulties in isolating patients who may have complex needs and have described problems with prolonged contagiousness due to delay in diagnosis and crowded living conditions as complicating factors (Lemaitre *et al.*, 1996). Even chemoprophylaxis with isoniazid is not straightforward due to interaction with other drugs such as carbamazepine (Wiggins *et al.*, 1989). A degree of clinical alertness and possible use of screening in high-risk areas may be required.

The literature, however, concentrates on describing the incidence and prevalence of conditions within institutions rather than on effective methods of control or prevention. Advice is often based on expert opinion extrapolated from these studies. One example of this is hepatitis. The high prevalence of hepatitis B has been well documented in institutional settings for people with ID (Cramp *et al.*, 1996; Lohiya *et al.*, 1986; Scanlan and Khan, 1989; Vellinga *et al.*, 1999) and has been associated with duration of stay (Arredo *et al.*, 1998). Although hepatitis C does not appear to be a problem (Cunningham *et al.*, 1994), it has been suggested that residents in these settings are also at increased risk of hepatitis A even in areas of moderate endemicity (Gil *et al.*, 1999). Although effective immunisations are available for hepatitis A and B studies are often limited to their use in single institutions. One study in Southampton, UK suggested that screening and immunisation for hepatitis B was necessary and cost-effective (Arulrajan *et al.*, 1992) whereas another in Northern Ireland found a low prevalence of infection that did not suggest the need for a vaccination programme (Kee *et al.*, 1989). Vaccination for staff and 'at risk' residents has also been recommended (Stehr-Green *et al.*, 1991). However, concerns have been raised about the long-term duration of protection for vaccinated individuals, particularly those with DS and a significant number of 'non-responders' to vaccination (Hayashi *et al.*, 1991; Van Damme *et al.*, 1990). Response to vaccination may also decrease with age (Cooper *et al.*, 1986). A more recent review proposes vaccination of all sero-negative residents as well as new entrants, after which no booster is needed (Vellinga *et al.*, 1999). To be cost-effective, advice may need to be refined in individual hospitals or institutions based on the make-up of the resident population and local prevalence (Leonard *et al.*, 1991).

A national survey of sexual behaviour and sexual behaviour policies in residential institutions in the USA found that sexual relationships between residents occurred sometimes or often within 63% of the facilities (Gust *et al.*, 2003). Over 5% of administrators reported sexually transmitted infections in at least one resident in the year preceding the survey. Monitoring of sexually transmitted infections and effective sex education was suggested but the research is unclear as how best to achieve this.

Conclusion

There are considerable difficulties in writing a review of ID and infectious diseases not least because of the very wide spectrum of syndromes, disabilities and co-morbidities covered by the term. The number and variety of infectious diseases are also immense.

The research on the subject is often descriptive of the prevalence or incidence of infections in defined populations rather than orientated to preventive or therapeutic interventions. In particular, published research tends to show bias towards the priorities of developed countries and the smaller volume of research from developing countries often exposes significant existing health inequalities. Despite this there is good evidence that primary prevention of infectious disease by vaccination has the potential to significantly decrease the burden of disability in the developing world. One author suggests that there should be a 'world cognitive impairment watch' whereby paediatric specialists work with the United Nations to assess and assist countries with prevention programmes (Olness, 2003).

However, there are also some useful messages for clinicians. For those caring for individuals with ID it is important to be aware of increased vulnerability to infection and possible atypical presentation that may lead to delay both in diagnosis and prompt intervention. In a hospital or institutional setting this should be coupled with an awareness of prevention by good hygiene or vaccination and some forward planning for the management of possible outbreaks of infectious disease.

References

Abramovic, M., Hadzimurtezic, Z., Jokic, I., Milosavljevic, D. and Zaric, S. (1990). Recent experience in the treatment of pulmonary tuberculosis in mentally retarded persons. *Plucne Bolesti*, 42(3–4), 234–8.

Anneren, G., Magnusson, C. G., Lilja, G. and Nordvall, S. L. (1992). Abnormal serum IgG subclass pattern in children with Downs's syndrome. *Arch Dis Child*, 67(5), 628–31.

Arredo, A., Latorre, M. D., Pac, M. R. *et al.* (1998). Hepatitis A, B, and C in an occupational centre for the mentally handicapped. *Enferm Infecs Microbiol Clin*, 16(8), 370–3.

Arulrajan, A. E., Tyrie, C. M., Phillips, K. and O'Connell, S. (1992). Hepatitis B screening and immunisation for people with a mental handicap in Southampton: costs and benefits. *J Intellect Disabil Res*, 36(3), 259–64.

Baird, P. A. and Sadovnick, A. D. (1988). Causes of death to age 30 in Down syndrome. *Am J Hum Genet*, 43(3), 239–48.

Basualdo, W. and Arbo, A. (2004). Invasive Haemophilus influenzae type b infection in children in Paraguay. *Arch Med Res*, 35(2), 126–33.

Bell, J. A., Pearn, J. H. and Firman, D. (1989). Childhood deaths in Down's syndrome. Survival curves and causes of death from a total population study in Queensland, Australia, 1976 to 1985. *J Med Genet*, 26(12), 764–8.

Bhate, S. and Wilkinson, S. (2006). Aetiology of learning disability. *Psychiatry*, 5(9), 298–301.

Brosco, J. P., Mattingly, M. and Sanders, L. M. (2006). Impact of specific medical interventions on reducing the prevalence of mental retardation. *Arch Pediatr Adolesc Med*, 160(3), 302–9.

Brujin, M., Van Der Aa, L. B., van Rijn, R. R., Bos, A. P. and van Woensel, B. M. (2007). High incidence of acute lung injury in children with Down syndrome. *Intensive Care Med*, 33(12), 2179–82.

Butler, J. V., Whittington, J. E., Holland, A. J., *et al.* (2002). Prevalence of, and risk factors for, physical ill-health in people with Prader-Willi syndromes: a population based study. *Dev Med Child Neurol*, 44(4), 248–55.

Cannon, M. J. and Davis, K. F. (2005). *Washing our Hands of the Congenital Cytomegalovirus Epidemic*. BMC Public Health.5:70.\ Published Online 2005 June 20. doi: 10.1186/1471-2458-5-70.

Centers for Disease Control and Prevention (2005). Elimination of rubella and congenital rubella syndrome: United States 1969–2004. *MMWR Morb Mortal Wkly Rep*, 54(11), 279–82.

Choi, J. K. (2008). Hematopoietic disorders in Down syndrome. *Int J Clin Exp Pathol*, 1(5), 387–95.

Cichon, P., Crawford, L. and Grimm, W. D. (1998). Early-onset periodontitis associated with Down's syndrome-clinical interventional study. *Ann Periodontol*, 3(1), 370–80.

Clark, L. L. and O'Toole, M. S. (2007). Intellectual impairment and sexual health: information needs. *Br J Nurs*, 16(3), 154–6.

Clarke, D., Vemuri, M., Gunatilake, D. and Tewari, S. (2008). Helicobacter pylori infection in five inpatient units for people with intellectual disability and psychiatric disorder. *J Appl Res Intellect Disabil*, 21(1), 95–8.

Colugnati, F. A. B., Staras, S. A., Dollard, S. C. and Cannon, M. J. (2007). Incidence of cytomegalovirus infection among the general population and pregnant women in the United States. *BMC Infect Dis*, 2(7), 71.

Cooper, B. W., Klimek, J. J., Upadhyaya, A. and Devine, S. (1986). Poor seroconversion rate after hepatitis B vaccination in high risk institutionalised mentally retarded patients. *Am J Infect Control*, 14(5), 204–8.

Cramp, M. E., Grundy, H. C., Perinpanayagum, R. M. and Barnado, D. E. (1996). Seroprevalence of hepatitis B and C virus in two institutions caring for mentally handicapped adults. *J R Soc Med*, 89(7), 401–2.

Cunningham, S. J., Cunningham, R., Izmeth, M. G., Baker, B. and Hart, C. A. (1994). Seroprevalence of hepatitis B and C in a Merseyside hospital for the mentally handicapped. *Epidemiol Infect*, 112(1), 195–200.

Damato, E. G. and Winnen, C. W. (2002). Cytomegalovirus infection: perinatal implications. *J Obstet Gynecol Neonatal Nurs*, 31(1), 86–92.

Dawood, N., Bhagwanjee, A., Govender, K. and Chohan, E. (2006). Knowledge, attitudes and sexual practices of adolescents with mild retardation in relation to HIV/AIDS. *Afr J AIDS Res*, 5(1), 1–10.

Dennis, J. and Elliman, D. (2007). Basic medical surveillance essentials for people with Down's syndrome. Cardiac disease: congenital and acquired. Available from: http://www.dsmig.org.uk/library/articles/guideline-cardiac-5.pdf (last accessed December 2008).

Dennis, J. and Elliman, D. Down's syndrome: immunisation. Available from: http://www.dsmig.org.uk/library/articles/keypoints-immunisation.pdf (last accessed December 2008).

De Schryver, A., Cornelis, K., van Winckel, M. et al. (2008). The occupational risk of Helicobacter pylori infection among workers in institutions for people with intellectual disability. *Occup Environ Med*, 65(9), 587–91.

Duff, M., Scheppers, M., Copper, M., Hoghton, M. and Baddely, P. (2001). Helicobacter pylori: has the killer escaped from the institution? A possible cause of increased stomach cancer in a population with intellectual disability. *J Intellect Disabil Res*, 45(Pt 3), 219–25.

Durkin, M. (2002). The epidemiology of developmental disabilities in low-income countries. *Ment Retard Dev Disabil Res Rev*, 8(3), 206–11.

Enright, F., McMahon, B. and Washington, A. (2006). Varicella outbreak in a residential home. *Ir Med J*, 99(5), 133–5.

Ezeamama, A. E., Friedman, J. F., Acosta, L. P. et al. (2005). Helminth infection and cognitive impairment among Filipino children. *Am J Trop Med Hyg*, 72(5), 540–8.

Foster, C. J., Biggs, R. L., Melvin, D. et al. (2006). Neurodevelopmental outcomes in children with HIV infection under 3 years of age. *Dev Med Child Neurol*, 48(8), 677–82.

Fuccio, L., Laterza, L., Zagari, R. M. et al. (2008). Treatment of Helicobacter pylori infection. *BMJ* 337, 746–50.

Gatti, S., Lopes, R., Cevini, C. et al. (2000). Intestinal parasitic infections in an institution for the mentally retarded. *Ann Trop Med Parasitol*, 94 (5), 453–60.

Gil, A., Gonzalez, A., Dal-Re, R. et al. (1999). Prevalence of hepatitis A in an institution for the mentally retarded in an intermediate endemicity area: influence of length of institution alisation. *J Infect*, 38(2), 120–3.

Gilad, J., Borer, A., Smolyakov, R. et al. (2006). Impaired neutrophil functions in the pathogenesis of an outbreak of recurrent furunculosis caused by methicillin-resistant Staphylococcus aureus among mentally retarded adults. *Microbes Infect*, 8(7), 1801–5.

Goetghebuer, T., West, T. E., Wermenbol, V. et al. (2000). Outcome of meningitis caused by Streptococcus pneumoniae and Haemophilus Influenzae type b in children in The Gambia. *Trop Med Int Health*, 5(3), 207–13.

Gust, D. A., Wang, S. A., Grot, J., Ransom, R. and Levine, W. C. (2003). National survey of sexual behavior and sexual behavior policies in facilities for individuals with mental retardation/developmental disabilities. *Ment Retard*, 41(5), 365–73.

Harris, L. L. (1999). Neuropsychological functioning among school-aged children with perinatally-acquired HIV infection. *Diss Abs Int B Sci Eng*, 64(4), 1853.

Hawkes, R. A., Boughton, C. R., Schroeder, D. R., Decker, R. H. and Overby, L. R. (1980). Hepatitis B infection in institutionalized Down's syndrome inmates: a longitudinal study with five hepatitis B virus markers. *Clin Exp Immunol*, 40(3), 478–86.

Hayashi, J., Noguchi, A., Nakashima, K., Morofuji, M. and Kashiwagi, S. (1991). Long term observation of the effect of intradermal hepatitis B vaccination on mentally retarded patients. *Eur J Epidemiol*, 7(6), 649–53.

Heijtink, R. A., De Jong, P., Schalm, S. W. and Masurel, N. (1984). Hepatitis B vaccination in Down's syndrome and other mentally retarded patients. *Hepatology*, 4(4), 611–14.

Hornig, M., Briese, T., Buie, T. *et al.* (2008). Lack of association between measles virus vaccine and autism with enteropthy: a case-control study. *PLoS ONE*, 3(9), e3140.

Huang, H. Y., Jou, R., Chiang, C. Y. *et al.* (2007). Nosocomial transmission of tuberculosis in two hospitals for mentally handicapped patients. *J Formos Med Assoc*, 106(12), 999–1006.

Jardim-Botelho, A., Raff, S., Rodrigues Rde, A. *et al.* (2008). Hookworm, Ascaris lumbricoides infection and polyparisitism associated with poor cognitive performance in Brazilian school children. *Trop Med Int Health*, 13(8), 994–1004.

Jones, J., Lopez, A. and Wilson, M. (2003). Congenital toxoplasmosis. *Am Fam Physician*, 67(10), 2131–30.

Karino, T., Osuki, K., Nakano, E. and Okimoto, N. (2001). [A pertussis outbreak in a ward for severely retarded.] *Kansenshogaku Zasshi*, 75(11), 916–22.

Kaye, J., del Mar Melero-Montes, M. and Hershel, J. (2001). Mumps, measles and rubella vaccine and the incidence of autism recorded by general practitioners: a time trend analysis. *BMJ*, 322, 460–3.

Kee, F., McGinnity, M., Marriott, C. *et al.* (1989). Hepatitis B screening in a northern Irish mental handicap institution: relevance to Hepatitis B vaccination. *J Hosp Infect*, 14(3), 227–32.

Kenneson, A. and Cannon, M. J. (2007). Review and meta-analysis of the epidemiology of congenital cytomegalovirus infection. *Rev Med Virol*, 17(4), 253–76.

Leary, P. M., Riordan, G., Schlegel, B. and Morris, S. (1999). Childhood secondary (symptomatic) epilepsy, seizure control and intellectual handicap in a non tropical region of South Africa. *Epilepsia*, 40(8), 1110–13.

Lemaitre, N., Sougakoff, W., Coetmeur, D. *et al.* (1996). Nosocomial transmission of tuberculosis among mentally- handicapped patients in a long term care facility. *Tuber Lung Dis*, 77(6), 531–6.

Leonard, J., Holtgrave, D. R. and Johnson, R. P. (1991). Cost-effectiveness of Hepatitis B screening in a mental institution. *J Fam Pract*, 32(1), 45–8.

Levitt, G. A., Stiller, C. A. and Chessells, J. M. (1990). Prognosis of Down's syndrome with acute leukaemia. *Arch Dis Child*, 65(2), 212–16.

Lohiya, G. S. (1993). Human immunodeficiency virus type 1 antibody in 6703 institutionalised mentally retarded clients: an unlinked serosurvey at seven California developmental centers. *AIDS Res Hum Retroviruses*, 9(3), 247–9.

Lohiya, S., Lohiya, G. and Caires, S. (1986). Epidemiology of hepatitis B infection in institutionalized mentally retarded clients. *Am J Public Health*, 76(7), 799–802.

MacDonald, R. A. R., Murray, J. L. and Levenson, V. L. (1999). Intellectual disability and HIV infection: a service related study of policies and staff attitudes. *J Appl Res Intellect Disabil*, 12(4), 348–57.

Mandell, D. S., Eleey, C. C., Cederbaum, J. A. *et al.* (2008). Sexually transmitted infection among adolescents receiving special education services. *J Sch Health*, 78(7), 382–8.

Manes, G., Zanetti, M. V., Piccirillo, M. M. *et al.* (2005). Accuracy of a new monoclonal stool antigen test in post-eradication assessment of helicobacter pylori infection: comparison with the polyclonal stool antigen test and urea breath test. *Dig Liver Dis*, 37(10), 751–5.

Mayor, S. (2003). Researcher from study alleging link between MMR and autism warns of measles epidemic. *BMJ*, 327(7423), 1069.

McConnell, V., Derham, R., McManus, D. and Morrison, P. J. (2004). Mosaic monosomy 14: clinical features and recognizable facies. *Clin Dysmorphol*, 13(3), 155–60.

McGillivray, J. A. (1999). Level of knowledge and risk of contracting HIV/AIDS among young adults with mild/moderate intellectual disability. *J Appl Res Intellect Disabil*, 12(2), 113–26.

McIntosh, E. D. (2005). Pediatric infections: prevention of transmission and disease-implications for adults. *Vaccine*, 23(17–18), 2087–9.

Meyer, U., Nyffeler, M., Engler, A. *et al.* (2006). The time of prenatal immune challenge determines the specificity of inflammation-mediated brain and behavioral pathology. *J Neurosci*, 26(18), 4752–62.

Monteno, C., Smit, I., Mills, J. and Huskisson, J. (2000). Nutritional status of patients in a long-stay hospital for people with mental handicap. *S Afr Med J*, 90(11), 1135–40.

Montoya, J. G. and Remington, J. S. (2008). Management of Toxoplasma Gondii infection during pregnancy. *Clin Infect Dis*, 47(4) 554–66.

Morad, M., Merrick, J. and Nasri, Y. (2002). Prevalence of Helicobacter pylori in people with intellectual disability in a residential care centre in Israel. *J Intellect Disabil Res*, 46(2), 141–3.

Morgan, J. (2007). Why is periodontal disease more prevalent and more severe in people with Down syndrome? *Spec Care Dentist*, 27(5), 196–201.

Neri, S. V., Bradley, E. H. and Groce, N. E. (2007). Frequency of HIV testing among persons with disabilities: results from the National Health Interview Survey, 2002. *AIDS Educ Prev*, 19(6), 545–54.

Nespoli, L., Burgio, G. R., Ugazio, A. G. and Maccaino, R. (1993). Immunological features of Down's syndrome: a review. *J Intellect Disabil Res*, 37(6), 543–51.

Noorda, J. and Hoebe, C. J. (2004). Fatal outbreak of chicken pox (varicella-zoster virus infection) among institutionalized adults with learning difficulties. *Commun Dis Public Health*, 7(3), 162–3.

Noyola, D. E., Demmler, G. J., Nelson, C. T. *et al.* (2001). Early predictors of neurodevelopmental outcome in symptomatic congenital cytomegalovirus infection. *J Pediatr*, 138(3) 325–31.

Nurmi, T., Leinonen, M., Haiva, V. M., Tiilikainen, A. and Kouvalainen, K. (1982). Antibody response to pneumococcal vaccine in patients with trisomy 21 (Down's syndrome). *Clin Exp Immunol*, 48(2), 485–90.

Ogunmodede, F., Scheftel, J., Jones, J. L. and Lynfield, R. (2005). Toxoplasmosis prevention knowledge among pregnant women in Minnesota. *Minn Med*, 88(2), 32–4.

Olness, K. (2003). Effects on brain development leading to cognitive impairment: a worldwide epidemic. *J Dev Behav Pediatr*, 24(2), 120–30.

Ono, K., Tsuji, H., Torita, S. *et al.* (1999). [Invasive amebiasis at an institution for the mentally retarded in Hyogo prefecture.] *Rinsho Byori*, 47(7), 669–75.

Owens, S. R. (2002). Injection of confidence: the recent controversy in the UK has led to falling MMR vaccination rates. *EMBO Rep*, 3(5), 406–9.

Peyron, F., Wallou, M., Liou, C. and Garner, P. (1999). Treatments for toxoplasmosis in pregnancy. *Cochrane Database Syst Rev*, Issue 3. Art. No.: CD001684. DOI: 10.1002/14651858.CD001684.

Pincus, S. H., Schoenbaum, E. E. and Webbe, M. (1990). A seroprevalence survey for human immunodeficiency virus antibody in mentally retarded adults. *N Y State J Med*, 90(3), 139–42.

Prada, N., Nasi, M., Troiano, L. *et al.* (2005). Direct analysis of thymic function in children with Down's syndrome. *Immun Ageing*, 2(1), 4.

Pueschel, S., Anneren, G., Durlach, R. *et al.* (1995). Guidelines for optimal medical care of Persons with Down syndrome. International League of Societies for Persons with Mental Handicap. *Acta Paediatr*, 84(7), 823–7.

Puri, B. K., Lekh, S. K., Langa, A., Zaman, R. and Singh, I. (1995). Mortality in a hospitalized mentally handicapped population: a ten year survey. *J Intellect Disabil Res*, 39(5), 442–6.

Renner, F., Andrie, M., Horak, W. and Rett, A. (1985). Hepeatitis A and B in non institutionalized mentally retarded patients. *Hepatogastroenterology*, 32(4), 175–7.

Revello, M. G. and Gerna, G. (2004). Pathogenesis and prenatal diagnosis of human cytomegalovirus infection. *J Clin Virol*, 29(2), 71–83.

Scanlan, S. and Khan, S. A. (1989). Hepatitis B in a residential population with mental handicap. *Ir Med J*, 82(2), 80–2.

Schleiss, M. R. (2008). Congenital cytomegalovirus infection: update on management strategies. *Curr Treat Options Neurol*, 10(3), 186–92.

Scotti, J. R., Speaks, L. V., Masia, C. L. and Boggess, J. T. (1996). The educational effects of providing AIDS risk information to persons with developmental disabilities: an exploratory study. *Educ Train Ment Retard Dev Disabil*, 31(2), 115–22.

Simpore, J., Savadogo, A., Ilboudo, D. *et al.* (2006). Toxoplasma gondii HCV and HBV seroprevalence and co-infection among HIV positive and negative pregnant women in Burkina Faso. *J Med Virol*, 78(6), 730–3.

Siriv: chayakul, C., Pojjaroen-Anant, C., Wisetsing, P. *et al.* (2003). Prevalence of intestinal parasite infection among Thai people with mental handicaps. *Southeast Asian J Trop Med Public Health*, 34(2), 259–63.

Stehr-Green, P., Wilson, N., Miller, J. and Lowther, A. (1991). Risk factors for Hepatitis B at a residential institution for intellectually handicapped persons. *N Z Med J*, 104(925), 514–16.

Steketee, R. W., Wassilak, S. G., Adkins, W. N. Jr. *et al.* (1988). Evidence for a high attack rate and efficacy of erythromycin prophylaxis in a pertussis outbreak in a facility for the developmentally disabled. *J Infect Dis*, 157(3), 434–40.

Stephenson, L. S. (2001). Optimising the benefits of anthelmintic treatment in children. *Paediatr Drugs*, 3(7), 495–508.

Straetmans, J. M. J. A. A., van Schrojenstein Lantman-de, Valk, H. M. J., Schellevis, F. G. and Dianant, G.-J. (2007). Health problems of people with intellectual disabilities: the impact for general practice. *Br J Gen Pract*, 57(534), 64–6.

Su, S. B., Guo, H. R., Chuang, Y. C., Chen, K. T. and Lin, C. Y. (2007). Eradication of amebiasis in a large institution for adults with mental retardation in Taiwan. *Infect Control Hosp Epidemiol*, 28(6), 679–83.

Taylor, B., Miller, E., Lingam, R. *et al.* (2002). Measles mumps and rubella vaccination and bowel problems or developmental regression in children with autism: population study. *BMJ*, 324(7334), 393–6.

Thiebaut, R., Leproust, S., Chene, G. and Gilbert, R. (2007). Effectiveness of prenatal treatment for congenital toxoplasmosis: a meta-analysis of individual patients' data. *Lancet*, 369(9556), 115–22.

Thompson, D. (1994). The sexual experiences of men with learning disabilities having sex with men-issues for HIV prevention. *Sex Disabil*, 12(3), 221–42.

Van Damme, P., Vranckx, R. and Meheus, A. (1990). Immunogenicity of a recombinant DNA hepatitis B vaccine in institutionalized patients with Down's syndrome. *Vaccine*, 8 Suppl: S53–5; discussion S60–2.

van Schrojenstein Lantman-de Valk, H. M., Haveman, M. J. and Crebolder, H. F. (1996). Comorbidity in people with Down's syndrome: a criteria-based analysis. *J Intellect Disabil Res*, 40(5), 385–99.

Vellinga, A., van Damme, P. and Meheus, A. (1999). Hepatitis B and C in institutions for individuals with intellectual disability. *J Intellect Disabil Res*, 43(6), 445–53.

Wakefield, A. J., Murch, S. H. *et al.* (1998). Ileal-lymphoid-nodular hyperplasia, non-specific colitis and pervasive developmental disorder in children. *Lancet*, 351, 637–41.

Wallace, R. A. (2007). Clinical audit of gastrointestinal conditions occurring among adults with Down syndrome attending a specialist clinic. *J Intellect Dev Disabil*, 32(1), 45–50.

Wallace, R. A., Webb, P. M. and Schluter, P. J. (2002). Environmental, medical, behavioural, and disability factors associated with Helicobacter pylori infection in adults with intellectual disability. *J Intellect Disabil Res*, 46(Pt 1), 51–60.

Wallace, R. A., Schluter, P. J., Forgon-Smith, R., Wood, R. and Webb, P. M. (2003a). Diagnosis of Helicobacter pylori infection in adults with intellectual disability. *J Clin Microbiol*, 41(10), 4700–4.

Wallace, R. A., Schluter, P. J. and Webb, P. M. (2003b). Helicobacter pylori and hepatitis A and B infections in carers of adults with intellectual disability. *J Occup Health Saf Aust NZ*, 19(1), 99–108.

Wallace, R. A., Schluter, P. J. and Webb, P. M. (2004a). Effects of Helicobacter pylori eradication among adults with intellectual disability. *J Intellect Disabil Res*, 48(Pt 7), 646–54.

Wallace, R. A., Schluter, P. J. and Webb, P. M. (2004b). Recurrence of Helicobacter

infection in adults with intellectual disability. *Intern Med J*, 34(3), 132–3.

WHO Scientific Group (1995). Primary immunodeficiency diseases. Report of Who Scientific Group. *Clin Exp Immunol*, 99(1), 1–24.

Wiggins, J., Hearn, G. and Skinner, C. (1989). Recent experience in the control and management of tuberculosis in a mental handicap hospital. *Respir Med*, 83(4), 315–19.

Wloch, M. K., Smith, L. R., Boutsaboualov, S. *et al.* (2008). Safety and immunogenicity of bivalent cytomegalovirus DNA vaccine in healthy adult subjects. *J Infect Dis*, 197(12), 1634–42.

Wong, S. Y., Lim, W. W., Que, T. L. and Au, D. M. (2005). Reflection on SARS precautions in a severe intellectual disabilities hospital in Hong Kong. *J Intellect Disabil Res*, 49(5), 379–84.

Immune system diseases

5

Jennifer Torr and Lynette Lee

Introduction

Immune system diseases are varied and complex but may be broadly classified into disorders of immunodeficiency, cell-mediated and humoral, or the abnormal immune responses of hypersensitivity or allergic responses and autoimmune diseases. Although not covered in this chapter secondary immunodeficiency may be related to stress, poor nutrition, medication and other factors that may be particularly relevant to people with intellectual disability (ID). This chapter will focus on the role of immune system diseases in the pathogenesis of neurodevelopmental disorders and immune disorder associated with specific genetic syndromes of ID.

Method

The electronic database MEDLINE (1960 to last update June 2008) was searched to find 513 papers on the association between ID and immune system disorders. A broad search strategy included references from papers identified in the electronic search. The electronic search employed the specialised MeSH terms and keywords: (intellectual disabilities or mental retardation or learning disabilities or developmental disabilities or autistic disorder or down syndrome or chromosome 18) and (immune system diseases or immunodeficiency or autoimmune diseases).

The focus was on epidemiological and clinical studies of immune system disorders in ID in general as well as specific syndromes of ID, in particular genetic disorders. All abstracts found were screened, relevant abstracts read, and potentially relevant articles inspected in more detail. The review was restricted to English language papers or papers with English language abstracts.

Results

A summary of the search results is shown in Table 5.1.

Most studies were observational case studies or series, based on clinical or institutional populations with specific genetic syndromes, often with comparative or control groups. There were some epidemiological studies on the association between immune system disorder and the aetiology of ID. There were no epidemiological studies identified regarding the prevalence of immune system disorders in people with ID in general. Due to the vast scope of the topic, the discussion has at times been selective and illustrative, rather than exhaustive.

Intellectual Disability and Ill Health: A Review of the Evidence, ed. Jean O'Hara, Jane McCarthy and Nick Bouras. Published by Cambridge University Press. © Cambridge University Press 2010.

Table 5.1. Search results

		With evidence-based medicine screen
MEDLINE	513	182

Where the literature on a topic is complex, review articles have been cited. The evidence base relating to the medical treatment of immune system disorders was not included in this review.

Discussion

The immune system and the pathogenesis of neurodevelopmental disorders
Immune system disorders are implicated in the pathogenesis of neurodevelopmental disorders through complex mechanisms that have yet to be elucidated. (Please refer to Chapter 17 on Neurodevelopmental disorders.)

Maternal immune response and neurodevelopmental disorder

There is a body of research pertaining to the relationship of maternal antibodies to brain antigens, the development of the fetal central nervous system (CNS) and a range of neurodevelopmental disorders (Adinolfi, 1993; Crawford *et al.*, 1992; Dalton *et al.*, 2003; Gualtieri, 1987; Gualtieri and Hicks, 1985; McAllister *et al.*, 1997; Vincent *et al.*, 2003). Maternal systemic erythematosus is associated with neurodevelopmental disorders, especially in male offspring (Flannery and Liederman, 1994; Lahita, 1988; McAllister *et al.* 1997). Maternal neuronal antibodies have been demonstrated to be the likely causative agent in some cases of autism (Dalton *et al.*, 2003; Warren *et al.*, 1990).

Immune response and neurodevelopmental disorder

Immune reactions during gestation, infancy and early childhood are also implicated in neurodevelopmental disorders. Leviton *et al.* (2005) propose that fetal exposure to infection can set in train immunological and inflammatory responses that can damage brain white matter in the fetus and newborn. There is some evidence for immune system dysfunction in the pathogenesis of the symptoms of attention deficit hyperactivity disorder (Marshall 1989; Niederhofer and Pittschieler, 2006; Roth *et al.* 1991). Grave's disease in early childhood, though rare, can result in developmental delay that may be corrected with treatment, but may also be associated with persisting intellectual deficits (Segni *et al.*, 1999). Left-handedness, mixed dominance and dyslexia are associated with autoimmune thyroid disease in men (Wood and Cooper, 1992).

Immunity and autistic spectrum disorders

The role of the measles, mumps and rubella (MMR) vaccine in the pathogenesis of autistic spectrum disorders (ASD) is controversial. Anecdotal parental reports of a temporal association between the MMR vaccine and the onset of gastrointestinal symptoms and developmental regression have raised a number of hypotheses of pathogenic mechanisms including initiation of autoimmune response, toxicity of vaccine media such as the mercury-containing preservative thimerosal and chronic infection with the attenuated measles virus (Krause *et al.*, 2002). However, a Cochrane review concluded that MMR vaccination was unlikely to be associated with ASD (Demicheli *et al.*, 2008).

Abnormal peripheral immune responses are associated with ASD (Burger and Warren, 1998). Immunological dysfunction is reported in up to 60% of individuals with ASD (Pardo and Eberhart, 2007) including aberrant gastrointestinal immune responses (Jyonouchi *et al.*, 2002, 2005; Schneider *et al.*, 2006), abnormal inflammatory and innate immune responses (Croonenberghs *et al.*, 2002; Jyonouchi *et al.*, 2002), altered levels of immunoglobulins, abnormal T cell-mediated immunity and deficient complement activity (Krause *et al.*, 2002). In addition, innate neuroimmune abnormalities in the brain tissue and cerebrospinal fluid of people with ASD have now been demonstrated raising the potential for future treatments (Pardo and Eberhart, 2007; Pardo *et al.*, 2005; Vargas *et al.*, 2005).

There are associations between autoimmune disease in family members and probands with ASD. When three family members had autoimmune disease the odds ratio for ASD increased to 5.5 compared with controls (Comi *et al.*, 1999). Autoantibodies against proteins in the nervous system, including neuron-axon filament proteins (Singh *et al.*, 1988), cerebellar neurofilaments (Plioplys *et al.*, 1989), myelin basic protein (Singh *et al.*, 1993), brain endothelia (Connolly *et al.*, 1999) and other neuronal and glial proteins (Singh *et al.*, 1997), have all been found in individuals with ASD, suggesting that autoantibodies targeting the brain may be causative in ASD (Krause *et al.*, 2002).

HIV infection and neurodevelopmental disorder

Vertical transmission or childhood infection with HIV can result in neurodevelopmental deficits that range from mild to severe (Chase *et al.*, 2000; Drotar *et al.*, 1999; McGrath *et al.*, 2006). The virus may infect brain macrophages, microglia and astrocytes and secretions from these infected cells are thought to be neurotoxic. Neurodevelopmental damage may be compounded by factors associated with HIV infection such as impoverishment, poor nutrition and lack of access to medical care and treatments (Willen, 2006). Opportunistic CNS infections and progressive multifocal leukoencephalopathy are less common in children and adolescents than in adults (Mitchell, 2001). There is evidence that aggressive antiretroviral treatment may limit progression of encephalopathy, however, abnormal neurological findings may persist (Exhenry and Nadal, 1996; Foster *et al.*, 2006). (Please refer to Chapter 4 on Infectious diseases.)

Genetic syndromes and the immune system

Down syndrome

Down syndrome (DS) occurs in 1 in 600 to 1000 live births, representing about 10% of the population with ID (Sullivan *et al.*, 2007), and is due to Trisomy 21 in 95% of cases; the remaining 5% being due to mosaicism and translocations (Stoll *et al.*, 1998). Triplication of chromosome 21, the smallest autosome encoding 225 genes (Hattori *et al.*, 2000), results in dysregulation of gene expression affecting biological processes in all body systems, including the immune system. Immune system abnormalities in DS are characterised by immunodeficiency (both cell-mediated and humoral), myeloproliferative disorders and leukaemia, and high prevalence of autoimmune diseases.

Immune deficiency

John Langdon Down first noted that people with DS were highly susceptible to infection (Down, 1866). Putting this susceptibility into perspective, in the 1950s, deaths from respiratory and other infections were 124 and 62 times greater, respectively, than for the general population (Oster *et al.*, 1975; Ugazio *et al.*, 1990). Respiratory infections remain a leading cause of death in DS with a standardised mortality ratio of 7.6 (Yang *et al.*, 2002).

In DS, the thymus is typically hypoplastic with abnormal anatomical structure (including thin cortex, poor corticomedullary demarcation, increased Hassal corpuscles and abnormal histology of lymphoid and epithelial compartments), cortical thymocyte depletion, abnormal proliferation, differentiation and maturation of thymocytes resulting in reduced numbers of circulating immunocompetent T lymphocytes, and other functional abnormalities including lack of thymic humoral factors and dysregulation of cytokines (Aita and Amantea, 1991; Duse *et al.*, 1980; Fabris *et al.*, 1984; Fonseca *et al.*, 1989; Murphy *et al.*, 1992, 1993 Musiani *et al.*, 1990; Ugazio, 1981). The T-lymphocyte CD4+/CD8+ is inverted with a marked increase in the percentage of suppressor-cytotoxic CD8+ lymphocytes and an abnormally high number of functionally deficient natural killer cells (Ugazio, *et al.*, 1990).

There is no clear evidence for phenotypic abnormalities of B lymphocytes; however, humoral immunity undergoes 'precocious ageing' (Nespoli *et al.*, 1993). From adolescence there is a tendency for high levels of immunoglobulin (Ig)G and low levels of IgM. There is also evidence of low IgA in utero (Cederqvist *et al.*, 1981). Specific humoral responses to vaccine antigens, including influenza, pneumococcus, tetanus and hepatitis B vaccines, have been found to be low in some studies and normal in others (Ugazio *et al.*, 1990). However, although the measured immune response to hepatitis B vaccine is lower than in controls, people with DS do develop protective levels of antibodies after vaccination but the decline in antibodies over time is greater (Vellinga *et al.*, 1999). The prevalence of hepatitis B surface antigen (HBsAg) is 1.5–16.8 times greater in individuals with DS than in those with other causes of ID, with prevalence rates varying from 12% to 25% in institutional settings. People with DS positive for HBsAg are much more likely to be HBeAg positive (22–78%), and therefore more infective, than those with other ID positive for HBsAg (0–12%) (Vellinga *et al.*, 1999). Inactivated hepatitis A vaccine has been found to be safe in children with DS living at home and seroconversion rates are not significantly different to controls (Ferreira *et al.*, 2004). Hepatitis B vaccination has been recommended for all people with DS. Hepatitis A vaccination has also been recommended because of the potentially severe complications of infection with both hepatitis B and A (Vellinga *et al.*, 1999). Given the high rates of death from pneumonia and other infections there is surprisingly little guidance in the literature about vaccination of people with DS.

Autoimmune disease

The prevalence of autoimmune antibodies and diseases are increased in DS. These include thyroiditis (15%), coeliac disease (6%), Type I diabetes mellitus (1%) and idiopathic juvenile arthritis (1%) (Gillespie *et al.*, 2006; Quartino 2006).

Less common autoimmune diseases include pernicious anaemia, alopecia areata and chronic active hepatitis (Du Vivier and Munro, 1975; Kaushik *et al.*, 2000; O'Mahony *et al.*, 1990). Multiple autoimmune diseases may be co-morbid (McCulloch *et al.* 1982). In the general population the recessive autoimmune polyendocrine syndrome type 1 (APS1) is caused by mutations in the gene *AIRE* on chromosome 21. Autoimmune polyendocrine syndrome type 1 diseases and autoantibodies unique for APS1 are common in DS suggesting dysregu-lation of the *AIRE* gene (Soderbergh *et al.*, 2006).

Thyroid abnormalities have been reported in 28–64% and thyroid autoantibodies found in 29–40% of people with DS indicating an autoimmune basis to some, but not all, of the thyroid dysfunction (Ivarsson *et al.*, 1997; Nicholson *et al.*, 1994; Zori *et al.*, 1990). Autoim-mune thyroiditis in DS has been reported in infants as young as five months (Shalitin and Phillip, 2002) and includes Hashimoto's thyroiditis (a chronic lymphocytic thyroiditis lead-ing to hypothyroidism) and the less common Grave's disease resulting in hyperthyroidism (Abdullah *et al.*, 1994; Karlsson *et al.*, 1998; Nicholson *et al.*, 1994; Zori *et al.*, 1990).

Myeloproliferative disorders and leukaemia

Standardised incidence ratio (SIR) for leukaemia in DS for all ages is 8, but for children under five years SIR for leukaemia is 60 (Sullivan *et al.*, 2007). Children with DS have a 10- to 20-fold increase in acute lymphoblastic and myeloid leukaemias (ALL and AML). Transient myeloproliferative disorder/leukaemia occurs in 10% of newborns with DS, it may be an incidental finding (25%) or severe and potentially fatal (20%). There is usually spontaneous remission within the first three months of life although 20–30% convert to acute megakaryo-blastic leukaemia (AMKL) in early childhood in DS. There is a 500-fold increase in AMKL, a biologically distinct leukaemia, in DS. Chemotherapy is curative in 70–100% of AMKL in DS compared with poorer outcomes for children without DS with AMKL (Bradbury, 2005; Hitzler and Zipursky, 2005; Massey *et al.*, 2006; Ravindranath, 2003). (Please refer to Chapter 12 on Neoplasms.)

Chromosome 22q11 deletion syndromes

Di George syndrome, velo-cardio-facial syndrome (VCFS) and co-truncal anomaly face syn-drome represent the highly variable clinical presentations of chromosome 22q11.2 deletions. Common features include abnormalities of the face, pharynx, larynx, heart, kidney, parathy-roid glands, thymus, skeleton, brain and immune system, together with cognitive impair-ments and ID, psychiatric disorders including ASD (14%), a range of anxiety and depressive disorders (19%) and schizophrenia (25–30%) (Goldmuntz, 2005; McDonald-McGinn *et al.*, 1999)

About 80% of individuals with a 22q11 deletion have immune system abnormalities, espe-cially mild to moderate reduction in T cell production due to thymic hypoplasia (~70%). Infants identified with 22q11 deletion should be tested for T cell markers, as in rare cases (<0.5%) there is a complete absence of T cells requiring a thymic transplant. Other immune abnormalities include impaired T cell functioning (~20%); humoral deficits (~25%), includ-ing IgA deficiency (10–15%); other immunodeficiency (~25%); and autoimmune disease. Live vaccines should be avoided in the first year of life. Clinically, individuals with a 22q11 deletion commonly experience frequent and prolonged viral infections with bacterial super-infections of the upper and lower respiratory tracts (Goldmuntz, 2005; Jawad *et al.*, 2001; McDonald-McGinn *et al.*, 1999; Sullivan *et al.*, 1998). The frequency of juvenile rheumatoid arthritis is reported to be 150 times greater than for the general population (McDonald-McGinn *et al.*, 1999).

Chromosome 18

The 18q deletion syndrome is characterised by short stature, hypotonia and ID. Immuno-globulin A deficiency has also been reported in 18q deletion syndrome, familial cryptic chromosome (18q; 10p) translocations, ring chromosome 18 and 18p deletion. The locus 18q22.3-q23 gene region is postulated to be locus of IgA deficiency in 18q deletion syndrome (Dostal *et al.*, 2007). Immunoglobulin A deficiency increases the risk of recurrent respiratory and gastrointestinal infections and is associated with autoimmune disease (Dostal *et al.*, 2007; Lomenick *et al.*, 2005). Autoimmune diseases, including autoimmune hypothyroidism, arthritis, pernicious anaemia, hypoparathyroidism and diabetes mellitus appear to be common in 18q deletion syndrome (Lomenick *et al.*, 2005). Autoimmune thyroiditis was reported in 7 out of 11 case reports of autoimmune diseases in 18q deletion syndrome, however, only 3 of these 11 reported cases had IgA deficiency (Lomenick *et al.*, 2005).

Chromosome instability syndromes

A number of heterogeneous chromosome instability, or breakage, syndromes are associated with various types of immunodeficiencies and include ataxia telangiectasia (AT), Nijmegen breakage syndrome (NBS), immunodeficiency, centromere instability and facial anomalies syndrome (ICF syndrome) and DNA ligase IV mutations (Ben-Omran *et al.*, 2005; Carney, 1999; Fasth *et al.*, 1990; Hagleitner *et al.*, 2008; O'Driscoll *et al.*, 2001; Yamada *et al.*, 2001).

Ataxia telangiectasia, a single gene defect on 11q22–23, is characterised by early childhood cerebellar motor degeneration, spider facial and ocular veins, immunodeficiency, cancer susceptibility and mild ID in a third of adolescents. Immunodeficiencies include hypoplastic thymus, low T cell levels, low serum levels of IgA, IgE and IgG2 and poor in vivo responses to pneumococcal polysaccharides. Young children have high risk for B cell lineage acute lymphocytic leukaemia and B cell lymphomas. Adolescents are prone to T cell lymphomas and T cell prolymphocytic leukaemia. Premature death is related to overwhelming sinopulmonary infections or incurable cancers, including leukaemia (Chun and Gatti, 2004; Gilad *et al.*, 1998; Moin *et al.*, 2007).

Nijmegen breakage syndrome (NBS), once thought to be a variant of AT, is a rare autosomal recessive condition of the *NBSI* gene on 8q21 characterised by phenotypic variation, spontaneous chromosome instability, microcephaly, ID, humoral immunodeficiency and high rates of malignancies, especially B cell lymphomas (Curry *et al.*, 1989; Michallet *et al.*, 2003; Seeman *et al.*, 2004; Stoppa-Lyonnet *et al.*, 1992; van der Burgt *et al.*, 1996; Weemaes *et al.*, 1981). Ligase IV syndrome (LIG4 syndrome) is phenotypically similar to NBS but results from mutations of *LIG4* gene on chromosome 13q22-q24. They are typically pancytopaenic (Ben-Omran *et al.*, 2005; O'Driscoll *et al.*, 2001). Immunodeficiency, centromere instability and facial anomalies syndrome is another rare autosomal recessive disorder with varying severity of ID, resulting from mutations in the *DNMT3B* gene, encoding DNA methyltransferase. Immunodeficiency is due to variable reductions in serum immunoglobulin levels which results in fatal infections in adulthood (Gimelli *et al.*, 1993; Hagleitner *et al.*, 2008; Jin *et al.*, 2008; Luciani *et al.*, 2005).

Phenylketonuria

Phenylketonuria (PKU) is a genetic error of metabolism (please refer to Chapter 2 on Congenital causes). Low levels of IgG, IgM and IgA have been reported in untreated PKU or those with poor dietary compliance and are postulated to be due to amino acid deficiencies, especially tyrosine, an important amino acid in antibodies (Giovannini *et al.*, 1988; Passwell *et al.*, 1976). Children with PKU treated from infancy had the same IgM and IgA levels as, but lower IgG and higher IgE levels than, normal controls. Immunoglobulin E levels have been found to be higher in children who started dietary treatment after six months of age rather than within the first month of life. Eczema is a recognised clinical manifestation of untreated PKU (Riva *et al.*, 1994). Other allergic conditions have been reported in individuals with untreated PKU including allergy to cow's milk (Dockhorn, 1970) and atopic asthma associated with allergies to grass and mites (Tolokh *et al.*, 1989). Although allergic sensitisation was found to be greater in children with treated PKU they had the same rates of eczema and lower rates of asthma than the control group. It would seem that early implementation and ongoing compliance of dietary treatment of PKU is important in normalising immune function (Riva *et al.*, 1994).

Conclusion

Immune system disorders implicated in the pathogenesis of neurodevelopmental disorders and ID include maternal or early life autoimmune responses to the developing brain; dysregulated immune and inflammatory responses to bacterial infections in utero and the neonatal period; and neurotoxic effects of HIV, and associated secondary infections, in infancy and childhood. Immune system disorders, such as allergies, autoimmune diseases, cell-mediated and/or humoral immunodeficiencies, and predisposition to cancers, are important findings in a range of genetic syndromes of ID, and are a cause of much morbidity and premature death.

The identification and prevention of immune-mediated neurodevelopmental disability is not yet a reality. However, the identification and management of immune system diseases in individuals with specific genetic syndromes could prevent much morbidity and early mortality. More research and clinical guidance is needed to inform vaccination schedules of groups at risk of immunodeficiency syndromes. There also needs to be more guidance on the inclusion of specific tests in general health screening for genetic syndromes.

References

Abdullah, M. A., Salman, H., Al-Habib, S., Ghareeb, A. and Abanamy A. (1994). Antithyroid antibodies and thyroid dysfunction in Saudi children with Down syndrome. *Ann Saudi Med*, 14(4), 283–5.

Adinolfi, M. (1993). Fetal exposure to maternal brain antibodies and neurological handicap. In *Dyslexia and Development: Neurobiological Aspects of Extra-ordinary Brains*, ed. A. M. Galaburda. Cambridge, MA: Harvard University Press, pp. 155–67.

Aita, M. and Amantea, A. (1991). Distribution of anti-keratins and anti-thymostimulin antibodies in normal and in Down's syndrome human thymuses. *Thymus*, 17(3), 155–66.

Ben-Omran, T. I., Cerosaletti, K., Concannon, P., Weitzman, S. and Nezarati, M. M. (2005). A patient with mutations in DNA Ligase IV: clinical features and overlap with Nijmegen breakage syndrome. *Am J Med Genet A*, 137(3), 283–7.

Bradbury, J. (2005). High leukaemia cure rate in Down's syndrome explained. *Lancet Oncol*, 6(3), 134.

Burger, R. A. and Warren, R. P. (1998). Possible immunogenetic basis for autism. *Ment Retard Dev Disabil Res Rev*, 4(2), 137–41.

Carney, J. P. (1999). Chromosomal breakage syndromes. *Curr Opin Immunol*, 11(443–7).

Cederqvist, L. L., Spigelman, S. and Litwin, S. D. (1981). Decreased cord blood IgM and IgA in trisomy 21. *Am J Reprod Immunol*, 1(2), 62–4.

Chase, C., Ware, J., Hittelman, J. *et al.* (2000). Early cognitive and motor development among infants born to women infected with human immunodeficiency virus. Women and Infants Transmission Study Group. *Pediatr Int*, 106(2), E25.

Chun, H. H. and Gatti, R. A. (2004). Ataxia-telangiectasia, an evolving phenotype. *DNA Repair (Amst)*, 3(8–9), 1187–96.

Comi, A. M., Zimmerman, A. W., Frye, V. H., Law, P. A. and Peeden, J. N. (1999). Familial clustering of autoimmune disorders and evaluation of medical risk factors in autism. *J Child Neurol*, 14(6), 388–94.

Connolly, A. M., Chez, M. G., Pestronk, A. *et al.* (1999). Serum autoantibodies to brain in Landau-Kleffner variant, autism, and other neurologic disorders. *J Pediatr*, 134(5), 607–13.

Crawford, S. G., Kaplan, B. J. and Kinsbourne, M. (1992). The effects of parental immunoreactivity on pregnancy, birth, and cognitive development: maternal immune attack on the fetus? *Cortex*, 28(3), 483–91.

Croonenberghs, J., Bosmans, E., Deboutte, D., Kenis, G. and Maes, M. (2002). Activation of the inflammatory response system in autism. *Neuropsychobiology*, 45(1), 1–6.

Curry, C. J., O'Lague, P., Tsai, J. *et al.* (1989). ATFresno: a phenotype linking ataxia-telangiectasia with the Nijmegen breakage syndrome. [Erratum appears in *Am J Hum Genet*, 1989 Oct;45(4),663.] *Am J Hum Genet*, 45(2), 270–5.

Dalton, P., Deacon, R., Blamire, A. *et al.* (2003). Maternal neuronal antibodies associated with autism and a language disorder. *Ann Neurol*, 53(4), 533–7.

Demicheli, V., Jefferson, T., Rivetti, A. and Price, D. (2008). Vaccines for measles, mumps and rubella in children [Systematic Review]. *Cochrane Database Syst Rev* (3).

Dockhorn, R. J. (1970). Milk allergy in an infant with phenylketonuria. *Ann Allergy*, 28, 33–5.

Dostal, A., Linnankivi, T., Somer, M. *et al.* (2007). Mapping susceptibility gene locus for IgA deficiency at del(18)(q22.3–q23): report of familial cryptic chromosome t(18q; 10p) translocations. *Int J Immunogen*, 34(3), 143–7.

Down, J. L. H. (1866). Observation on an ethnic classification of idiots. *London Hosp Clin Lect Rep*, 3, 259–62.

Drotar, D., Olness, K., Wiznitzer, M. *et al.* (1999). Neurodevelopmental outcomes of Ugandan infants with HIV infection: an application of growth curve analysis. *Health Psychol*, 18(2), 114–21.

Du Vivier, A. and Munro, D. D. (1975). Alopecia areata, autoimmunity, and Down's syndrome. *Br Med J*, 1(5951), 191–2.

Duse, M., Brugo, M. A., Martini, A. *et al.* (1980). Immunodeficiency in Downs syndrome: low levels of serum thymic factor in trisomic children. *Thymus*, 2(3), 127–32.

Exhenry, C. and Nadal, D. (1996). Vertical human immunodeficiency virus-1 infection: involvement of the central nervous system and treatment. *Eur J Pediatr*, 155(10), 839–50.

Fabris, N., Amadio, L., Licastro, F. *et al.* (1984). Thymic hormone deficiency in normal aging and Downs syndrome is there a primary failure of the thymus? *Lancet*, 1(8384), 983–6.

Fasth, A., Forestier, E., Holmberg, E. *et al.* (1990). Fragility of the centromeric region of chromosome 1 associated with combined immunodeficiency in siblings. A recessively inherited entity? *Acta Paediatr Scand*, 79(6–7), 605–12.

Ferreira, C. T., Leite, J. C., Taniguchi, A. *et al.* (2004). Immunogenicity and safety of an inactivated hepatitis A vaccine in children with Down syndrome. *J Pediatr Gastroenterol Nutr*, 39(4), 337–40.

Flannery, K. A. and Liederman, J. (1994). A test of the immunoreactive theory for the origin of neurodevelopmental disorders in the offspring of women with immune disorder. *Cortex*, 30(4), 635–46.

Fonseca, E. C., Lannes-Vieira, J., Villa-Verde, D. M. and Savino, W. (1989). Thymic extracellular matrix in Down's syndrome. *Braz J Med Biol Res*, 22(8), 971–4.

Foster, C. J., Biggs, R. L., Melvin, D. *et al.* (2006). Neurodevelopmental outcomes in children with HIV infection under 3 years of age. *Dev Med Child Neurol*, 48(8), 677–82.

Gilad, S., Chessa, L., Khosravi, R. *et al.* (1998). Genotype-phenotype relationships in ataxia-telangiectasia and variants. *Am J Hum Genet*, 62(3), 551–61.

Gillespie, K. M., Dix, R. J., Williams, A. J. K *et al.* (2006). Islet autoimmunity in children with Down's syndrome. *Diabetes*, 55(11), 3185–8.

Gimelli, G., Varone, P., Pezzolo, A., Lerone, M. and Pistoia, V. (1993). ICF syndrome with variable expression in sibs. *J Med Genet*, 30(5), 429–32.

Giovannini, M., Agostoni, C., Galluzzo, C. *et al.* (1988). Low serum concentrations of immunoglobulin G, A, and M in children on low antigenic charge diets. *Acta Paediatr Scand*, 77(2), 306–7.

Goldmuntz, E. (2005). DiGeorge syndrome: new insights. *Clin in Perinatol*, 32(4), 963–78.

Gualtieri, C. and Hicks, R. E. (1985). An immunoreactive theory of selective male affliction. *Behav Brain Sci*, 8(3), 427–77.

Gualtieri, C. T. (1987). Fetal antigenicity and maternal immunoreactivity. Factors in mental retardation. *Monogr Am Assoc Ment Defic*, (8), 33–69.

Hagleitner, M. M., Lankester, A., Maraschio, P. *et al.* (2008). Clinical spectrum of immunodeficiency, centromeric instability and facial dysmorphism (ICF syndrome). *J Med Genet*, 45(2), 93–9.

Hattori, M., Fujiyama, A., Taylor, T. D. *et al.* (2000). The DNA sequence of human chromosome 21. *Nature*, 405, 311–19.

Hitzler, J. K. and Zipursky, A. (2005). Origins of leukaemia in children with Down syndrome. *Nat Rev Cancer*, 5(1), 11–20.

Ivarsson, S. A., Ericsson, U. B., Gustafsson, J. *et al.* (1997). The impact of thyroid autoimmunity in children and adolescents with Down syndrome. *Acta Paediatr*, 86(10), 1065–7.

Jawad, A. F., McDonald-Mcginn, D. M., Zackai, E. and Sullivan, K. E. (2001). Immunologic features of chromosome 22q11.2 deletion syndrome (DiGeorge syndrome/velocardiofacial syndrome). *J Pediatr*, 139(5), 715–23.

Jin, B., Tao, Q., Peng, J. *et al.* (2008). DNA methyltransferase 3B (DNMT3B) mutations in ICF syndrome lead to altered epigenetic modifications and aberrant expression of genes regulating development, neurogenesis and immune function. *Hum Mol Genet*, 17(5), 690–709.

Jyonouchi, H., Sun, S. and Itokazu, N. (2002). Innate immunity associated with inflammatory responses and cytokine production against common dietary proteins in patients with autism spectrum disorder. *Neuropsychobiology*, 46(2), 76–84.

Jyonouchi, H., Geng, L., Ruby, A. and Zimmerman-Bier, B. (2005). Dysregulated innate immune responses in young children with autism spectrum disorders: their relationship to gastrointestinal symptoms and dietary intervention. *Neuropsychobiology*, 51(2), 77–85.

Karlsson, B., Gustafsson, J., Hedov, G., Ivarsson, S. A. and Anneren, G. (1998). Thyroid dysfunction in Down's syndrome: relation to age and thyroid autoimmunity. *Arch Dis Child*, 79(3), 242–5.

Kaushik, S. P., Kaye, G. and Clarke, A. C. (2000). Autoimmune hepatobiliary disease in trisomy 21. *J Clin Gastroenterol*, 30(3), 330–2.

Krause, I., He, X.-S., Gershwin, M. E. and Shoenfeld, Y. (2002). Brief report: immune factors in autism: a critical review. *J Autism Dev Disord*, 32(4), 337–45.

Lahita, R. G. (1988). Systemic lupus erythematosus: learning disability in the male offspring of female patients and relationship to laterality. *Psychoneuroendocrinology*, 13(5), 385–96.

Leviton, A., Dammann, O. and Durum, S. K. (2005). The adaptive immune response in neonatal cerebral white matter damage. *Ann Neurol*, 58(6), 821–8.

Lomenick, J. P., Smith, W. J. and Rose, S. R. (2005). Autoimmune thyroiditis in 18q deletion syndrome. *J Pediatr*, 147(4), 541–3.

Luciani, J. J., Depetris, D., Missirian, C. et al. (2005). Subcellular distribution of HP1 proteins is altered in ICF syndrome. *Eur J Hum Genet*, 13(1), 41–51.

Marshall, P. (1989). Attention deficit disorder and allergy: a neurochemical model of the relation between the illnesses. *Psychol Bull*, 106(3), 434–46.

Massey, G. V., Zipursky, A., Chang, M. N. et al., Children's Oncology Group. (2006). A prospective study of the natural history of transient leukemia (TL) in neonates with Down syndrome (DS): Children's Oncology Group (COG) study POG-9481. *Blood*, 107(12), 4606–13.

McAllister, D. L., Kaplan, B. J., Edworthy, S. M. et al. (1997). The influence of systemic lupus erythematosus on fetal development: cognitive, behavioral, and health trends. *J Int Neuropsychol Soc*, 3(4), 370–6.

McCulloch, A. J., Ince, P. G. and Kendall-Taylor, P. (1982). Auto immune chronic active hepatitis in Downs syndrome. *J Med Genet*, 19(3), 232–4.

McDonald-McGinn, D. M., Kirschner, R., Goldmuntz, E. et al. (1999). The Philadelphia story: the 22q11.2 deletion: report on 250 patients. *Genet Couns*, 10(1), 11–24.

McGrath, N., Fawzi, W. W., Bellinger, D. et al. (2006). The timing of mother-to-child transmission of human immunodeficiency virus infection and the neurodevelopment of children in Tanzania. *Pediatr Infect Dis J*, 25(1), 47–52.

Michallet, A. S., Lesca, G., Radford-Weiss, I. et al. (2003). T-cell prolymphocytic leukemia with autoimmune manifestations in Nijmegen breakage syndrome. *Ann Hematol*, 82(8), 515–17.

Mitchell, W. (2001). Neurological and developmental effects of HIV and AIDS in children and adolescents. *Ment Retard Dev Disabil Res Rev*, 7(3), 211–16.

Moin, M., Aghamohammadi, A., Kouhi, A. et al. (2007). Ataxia-telangiectasia in Iran: clinical and laboratory features of 104 patients. *Pediatr Neurol*, 37(1), 21–8.

Murphy, M., Friend, D. S., Pike-Nobile, L. and Epstein, L. B. (1992). Tumor necrosis factor-alpha and Ifn-gamma expression in human thymus localization and overexpression in Down syndrome trisomy 21. *J Immunol*, 149(7), 2506–12.

Murphy, M., Insoft, R. M., Pike-Nobile, L., Derbin, K. S. and Epstein, L. B. (1993). Overexpression of LFA-1 and ICAM-1 in Down syndrome thymus: implications for abnormal thymocyte maturation. *J Immunol*, 150(12), 5696–703.

Musiani, P., Valitutti, S., Castellino, F. *et al.* (1990). Intrathymic deficient expansion of T cell precursors in Down syndrome. *Am J Med Genet, Suppl*, 7, 219–24.

Nespoli, L., Burgio, G. R., Ugazio, A. G. and Maccario, R. (1993). Immunological features of Down's syndrome: a review. *J Intellect Disabil Res*, 37(6), 543–51.

Nicholson, L. B., Wong, F. S., Ewins, D. L. *et al.* (1994). Susceptibility to autoimmune thyroiditis in Down's syndrome is associated with the major histocompatibility class II DQA 0301 allele. *Clin Endocrinol*, 41(3), 381–3.

Niederhofer, H. and Pittschieler, K. (2006). A preliminary investigation of ADHD symptoms in persons with celiac disease. *J Attent Disord*, 10(2), 200–4.

O'Driscoll, M., Cerosaletti, K. M., Girard, P. M. *et al.* (2001). DNA ligase IV mutations identified in patients exhibiting developmental delay and immunodeficiency. *Molecular Cell*, 8(6), 1175–85.

O'Mahony, D., Whelton, M. J. and Hogan, J. (1990). Down syndrome and autoimmune chronic active hepatitis: satisfactory outcome with therapy. *Ir J Med Sci*, 159(1), 21–2.

Oster, J., Mikkelsen, M. and Nielsen, A. (1975). Mortality and life-table in Down's syndrome. *Acta Paediatr Scand*, 64(2), 322–6.

Pardo, C. A. and Eberhart, C. G. (2007). The neurobiology of autism. *Brain Pathol*, 17(4), 434–47.

Pardo, C. A., Vargas, D. L. and Zimmerman, A. W. (2005). Immunity, neuroglia and neuroinflammation in autism. *Int Rev Psychiatry*, 17(6), 485–95.

Passwell, J., Gazit, E., Efter, T. *et al.* (1976). Immunologic studies in phenylketonuria. *Acta Paediatr Scand*, 65(6), 673–7.

Plioplys, A. V., Greaves, A. and Yoshida, W. (1989). Anti-CNS antibodies in childhood neurologic diseases. *Neuropediatrics*, 20(2), 93–102.

Quartino, A. R. (2006). Down syndrome specificity in health issues. In *Down Syndrome: Neurobehavioural Specificity*, ed. J. E. Rondal and J. Perera. Chichester: John Wiley and Sons Ltd, pp. 53–66.

Ravindranath, Y. (2003). Down syndrome and acute myeloid leukemia: the paradox of increased risk for leukemia and heightened sensitivity to chemotherapy. *J Clin Oncol*, 21(18), 3385–7.

Riva, E., Fiocchi, A., Agostoni, C. *et al.* (1994). PKU-related dysgammaglobulinaemia: the effect of diet therapy on IgE and allergic sensitization. *J Inherit Metab Dis*, 17(6), 710–7.

Roth, N., Beyreiss, J., Schlenzka, K. and Beyer, H. (1991). Coincidence of attention deficit disorder and atopic disorders in children: empirical findings and hypothetical background. *J Abnorm Child Psychol*, 19(1), 1–13.

Schneider, C. K., Melmed, R. D., Barstow, L. E. *et al.* (2006). Oral human immunoglobulin for children with autism and gastrointestinal dysfunction: a prospective, open-label study. *J Autism Dev Disord*, 36(8), 1053–64.

Seeman, P., Gebertova, K., Paderova, K., Sperling, K. and Seemanova, E. (2004). Nijmegen breakage syndrome in 13% of age-matched Czech children with primary microcephaly. *Pediatr Neurol*, 30(3), 195–200.

Segni, M., Leonardi, E., Mazzoncini, B., Pucarelli, I. and Pasquino, A. M. (1999). Special features of Graves' disease in early childhood. *Thyroid*, 9(9), 871–7.

Shalitin, S. and Phillip, M. (2002). Autoimmune thyroiditis in infants with Down's syndrome. *J Pediatr Endocrinol Metab*, 15(5), 649–52.

Singh, V. K., Fudenberg, H. H., Emerson, D. and Coleman, M. (1988). Immunodiagnosis and immunotherapy in autistic children. *Ann N Y Acad Sci*, 540, 602–4.

Singh, V. K., Warren, R. P., Odell, J. D., Warren, W. L. and Cole, P. (1993). Antibodies to myelin basic protein in children with autistic behavior. *Brain Behav Immun*, 7(1), 97–103.

Singh, V. K., Warren, R., Averett, R. and Ghaziuddin, M. (1997). Circulating autoantibodies to neuronal and glial filament proteins in autism. *Pediatr Neurol*, 17(1), 88–90.

Soderbergh, A., Gustafsson, J., Ekwall, O. *et al.* (2006). Autoantibodies linked to autoimmune polyendocrine syndrome type I are prevalent in Down syndrome. *Acta Paediatr*, 95(12), 1657–60.

Stoll, C., Alembik, Y., Dott, B. and Roth, M. P. (1998). Study of Down syndrome in 238,942 consecutive births. *Ann Genet*, 41(1), 44–51.

Stoppa-Lyonnet, D., Girault, D., LeDeist, F. and Aurias, A. (1992). Unusual T cell clones in a patient with Nijmegen breakage syndrome. *J Med Genet*, 29(2), 136–7.

Sullivan, K. E., Jawad, A. F., Randall, P. *et al.* (1998). Lack of correlation between impaired T cell production, immunodeficiency, and other phenotypic features in chromosome 22q11.2 deletion syndromes. *Clin Immunol Immunopathol*, 86(2), 141–6.

Sullivan, S. G., Hussain, R., Glasson, E. J. and Bittles, A. H. (2007). The profile and incidence of cancer in Down syndrome. *J Intellect Disabil Res*, 51(3), 228–31.

Tolokh, O. S., Kolganova, N. A., Apultsina, I. D. and Lebedin, I. (1989). [A case of atopic bronchial asthma associated with phenylketonuria.] *Ter Arkh*, 61, 127–8.

Ugazio, A. G. (1981). Down's syndrome: problems of immunodeficiency. *Hum Genet, Suppl*, 2, 33–9.

Ugazio, A. G., Maccario, R., Notarangelo, L. D. and Burgio, G. R. (1990). Immunology of Down syndrome: a review. *Am J Med Genet, Suppl*, 7, 204–12.

van der Burgt, I., Chrzanowska, K. H., Smeets, D. and Weemaes, C. (1996). Nijmegen breakage syndrome. *J Med Genet*, 33(2), 153–6.

Vargas, D. L., Nascimbene, C., Krishnan, C., Zimmerman, A. W. and Pardo, C. A.

(2005). Neuroglial activation and neuroinflammation in the brain of patients with autism. *Ann Neurol*, 57(1), 67–81.

Vellinga, A., Van Damme, P. and Meheus, A. (1999). Hepatitis B and C in institutions for individuals with intellectual disability. *J Intellect Disabil Res*, 43(Pt 6), 445–53.

Vincent, A., Dalton, P., Clover, L., Palace, J. and Lang, B. (2003). Antibodies to neuronal targets in neurological and psychiatric diseases. *Ann N Y Acad Sci*, 992, 48–55.

Warren, R. P., Cole, P., Odell, J. D. *et al.* (1990). Detection of maternal antibodies in infantile autism. *J Am Acad Child Adolesc Psychiatry*, 29(6), 873–7.

Weemaes, C. M., Hustinx, T. W., Scheres, J. M. *et al.* (1981). A new chromosomal instability disorder: the Nijmegen breakage syndrome. *Acta Paediatr Scand*, 70(4), 557–64.

Willen, E. J. (2006). Neurocognitive outcomes in pediatric HIV. *Ment Retard Dev Disabil Res Rev*, 12(3), 223–8.

Wood, L. C. and Cooper, D. S. (1992). Autoimmune thyroid disease, left-handedness, and developmental dyslexia. *Psychoneuroendocrinology*, 17(1), 95–9.

Yamada, M., Matsuura, S., Tsukahara, M. *et al.* (2001). Combined immunodeficiency, chromosomal instability, and postnatal growth deficiency in a Japanese girl. *Am J Med Genet*, 100(1), 9–12.

Yang, Q., Rasmussen, S. A. and Friedman, J. M. (2002). Mortality associated with Down's syndrome in the USA from 1983 to 1997: a population-based study. *Lancet*, 359(9311), 1019–25.

Zori, R. T., Schatz, D. A., Ostrer, H. *et al.* (1990). Relationship of autoimmunity to thyroid dysfunction in children and adults with Down syndrome. *Am J Med Genet, Suppl*, 7, 238–41.

Cardiovascular disease

Joav Merrick and Mohammed Morad

Introduction

Cardiovascular disease (CVD) is today the leading cause of death worldwide surpassing all forms of cancer combined, and has resulted in a great deal of research on risk reduction and prevention with an increased emphasis on preventing atherosclerosis by modifying risk factors, such as healthy eating, exercise and avoidance of smoking. Research has focused on the general population and little is known about the population with intellectual disability (ID) (Draheim, 2006).

Method

A search in MEDLINE (1967–2008) was made to find studies on the association between intellectual disabilities and cardiovascular disease. A search strategy also included the MeSH terms mental retardation and cardiovascular diseases together with a hand search of journals and other material relevant to ID.

Results

A Google Scholar search for cardiovascular disease and mental retardation found 41 papers, while for cardiovascular disease and intellectual disability we found only 4 papers. The MED-LINE/PubMed search for cardiovascular disease and mental retardation yielded 12 papers, while cardiovascular disease and intellectual disability resulted in 3 papers (see Table 6.1). All abstracts were read and relevant articles inspected in more detail and used for this chapter.

Discussion

Congenital heart disease

Congenital heart disease (CHD) refers to disease that develops before birth (problems with the heart muscle, chambers or valves), such as coarctation of the aorta, atrial or ventricular septal defect. Some are apparent at birth, while others will only be detected later in life. In the general population CHD is rare (under one per cent), but several syndromes associated with ID have much higher prevalence of CHD (Akker et al., 2006).

DiGeorge syndrome, Turner syndrome, Williams syndrome, Alagille syndrome, VAC-TERL association and CHARGE (Coloboma, Heart disease, Atresia of choanae, Retarded mental development and growth, Genital hypoplasia, Ear anomalies and deafness)

Intellectual Disability and Ill Health: A Review of the Evidence, ed. Jean O'Hara, Jane McCarthy and Nick Bouras. Published by Cambridge University Press. © Cambridge University Press 2010.

Table 6.1. Search results for cardiovascular
disease and ID

Before evidence-based screening	4463
After evidence-based screening	60

association are just some of the syndromes associated with cardiovascular abnormalities
(Dooley, 2006; Pober *et al.*, 2008), but CHD is especially seen in people with Down syndrome, where the prevalence of CHD is as high as 40–60% (Akker *et al.*, 2006; Dooley, 2006).
In Down syndrome the most common malformation is atrioventricular canal defect, which
resulted in a high mortality rate until the 1970s, when it was first decided to operate on these
children. More advanced technology has also increased survival rates tremendously (Dooley,
2006).

When children with CHD enter adulthood there is an increased risk of aortic and mitral
insufficiency, which is the reason that preventive antibiotic treatment is warranted with dental treatment, ENT procedures and ear tube insertion (Dooley, 2006).

Prevalence

In a study from the Netherlands of 436 people with ID (all ages but most were 40–9 years of
age) in residential care the total prevalence of cardiac disease was found to be 14%, higher
than the 9% in the general Dutch population with 1% CHD (Akker *et al.*, 2006).

A study of 1371 people with ID aged 40 years and older living in community settings
from two regions in New York State (Janicki *et al.*, 2002) and a study from Israel of 2282
people living in residential care (Merrick *et al.*, 2004) both found 7% with heart disease. This
prevalence was lower than in the general American and Israeli populations. A smaller recent
study from Australia among 155 adults over 40 years of age attending a specialist ageing clinic
found a prevalence of 5% (Wallace and Schluter, 2008). The prevalence of CVD in people with
ID in some studies seems more prevalent than the general population, while other larger
studies have found a prevalence lower than the general population (Draheim, 2006).

Risk factors

Rimmer *et al.* (1994) found that adults with ID residing in community settings had the same
cardiovascular risk profile as the general population. In a large study from Israel the apparently low frequency of CVD resulted in further analysis (Merrick *et al.*, 2004). The most
frequently occurring CVD was hypertension (11%), with a high of 28% in the 60–9 year age
group and no gender difference. Coronary heart disease, congestive heart failure, acquired
valvular disease and CHD occurred in fewer than 8% of participants at any age. Almost 13%
of the Israeli cohort had hyperlipidaemia and 7% had diabetes. The frequency of hyperlipidaemia and Type 2 diabetes increased with age. This study had lower frequencies of hyperlipidaemia, hypertension and diabetes than the general Israeli population. The proportion
that performed no weekly exercise remained at about 52% regardless of age.

Gender differences

In the general population, a study by the Institute of Medicine, Washington DC provided the first systematic review of gender differences in CVD and found important differences in prevention, diagnosis, testing and disease management between men and women

Table 6.2. Cardiovascular risk factors (in %) by level of ID (all factors significant at the 0.0001 level)

Risk factors	Mild	Moderate	Severe	Profound	χ^2
Heart disease	18.7	18.1	10.7	7	36.6
BMI > 27	45.7	45.1	27.1	15	194.7
Hyperlipidaemia	18	15.9	9.6	5.6	35.9
Diabetes	7.6	10	4.3	2.1	32.9
No weekly exercise	36.7	41.3	61	76.9	181.0
Hypertension	16.2	14.4	7.3	4.9	40.6

(Wizemann and Pardue, 2001). The report emphasised the need to carefully evaluate gender-based differences in medical research and incorporate these differences into clinical practice. It has since been clear that there are major differences in male and females in the pathophysiology, clinical presentation, diagnostic strategies, response to therapies and adverse outcomes of CVD.

In a Dutch study the prevalence of cardiac diseases in people with ID was higher in females than in males (17% versus 10%) (Akker *et al.*, 2006), while larger studies from New York (Janicki *et al.*, 2002) and Israel (Merrick *et al.*, 2004) found no gender differences, except in older age, where women displayed more CVD.

Age

Large studies of people with ID in New York (Janicki *et al.*, 2002) and Israel (Merrick *et al.*, 2004) showed that CVD increased significantly with age, with 45% of females and 38% of males aged 70 years and older having CVD. The rates of CVD were also higher in people who were more able, had a history of seizures or were obese (Janicki *et al.*, 2002). In a Dutch study (Akker *et al.*, 2006) those aged 50–9, 60–9 and 70 years and older had a higher risk of CVD (OR = 1.78, 2.73 and 4.84 respectively).

Level of intellectual disability

Several studies have found the prevalence of CVD in people with mild/moderate ID to be significantly higher than in those with severe ID (e.g. Akker *et al.*, 2006). Our study from Israel also showed this trend, as shown in Table 6.2 (Merrick *et al.*, 2004).

Mortality

In the general population there has been a decline in CVD mortality (American Heart Association, 2008) as a result of prevention and awareness of risk factors, but this picture has not been the same for people with ID (Draheim, 2006).

During 1930–80 a steady increase in mortality was observed in the population of people with ID with a leveling off from 1984 to 1993 (Draheim, 2006). Janicki *et al.* (1999) described mortality in New York over a ten-year period for 2752 people with ID aged 40 years and older. It was found that although individuals with ID still generally die at an earlier age than adults in the general population (average age at death for people with ID: 66.1 years), there were also many adults with ID who lived as long as their peers in the general population. It was also confirmed that adults with Down syndrome are living longer than was expected from experience over the past 100 years (average age at death was 55.8 years for persons with Down syndrome).

National data from Israel on mortality for people with ID in a residential care centre during 1991–7 showed that CVD was the main cause of death with 35.3% of all causes (Merrick, 2002).

Prevention

Prevention of CVD should be directed at modifying risk factors, although some factors, such as gender, age and family history, cannot be modified. Smoking cessation (or abstinence) is an effective and easily modifiable change and regular cardiovascular exercise (aerobic exercise) should complement healthy eating habits. The combination of healthy diet and exercise is a means to improve serum cholesterol levels and reduce risks of CVD.

These preventative measures should also be introduced for people with ID, who unfortunately are not always included in preventive programmes for the general population. Merrick *et al.* (2004) found that 52% of people in residential care did not perform any weekly exercise. It is important that the same preventive measures for CVD are introduced for people with ID.

Conclusion

Most of the earlier evidence on cardiovascular conditions among people with ID was from case reports or studies with small sample sizes. In recent years several large studies from different countries have shown that rates of CVD increase in older people with ID in a similar way to the general population (Janicki *et al.*, 1999; Merrick *et al.*, 2004).

There is a lack of larger scale, randomised controlled, longitudinal studies on interventions for people with ID to enlighten our knowledge in reducing cardiovascular risk factors in this population (Draheim, 2006).

The existing evidence should stimulate changes in health policy and practice with a greater emphasis on preventative health strategies for middle age and older adults with ID.

References

Akker, M., Maaskant, M. A. and Meijden, R. J. M. (2006). Cardiac diseases in people with intellectual disability. *J Intellect Disabil Res*, 50(7), 515–22.

American Heart Association (2008). *Heart Disease and Stroke Statistics, 2008 Update*. Dallas, TX: American Heart Association.

Dooley, K. J. (2006). History of management of congenital heart disease. In *Cardiology in Medical Care for Children and Adults with Developmental Disabilities*, ed. I. L. Rubin and A. C. Crocker. Baltimore: Paul H Brookes, pp. 373–9.

Draheim, C. C. (2006). Cardiovascular disease prevalence and risk factors of persons with mental retardation. *Ment Retard Dev Disabil Res Rev*, 12, 3–12.

Janicki, M. P., Dalton, A. J., Henderson, C. M. and Davidson, P. W. (1999). Mortality and morbidity among older adults with intellectual disability: health services considerations. *Disabil Rehabil*, 21(5–6), 284–94.

Janicki, M. P., Davidson, P. W., Henderson, C. M. *et al.* (2002). Health characteristics and health services utilization in older adults with intellectual disability living in community residences. *J Intellect Disabil Res*, 46(4), 287–98.

Merrick, J. (2002). Mortality of persons with intellectual disability in residential care in Israel 1991–1997. *J Intellect Dev Disabil*, 27(4), 265–72.

Merrick, J., Davidson, P. W., Morad, M. *et al.* (2004). Older adults with intellectual disability in residential care centers in Israel: health status and service utilization. *Am J Ment Retard*, 109(5), 413–20.

Pober, B. R., Johnson, M. and Urban, Z. (2008). Mechanisms and treatment of cardiovascular disease in Williams-Beuren syndrome. *J Clin Invest*, 118(5), 1606–15.

Rimmer, J. H., Braddock, D. and Fujiura, G. (1994). Cardiovascular disease risk factors in adults with mental retardation. *Am J Ment Retard*, 98, 510–18.

Wallace, R. A. and Schluter, P. (2008). Audit of cardiovascular disease risk factors among supported adults with intellectual disability attending an aging clinic. *J Intellect Dev Disabil*, 33(1), 48–58.

Wizemann, T. M. and Pardue, M. (eds.) (2001). *Exploring the Biological Contributions to Human Health: Does Sex Matter?* New York: National Academy Press.

7

Respiratory diseases

Muhunthan Thillai

Introduction

The relationship between intellectual disability (ID) and respiratory disease was hinted at in modern medicine long before the conduct of any formal research. A nineteen-century medical report from the 'lunatic asylum of Aberdeen' listed the cause of death of all patients who had died that year (Chalmers, 1841). Amongst them, a 23-year-old man with 'dementia since childhood', perhaps an early attempt at a diagnosis of ID. His cause of death was listed as 'pneumonia typhoides'.

The link was formally identified more than half a century ago when a study which began in 1958 reviewed the autopsy reports of 237 institutionalised patients with ID and concluded that pneumonia was the single highest cause of mortality, accounting for 40% of all deaths (Polednak, 1975).

The underlying causes of ID are often paired with specific respiratory conditions, e.g. premature infants with immature lungs and cerebral palsy or Prader-Willi syndrome and nocturnal hypoventilation.

The observed to expected mortality ratio in patients with ID is as high as 3:1 (Decouflé and Autry, 2002) but the increased incidence of respiratory morbidity is often preventable. A thorough understanding of this co-morbidity is vital to reduce mortality and improve the overall health of patients with ID.

Method

A search was made to find studies on the association between ID and respiratory tract diseases. A broad strategy involved searching databases including the Ovid/MEDLINE database, PubMed database, Cochrane Collaboration, US National Institute of Health Clinical Trials database and Meta-Register of Current Controlled Trials. British and American Thoracic Society guidelines were reviewed.

A combination of the following keywords and MeSH headings were used: academic disorder, auditory processing disorders, autism, cerebral palsy, Down syndrome, dyscalculia, dyslexia, dyspraxia, Fragile X syndrome, intellectual disability, intellectual disorder, language disorder, learning disabilities, learning disorders, learning disturbance, mental retardation, Prader-Willi syndrome, asthma, bronchial diseases, bronchiectesis, bronchitis, ciliary motility disorders, COPD, cough, critical care, emphysema, lung cancer, lung diseases, pleural diseases, pulmonary diseases, pulmonary embolus, respiratory tract diseases, respiratory

Intellectual Disability and Ill Health: A Review of the Evidence, ed. Jean O'Hara, Jane McCarthy and Nick Bouras. Published by Cambridge University Press. © Cambridge University Press 2010.

Table 7.1. Search results

Method of search	Number of references retrieved
MEDLINE	992
PubMed	6
Cochrane Library	3
Additional articles from references of retrieved articles	125

tract infections, respiratory tract neoplasms, rhinitis, sleep apnoea, thoracic diseases, tracheal disease.

The first search was made in May 2008 and updated in September 2008. The focus was on co-morbidity, case-control, cohort, cross-sectional and longitudinal studies. Searches were performed of the reference lists of selected articles. The search was not limited by language. All guidelines, policy documents and abstracts from peer-reviewed journals were read and relevant articles were inspected in more detail.

Results

The initial search yielded 1001 articles, and 125 additional publications were selected from the reference lists of retrieved articles (see Table 7.1). Of these 1126 articles, 772 were excluded because they did not fulfil the primary inclusion criterion, i.e. they were not studies examining the co-morbidity between ID and respiratory disease. Of the remaining 354 articles, 54 were selected for inclusion in this review.

Discussion

Lung disease at birth

The relationship between ID and respiratory disease begins at birth. A large multicentre trial looked at 4503 children with cerebral palsy born across Europe over 14 years (Jarvis *et al.*, 2003). Babies of 32–42 weeks gestation with a birth weight for gestational age below the 10th percentile were up to six times more likely to have ID.

Birth weight is an independent factor for both lung disease and ID. A retrospective study of 365 newborns classed as having very low birth weight (< 1500 g) from a neonatal unit in Singapore over five years found that 25% developed chronic lung disease in later childhood (Yeo *et al.*, 1997). Within this subgroup there was a significantly higher risk of poor neurological development with functional cognitive disability in 34.6% of infants at two years. A study tracking 45 children in the USA with very low birth weights found that by age seven they had significantly higher levels of psychological morbidity and lower intelligence than normal birth weight counterparts (Farel *et al.*, 1998).

Aside from the implicated relationship between low birth weight and ID, the link between respiratory disease in the newborn and the subsequent development of ID is more concrete. A study of developmental outcome in infants with very low birth weight in the USA reviewed 329 newborns and found that those with bronchopulmonary dysplasia were significantly more likely to have ID (Singer *et al.*, 1997). The authors argued that newborns with low birth weight and acute respiratory disease should be followed up intensively in order to pick up any ID at an early age.

A review of 193 premature babies born between 24 and 27 weeks gestation with low birth weights in Japan found that of all the problems associated with low birth weight, respiratory complications after birth had the greatest impact on long-term neurological morbidity and cognitive outcome (assessed using the Wechsler Intelligence Scale for Children) (Kono *et al.*, 2007).

The underlying respiratory cause of impaired intelligence from birth is the presence of apnoeic episodes leading to oxygen starvation in the newborn brain. A Canadian study used a multiple linear regression model to determine relationships between apnoea days and neurodevelopmental impairment by three years of age in 175 premature babies (Janvier *et al.*, 2004). They concluded that an increased number of days on which at least one apnoea occurred was significantly associated with long-term ID.

Brain white matter damage in the newborn is associated with subsequent ID but there is minimal evidence that bronchopulmonary dysplasia itself is associated with actual brain damage. It may be, as hypothesised by a team in Germany, that brain white matter damage is not fully identified by ultrasound imaging (Dammann *et al.*, 2004) or that factors other than lung disease such as postnatal steroid exposure or maternal inflammation may be more relevant in the pathogenesis of ID.

Pneumonia

People with severe ID may have problems with feeding, leading to an increased risk of aspiration pneumonia. This may be recurrent and, in a proportion of cases, fatal. Studies of inpatient morbidity have repeatedly shown that pneumonias are amongst the top cause of hospital admission for all patients with ID. A review of 168 inpatients with ID over three years in Taiwan concluded that the incidence of pneumonia was significantly higher than the other top causes of admission including gastrointestinal disorders, cellulitis, orthopaedic problems and epilepsy (Loh *et al.*, 2007).

The pathogenesis of this co-morbidity has been investigated by carrying out 24-hour oesophageal pH monitoring and video fluoroscopy. Morton *et al.* (1999) assessed 35 children with severe ID and feeding difficulties; a combination of gastric reflux, direct aspiration and upper airway motor problems were all to blame for the increased incidence of pneumonia. A study of 57 patients with cerebral palsy (the majority of whom had ID) in Oxford who had gastrostomy tubes inserted because of feeding difficulties found that the incidence of hospital admissions for all chest infections fell significantly from 0.5 to 0.09 (Sullivan *et al.*, 2006). The number of chest infections requiring antibiotics in a given six-month period fell from 1.8 at the time of gastrostomy insertion to 0.9 at 12 months.

Case-controlled trials investigating pneumonia in people with ID often pose ethical problems as discovered through a study of the incidence of pneumonia in 194 children with ID and cerebral palsy in the Netherlands (Veugelers *et al.*, 2005). Assessment of malnutrition and gastro-oesophageal reflux at baseline was considered unethical, since these conditions could be easily treated and their study design had to be significantly altered.

Evaluation tools to identify people with ID at high risk of pneumonia are used in some care settings. A group in Japan evaluated a series of factors by scoring eating and swallowing behaviour to produce a questionnaire with a high accuracy of detecting patients admitted to hospital who were at risk of aspiration pneumonia (Kanda *et al.*, 2005). A more in-depth analysis from Manchester in the UK reviewed data collected from speech and language therapists and found that speed of eating, cramming food and premature loss of the bolus into the pharynx were all significant predictors of asphyxiation and subsequent aspiration pneumonia (Samuels and Chadwick, 2006).

In addition to bacterial pneumonias, the incidence and severity of viral respiratory infections may be increased. A review of 174 children with influenza requiring inpatient admission to an Edinburgh hospital over four years found that 16 patients required intensive care support and a significant number of these (7) had coexisting moderate to severe ID (Ting *et al.*, 2006).

Acute respiratory distress and critical care morbidity

People with ID undergoing sedation or general anaesthesia need special care with regard to their respiratory function. As well as the inherent difficulties of explaining a complicated procedure, intra-operative patient monitoring may be difficult to gauge.

A review of the anaesthetic records of 73 patients with ID undergoing dental procedures in Japan found that they needed a significantly higher level of sedation with midazolam and propofol compared to controls (Miyawaki *et al.*, 2004). Conversely, a slow recovery of patients with ID from inhaled anaesthetics may be due to significantly lower minimum alveolar concentration of anaesthetic gases such as halothane (Frei *et al.*, 1997).

This population also has a higher risk of both intra-operative anaesthetic complications and post-operative respiratory disease. Okada *et al.* (2008) investigated 41 surgical patients with ID and found significantly higher levels (compared to controls) of pharyngeal and laryngeal oedema during anaesthesia as well as increased incidence of post-operative pneumonias, pleural effusions and sudden apnoeas.

Children with ID are over-represented in the critical care (ICU) population. An investigation of 309 children with ID admitted to a tertiary paediatric ICU in the USA during a 12-month period found that they represented 23% of all admissions (Graham *et al.*, 2004). Down syndrome (DS) was the most common cause of ID in their population and 53% of all patients with ID required ventilator support.

As well as increased incidence of admission to ICU, people with DS have higher incidence of lung disease. A review of all patients with DS ventilated on an ICU in the Netherlands over seven years found that compared to controls they had a significantly higher rate of acute lung injury and acute respiratory distress syndrome (58.3% and 46% respectively vs. 12.9% and 7% for the controls) (Bruijn *et al.*, 2007). The authors cited increased cellular apoptosis and increased accumulation of reactive oxygen radicals in DS as possible causes for the disparity.

A study of a small number of patients with ID admitted to a district general hospital in Japan over seven years concluded that chronic aspiration with gastro-oesophageal reflux was the primary factor triggering admission in the vast majority of cases (Yoshikawa *et al.*, 2005). Despite adequate care 3 out of 13 patients died.

The physiological processes associated with intubation and ventilation can make existing ID more severe (in terms of further impairment of intelligence), particularly in young children. Mechanical ventilation results in a greatly increased positive intrathoracic pressure which can diminish venous return and reduce cardiac output, compromising cardiac blood flow (Aly, 2005). Long-term mechanical ventilation can lead to systemic inflammation, further injuring already damaged brain tissue (Schultz *et al.*, 2003). The use of prolonged sedation (Aly, 2004), painful procedures (Avery and Glass, 1989) and even enhanced stresses and noise on ICU (Duncan *et al.*, 2002) have been shown to impede the developing brain in children with ID.

A group in Japan looked at methods of monitoring respiratory distress in patients with ID and found significantly elevated urinary levels of the oxidative stress marker 8-hydroxy-2'-deoxyguanosine (8-OHdG) in patients with respiratory failure compared to controls with ID alone (Tanuma *et al.*, 2008). They postulated that this marker could be used to monitor respiratory disease in this population. On leaving ICU, patients with ID are more likely to require tracheostomies for long-term respiratory care, leading to an increased risk of procedure-related complications such as tracheoarterial fistulae (Hamano *et al.*, 2008).

Sleep apnoea and hypoventilation

Obstructive sleep apnoea is due to collapse of the soft palate at night-time leading to apnoeic periods resulting in oxygen desaturation for prolonged periods of time. It is associated with snoring, excessive daytime sleepiness and decrease in cognitive functioning. A prospective study of 149 children in the USA found that those with a higher apnoea:hypopnoea proportion had higher levels of nocturnal hypoxaemia and lower levels of immediate recall and IQ (Kaemingk *et al.*, 2003). Sleep apnoea in young children may even lead to long-term decline in intelligence as well as neuropsychological morbidity (Halbower and Mahone, 2006).

People with ID may have disorders of central breathing leading to similar problems. Prader-Willi syndrome is classically associated with a range of sleep disturbances which are often exacerbated on initiation of growth hormone therapy (Clift *et al.*, 1994). The apnoea usually has a central cause but obesity in these individuals can lead to obstructive sleep apnoea. This central loss of ventilator control leads to abnormal respiratory responses to hyperoxia, hypoxia and hypercarbia (Menendez, 1999). The night-time apnoeic episodes can be prolonged and result in nocturnal desaturations significant enough to warrant continuous positive airway pressure (CPAP) treatment. Growth hormone therapy for Prader-Willi syndrome has been linked with respiratory deterioration (Wilson *et al.*, 2006) and even sudden death (Craig *et al.*, 2006) due to an increased metabolic rate resulting in a sudden increase in oxygen demand.

An investigation of 29 individuals with Prader-Willi syndrome in Australia using questionnaires designed to assess daytime sleepiness found that sleepiness as a direct consequence of nocturnal apnoeas had a significantly detrimental effect on quality of life (Richdale *et al.*, 1999).

An assessment of 233 children with ID and cerebral palsy found significantly higher levels of habitual snoring (63%) and nasal obstruction (20%) compared to the control population (Shintani *et al.*, 1998). More than half (58%) of the children had nocturnal oxygenation levels measured at less than 85%. Recognised methods of treatment in this population include intrathecal baclofen (McCarty *et al.*, 2001) and surgical options such as uvulopalatopharyngoplasty or tracheostomy (Kosko and Derkay, 1995).

Sleep apnoeas in individuals with DS occur at greater frequency than the general population due to malformations in the upper airway resulting in sustained desaturations to below 50% for prolonged periods of time (Ferri *et al.*, 1997). Management is complicated and requires more extensive sessions of night-time CPAP (Anzai *et al.*, 2006). Interestingly, sufferers of sleep apnoea with high intelligence may have greater protection against cognitive decline due to nocturnal apnoeas compared to those with average or low intelligence (Alchanatis *et al.*, 2005). Management with CPAP has been shown to result in significant improvements in the quality of life for patients with ID, particularly those with cerebral palsy (Hsiao and Nixon, 2008) and may also improve cognitive functioning (Ferini-Strambi *et al.*, 2003) in the short term.

Other co-morbidity

The relationship between autistic spectrum disorder (ASD) and respiratory disease is currently unclear. Maternal asthma and allergy is not thought by most researchers to play a part in the subsequent development of ASD (Croen *et al.*, 2005). Some research groups have described the suspected link between asthma, atopy and ASD in the context of an immune-based hygiene hypothesis whereby infant immune stimulation hypersensitises the developing immune system toward inflammatory or cytokine responses affecting brain structure and function, leading to ASD (Becker, 2007). The incidence of asthma and atopy in children with ASD may be hard to diagnose as skin prick testing and serum immunoglobulin (IgG) levels may misrepresent the true extent of disease in this population (Bakkaloglu *et al.*, 2008).

People with DS may have an increased incidence of airway abnormalities as reported by Bertrand *et al.* (2003). They reviewed the bronchoscopic findings in 24 individuals with DS (vs. 324 controls) and found a significant increase in airway abnormalities including laryngomalacia, tracheomalacia and tracheal bronchus. Individuals with DS also have higher nasal and upper airway morbidity including upper respiratory infections, sleep-disordered breathing, and nasal itching (Chen *et al.*, 2006). (Please refer to Chapter 5 on Immune system diseases.)

Certain diseases have specific associations with structural disease such as Fragile X syndrome (Visootsak *et al.*, 2005) and Noonan syndrome (Noonan, 1994), both of which are associated with chest wall deformities such as pectus excavatum. Fetal alcohol syndrome is associated with scoliosis leading to long-term impairment of lung function (Floyd *et al.*, 2005).

Common respiratory diseases themselves may lead to the development of ID. A review of the records of over 100 000 children in the USA as part of the National Survey of Child Health found that asthma was independently linked with a higher incidence of depression, behavioural disorders and ID (Blackman and Gurka, 2007).

Conclusion

There are a number of limitations to the reviewed evidence. The studies are primarily cross-sectional or observational (few are longitudinal) and the heterogeneity of ID makes it difficult to make broad comparisons about co-morbidity. Accepting this, there are still a number of conclusions to be drawn from the evidence to date.

Newborns with low birth weight and bronchodysplasia should be followed up carefully due to the strong association with subsequent ID. All people with ID are at higher risk of pneumonia and in some cases should be considered for early gastrostomy tube insertion. Those admitted to secondary care should be assessed for risk of aspiration.

Individuals with ID are over-represented on ICU and have higher incidence of both ventilation and acute lung injury. The underlying cause of admission to ICU needs to be reviewed systematically as failure of clinical staff to recognise deterioration on the ward (rather than an inherent increased incidence of critical illness) may be the reason for the increased admission. Clinical research involving large-scale retrospective analysis of the pre-ICU admission notes of all patients with ID will help to answer this question. The increased risk and severity of influenza provides argument that current vaccination policy for this population may need to be reviewed.

All patients with Prader-Willi syndrome, Down syndrome and cerebral palsy who exhibit excessive daytime sleepiness should be assessed for sleep apnoea as initiation of CPAP may result in sustained improvement in both cognitive functioning and quality of life. In terms of further research, clinical studies are urgently needed to assess methods of reducing apnoea at birth and thus curb long-term neurological impact. Interventions for assessment should include aggressive ventilation policies immediately after birth and use of newborn automated apnoea monitoring systems. Further work is also needed in optimising non-invasive ventilation to assess the long-term cognitive impact of CPAP.

Larger studies are needed into pneumonia risk assessment scores (which are not widely used at present) as well as further research into prevention of pneumonia in people with ID, such as the use of percutaneous feeding tubes or investigations into early warning alert systems for carers.

References

Alchanatis, M., Zias, N., Deligiorgis, N. *et al.* (2005). Sleep apnea-related cognitive deficits and intelligence: an implication of cognitive reserve theory. *J Sleep Res*, 14(1), 69–75.

Aly, H. (2004). Preemptive strike in the war on pain: is it a safe strategy for our vulnerable infants? *Pediatrics*, 114, 1335–7.

Aly, H. (2005). Mechanical ventilation and cerebral palsy. *Pediatrics*, 115(6), 1765–7.

Anzai, Y., Ohya, T. and Yanagi, K. (2006). [Treatment of sleep apnea syndrome in a Down syndrome patient with behavioral problems by noninvasive positive pressure ventilation: a successful case report.] *No To Hattatsu*, 38(1), 32–6.

Avery, G. B. and Glass, P. (1989). The gentle nursery: developmental intervention in the NICU. *J Perinatol*, 9, 204–6.

Bakkaloglu, B., Anlar, B., Anlar, F. Y. *et al.* (2008). Atopic features in early childhood autism. *Eur J Paediatr Neurol*, 6, 476–9.

Becker, K. G. (2007). Autism, asthma, inflammation, and the hygiene hypothesis. *Med Hypotheses*, 69(4), 731–40.

Bertrand, P., Navarro, H., Caussade, S., Holmgren, N. and Sánchez, L. (2003). Airway anomalies in children with Down syndrome: endoscopic findings. *Pediatr Pulmonol*, 36(2), 137–41.

Blackman, J. A. and Gurka, M. J. (2007). Developmental and behavioral comorbidities of asthma in children. *J Dev Behav Pediatr*, 28(2), 92–9.

Bruijn, M., Van Der Aa, L. B., van Rijn, R. R., Bos, A. P. and van Woensel, J. B. (2007). High incidence of acute lung injury in children with Down syndrome. *Intensive Care Med*, 33(12), 2179–82.

Chalmers, D. (1841). *Medical Report to the Managers of the Lunatic Asylum of Aberdeen for the Year Ending 30th April 1841*. Aberdeen: D. Chalmers and Co.

Chen, M. A., Lander, T. R. and Murphy, C. (2006). Nasal health in Down syndrome: a cross-sectional study. *Otolaryngol Head Neck Surg*, 134(5), 741–5.

Clift, S., Dahlitz, M. and Parkes, J. D. (1994). Sleep apnoea in the Prader-Willi syndrome. *J Sleep Res*, 3(2), 121–6.

Craig, M. E., Cowell, C. T., Larsson, P. *et al.* (2006). Growth hormone treatment and adverse events in Prader-Willi syndrome: data from KIGS (the Pfizer International Growth Database). *Clin Endocrinol (Oxf)*, 65(2), 178–85.

Croen, L. A., Grether, J. K., Yoshida, C. K., Odouli, R. and Van de Water, J. (2005). Maternal autoimmune diseases, asthma and allergies, and childhood autism spectrum disorders: a case-control study. *Arch Pediatr Adolesc Med*, 159(2), 151–7.

Dammann, O., Leviton, A., Bartels, D. B. and Dammann, C. E. (2004). Lung and brain damage in preterm newborns. Are they related? How? Why? *Biol Neonate*, 85(4), 305–13.

Decouflé, P. and Autry, A. (2002). Increased mortality in children and adolescents with developmental disabilities. *Paediatr Perinat Epidemiol*, 16(4), 375–82.

Duncan, A., Aly, H. and El-Mohandes, A. E. (2002). Noise levels in the neonatal intensive care unit (NICU): do we provide safe environment for the ill neonate? *Pediatr Res*, 52, 404A.

Farel, A. M., Hooper, S. R., Teplin, S. W., Henry, M. M. and Kraybill, E. N. (1998). Very-low-birthweight infants at seven years: an assessment of the health and neurodevelopmental risk conveyed by chronic lung disease. *J Learn Disabil*, 31(2), 118–26.

Ferini-Strambi, L., Baietto, C., Di Gioia, M. R. *et al.* (2003). Cognitive dysfunction in patients with obstructive sleep apnea (OSA): partial reversibility after continuous positive airway pressure (CPAP). *Brain Res Bull*, 61(1), 87–92.

Ferri, R., Curzi-Dascalova, L., Del Gracco, S. *et al.* (1997). Respiratory patterns during sleep in Down's syndrome: importance of central apnoeas. *J Sleep Res*, 6(2), 134–41.

Floyd, R. L., O'Connor, M. J., Sokol, R. J., Bertrand, J. and Cordero, J. F. (2005). Recognition and prevention of foetal alcohol syndrome. *Obstet Gynecol*, 106(5), 1059–64.

Frei, F. J., Haemmerle, M. H., Brunner, R. and Kern, C. (1997). Minimum alveolar concentration for halothane in children with cerebral palsy and severe mental retardation. *Anaesthesia*, 52(11), 1056–60.

Graham, J., Dumas, H. M., O'Brien, J. E. and Burns, J. P. (2004). Congenital neurodevelopmental diagnoses and an intensive care unit: defining a population. *Pediatr Crit Care Med*, 4, 321–8.

Halbower, A. C. and Mahone, E. M. (2006). Neuropsychological morbidity linked to childhood sleep-disordered breathing. *Sleep Med Rev*, 10(2), 79–81.

Hamano, K., Kumada, S., Hayashi, M. *et al.* (2008). Hemorrhage due to tracheoarterial fistula with severe motor and intellectual disability. *Pediatr Int*, 50(3), 337–40.

Hsiao, K. H. and Nixon, G. M. (2008). The effect of treatment of obstructive sleep apnea on quality of life in children with cerebral palsy. *Res Dev Disabil*, 29(2), 133–40.

Janvier, A., Khairy, M., Kokkotis, A. *et al.* (2004). Apnea is associated with neurodevelopmental impairment in very low birth weight infants. *J Perinatol*, 24(12), 763–8.

Jarvis, S., Glinianaia, S. V., Torrioli, M. G. *et al.* (2003). Cerebral palsy and intrauterine growth in single births: European collaborative study. *Lancet*, 362(9390), 1106–11.

Kaemingk, K. L., Pasvogel, A. E., Goodwin, J. L. *et al.* (2003). Learning in children and sleep disordered breathing: findings of the Tucson Children's Assessment of Sleep Apnea (tuCASA) prospective cohort study. *J Int Neuropsychol Soc*, 9(7), 1016–26.

Kanda, T., Murayama, K., Kondo, I. *et al.* (2005). [An estimation chart for the possibility of aspiration in patients with severe motor and intellectual disabilities: its reliability and accuracy]. *No To Hattatsu*, 37(4), 307–16.

Kono, Y., Mishina, J., Takamura, T. *et al.* (2007). Impact of being small-for-gestational age on survival and long-term outcome of extremely premature infants born at 23–27 weeks' gestation. *J Perinat Med*, 35(5), 447–54.

Kosko, J. R. and Derkay, C. S. (1995). Uvulopalatopharyngoplasty: treatment of obstructive sleep apnea in neurologically impaired pediatric patients. *Int J Pediatr Otorhinolaryngol*, 32(3), 241–6.

Loh, C. H., Lin, J. D., Choi, I. C. *et al.* (2007). Longitudinal analysis of inpatient care utilization among people with intellectual disabilities: 1999–2002. *J Intellect Disabil Res*, 51(2), 101–8.

McCarty, S. F., Gaebler-Spira, D. and Harvey, R. L. (2001). Improvement of sleep apnea in a patient with cerebral palsy. *Am J Phys Med Rehabil*, 80(7), 540–2.

Menendez, A. A. (1999). Abnormal ventilatory responses in patients with Prader-Willi syndrome. *Eur J Pediatr*, 158(11), 941–2.

Miyawaki, T., Kohjitani, A., Maeda, S. *et al.* (2004). Intravenous sedation for dental patients with intellectual disability. *J Intellect Disabil Res*, 48(8), 764–8.

Morton, R. E., Wheatley, R. and Minford, J. (1999). Respiratory tract infections due to direct and reflux aspiration in children with severe neurodisability. *Dev Med Child Neurol*, 41(5), 329–34.

Noonan, J. A. (1994). Noonan syndrome: an update and review for the primary paediatrician. *Clin Pediatr*, 33(9), 548–55.

Okada, M., Takata, K., Hoshikawa, T. *et al.* (2008). [Airway and respiratory management for anesthesia in the patients with severe motor and intellectual disabilities]. *Masui*, 57(1), 76–81.

Polednak, A. P. (1975). Respiratory disease mortality in an institutionalised mentally retarded population. *J Ment Defic Res*, 19(3–4), 165–72.

Richdale, A. L., Cotton, S. and Hibbit, K. (1999). Sleep and behaviour disturbance in Prader-Willi syndrome: a questionnaire study. *J Intellect Disabil Res*, 43(5), 380–92.

Samuels, R. and Chadwick, D. D. (2006). Predictors of asphyxiation risk in adults with intellectual disabilities and dysphagia. *J Intellect Disabil Res*, 50(5), 362–70.

Schultz, C., Tautz, J., Reiss, I. and Moller, J. C. (2003). Prolonged mechanical ventilation induces pulmonary inflammation in preterm infants. *Biol Neonate*, 84, 64–6.

Shintani, T., Asakura, K., Ishi, K. *et al.* (1998). [Obstructive sleep apnea in children with cerebral palsy]. *Nippon Jibiinkoka Gakkai Kaiho*, 101(3), 266–71.

Singer, L., Yamashita, T., Lilien, L. and Baley, C. M. (1997). A longitudinal study of developmental outcome of infants with bronchopulmonary dysplasia and very low birth weight. *Pediatrics*, 100(6), 987–93.

Sullivan, P. B., Morrice, J. S., Vernon-Roberts, A. *et al.* (2006). Does gastrostomy tube feeding in children with cerebral palsy increase the risk of respiratory morbidity? *Arch Dis Child*, 91(6), 478–82.

Tanuma, N., Miyata, R., Hayashi, M., Uchiyama, A. and Kurata, K. (2008). Oxidative stress as a biomarker of respiratory disturbance in patients with severe motor and intellectual disabilities. *Brain Dev*, 30(6), 402–9.

Ting, A., Aniruddhan, K., Hallam, N., Freeman, J. and McFadzean, J. (2006). Severe influenza in children with neurodevelopmental impairment – implications for vaccination policy. *J Infect*, 53(2), 144–6.

Veugelers, R., Calis, E. A., Penning, C. *et al.* (2005). A population-based nested case control study on recurrent pneumonias in children with severe generalized cerebral palsy: ethical considerations of the design and representativeness of the study sample. *BMC Pediatr*, 19, 5–25.

Visootsak, J., Warren, S. T., Anido, A. and Graham, J.M. Jr. (2005). Fragile X syndrome: an update and review for the primary paediatrician. *Clin Pediatr*, 44(5), 371–81.

Wilson, S. S., Cotterill, A. M. and Harris, M. A. (2006). Growth hormone and respiratory compromise in Prader-Willi syndrome. *Arch Dis Child*, 91(4), 349–50.

Yeo, C. L., Choo, S. and Ho, L. Y. (1997). Chronic lung disease in very low birthweight infants: a 5-year review. *J Paediatr Child Health*, 33(2), 102–6.

Yoshikawa, H., Yamazaki, S. and Abe, T. (2005). Acute respiratory distress syndrome in children with severe motor and intellectual disabilities. Triggering factors: *Brain Dev*, 27(6), 395–9.

Digestive system diseases

Robert W. Davis

Introduction

People with intellectual disability (ID) have the same range of gastrointestinal (GI) disorders as the general population, however, issues with cognition and communication mean that diagnoses are often missed (Beange *et al.*, 1995) and many treatable disorders remain unrecognised and untreated. This makes it even more important that clinicians are aware of the particular vulnerabilities of this group. Over the last three decades, research has highlighted the high prevalence of gastro-oesophageal reflux and oesophagitis in people with ID. This population has been well known for having lifelong problems with constipation. The aetiological groupings within the population with ID have their own vulnerabilities.

Method

An advanced OVID search with access to the MEDLINE, CINAHL, EMBASE and all evidence-based medicine reviews including the entire Cochrane library was conducted. There was no search of unpublished research findings.

The search period was from 1966 to 2008 using the MeSH terms: intellectual disabilities/ learning disabilities, mental retardation, Down syndrome, mentally disabled persons.

Combined with the MeSH terms: digestive system, gastrointestinal, constipation, *Helicobacter pylori*, gastro-oesophageal reflux disease, oesophagitis.

The search was conducted in November 2008 and updated in December 2008. The abstracts of all articles identified were screened and only those that provided direct research findings and evidence on epidemiology, aetiology, diagnostic tools and treatment were accepted and inspected in more detail.

Results

The results were combined and generated 55 710 articles for 'Down syndrome/ or mental retardation/ or mentally disabled persons/ or intellectual disability' and 265 368 articles for 'digestive system/ or gastrointestinal motility/ or gastrointestinal diseases/ or gastrointestinal tract/ or gastrointestinal haemorrhage/ or oesophageal stenosis/ or oesophagitis/ or oesophagitis, peptic/ or gastroesophageal reflux/ or constipation'.

Apart from the date limitations quoted, there were no limitations placed on the search and there were no language restrictions although we were unable to further analyse results for which there were no abstracts in English. These articles were further reviewed and

Intellectual Disability and Ill Health: A Review of the Evidence, ed. Jean O'Hara, Jane McCarthy and Nick Bouras. Published by Cambridge University Press. © Cambridge University Press 2010.

Table 8.1. Summary of literature search

Database	Articles identified in search	Inclusion in review
MEDLINE	434	37
CINAHL	60	6
PsycINFO	63	9
EMBASE	1	0
All EBM reviews	11	4

39 articles were included with evidence of high-quality population-based and institutional-based studies with or without comparison control groups. The literature search and databases used are summarised in Table 8.1.

Discussion

Prevalence studies

Gastrointestinal disorders

Sondheimer and Morris (1979) looked at the daily nursing records of 136 children with severe ID in institutions and showed that over the preceding 12 months, 20 (15%) had recurrent vomiting, and of these 15 had gastro-oesophageal reflux disease (GORD) diagnosed by X-ray examination, acid reflux test or both, with oesophagitis noted by endoscopy in 10 of 14 patients. Kuruvilla and Trewby (1989) reported similar rates in institutionalised adults with severe ID where 39 (10%) of 380 had problems with recurrent vomiting and upper GI symptoms. Wang *et al.* (2007) compared institution-based (n = 614) and community-based (n = 514) people with ID selected at random from a population of 73 758 using interviews of families and carers about health. In the community-based population GI problems were reported in 11.9%, compared to 13.7% in the institutionalised population. Adults with Down syndrome were more likely to have GI disorders and to have had hepatitis or to be carriers.

Gastrointestinal cancers

Sullivan *et al.* (2004) reviewed the incidence of cancer, cross-referencing data from a state registry of 9409 individuals with ID and a state cancer registry. The age standardised incidence ratios (SIR) of all cancers in people with ID were not significantly different from the general population. Males had significantly higher incidence of stomach cancers (SIR 3.19, 95% CI = 1.29–6.59) and colorectal cancers were higher in females (SIR 3.10, 95% CI = 1.43–5.88). A review of the literature by Satge *et al.* (2006) suggested that the incidence of GI cancer in Down syndrome overall was decreased with a possible increase in the risk of pancreatic and gall bladder cancer. (Please refer to Chapter 12 on Neoplasms.)

Constipation

Two large studies indicate a wide range in the prevalence of constipation in people with ID. A study by Bohmer *et al.* (2001) randomly selected a population of 215 with an IQ less than 50 (including 48 children under the age of 20) from a population of 1379 residents and found 69.3% had constipation. Morad *et al.* (2007) reviewed 2400 people with ID over 40 years of age using a questionnaire relating to treatment for constipation and found a prevalence of 8%. The wide difference relates to the definition of constipation (with Bohmer *et al.* (2001) including those on treatment), methodology (contrasting a single question to a more directed survey) and in part population (with Morad *et al.*'s (2007) study reviewing a more ambulant population). Both studies found that neurological disease, cerebral palsy, immobility and physical inactivity increased the risk of constipation with Bohmer *et al.* (2001) also finding use of anti-epileptics, H2-antagonists and proton pump inhibitors, food refusal and an IQ less than 35 as risk factors.

Gastro-oesophageal reflux disease (GORD)

Evidence of the high prevalence of reflux in people with ID in general and for aetiological groupings with specific vulnerabilities has built over the last three decades. A case series of eight patients between the ages of 12 and 15 with severe ID by Cadman *et al.* (1978) highlighted most of the features associated with GORD in people with ID in later literature. This included symptoms of recurrent vomiting and frequent haemetemesis and findings of spasticity, kyphoscoliosis and radiologically proven GORD. When Swischuk *et al.* (1981) reviewed 47 children (5 weeks to 14 years old) with marked dilated air-filled oesophagus on plain chest X-rays, 84% had a history of chronic vomiting or reflux. Snyder and Goldman (1990) found that ID was present in 7 of 10 patients diagnosed with Barrett's oesophagus (a rare and severe form of oesophagitis) amongst 1423 biopsies from 1173 patients.

A review by Halpern *et al.* (1991) of 704 children consecutively evaluated for GORD with oesophageal pH monitoring showed that 132 had neurological (central nervous system (CNS)) disease prior to evaluation and in those older than one year, higher rates of GORD (31/45 (69%)) in the group with CNS disease compared to the group without CNS disease (38/81 (47%)). Staiano *et al.* (1991) reviewed 25 children with different degrees of psychomotor retardation – severe (n = 13) or mild to moderate (n = 12) – and symptoms of GORD using oesophageal manometry and pH monitoring; 21 (84%) had GORD. The severe group with GORD (12/13) showed marked motility abnormalities that persisted after curing the GORD. The mild to moderate group with GORD (9/12) had normal motility or a less severe oesophageal motor dysfunction which improved after curing the GORD. Oesophageal motor dysfunction occurs frequently in people with psychomotor retardation and GORD increased with the severity of the disability.

Bohmer and Klinkenberg-Knol (2002) tested the oesophageal pH in 435 individuals (including 48 children) randomly selected from 1195 people with ID with IQ less than 50. Those with a pathological pH were followed up with endoscopy. The pH test failed for technical reasons in 49. In the remaining 386, 200 (51.8%) showed a normal pH while 186 (48.2%) showed a pathological pH. Scoliosis, cerebral palsy, anticonvulsant medication and benzodiazepines were more frequent in those with a pathological pH as were vomiting, haematemesis, rumination, depression and past endoscopic evidence of GORD. Endoscopy of all those with abnormal pH (186 patients) showed 126 (67.7%) had oesophagitis, with 47.3% grade I, 33.3% grade II and 19.4% grade III/IV. Barrett's oesophagitis was found in 14%.

Helicobacter pylori

People with ID appear to be particularly prone to *Helicobacter pylori* (*H. pylori*) infection (please refer to Chapter 4 on Infectious diseases). Bohmer *et al.* (1997) demonstrated positive blood tests in 82.8% of 338 people with ID compared to 27.2% of 254 employees of institutions for people with ID. The rate increased in the employees with degree of physical contact and time in the field. Luzza *et al.* (2004) showed 50% of 84 children with ID, aged 2–18 years, were sero-positive for *H. pylori* compared to 16% of 84 controls matched for age and gender. Wallace *et al.* (2002) demonstrated current infection in 67% of 168 people with ID from a single outpatient clinic. The rate varied significantly across settings; 87% of institutionalised people with ID, 79% of previously institutionalised people with ID and 44% of people with ID who had never been institutionalised having the infection at some stage. A study by Wallace *et al.* (2003) of 168 people with ID tested for *H. pylori* showed that at least one test of serology, helicobacter breath test and faecal antigen test was possible in all patients (23% faecal only, 27% serology only). Only 25% provided breath specimens. Failure to complete tests was associated with lower IQ and higher maladaptive behaviour scores.

Specific syndromes and disorders

Down syndrome

van Trotsenburg *et al.* (2006) reviewed co-morbidity in 163 neonates with Down syndrome (DS) using a combination of parent interviews and cross-check of files; 15 (9.2%) needed GI surgery. Gastrointestinal problems were second only to cardiovascular problems as a reason for admission in the first three years of life. Motor development was significantly delayed in those with GI surgery. Wallace (2007) reported on an audit of 57 adults with DS, average age of 37, where 56 had at least one GI problem,12% were likely to have coeliac disease (positive specific immunoglobulin A (IgA) antibody tests or endoscopically proven), 9% reflux, 67% positive *H. pylori*, 25% hepatitis B, 19% had unexplained constipation and 19% diarrhoea.

In 187 people with DS, Buchin *et al.* (1986) identified 27 with major GI disorders, most commonly duodenal stenosis (9), GORD (5), imperforate anus (5) and Hirschsprung's disease (4). The mortality for the whole group was 11% (20 individuals). Mortality in those with duodenal stenosis was particularly high (5 out of 9, or 56%). Thompson *et al.* (1999) reviewed 24 infants with DS and atrio-septal defect who had symptoms of reflux and a positive oesophageal pH test. All 10 receiving standard medical treatment that included an H2 receptor antagonist required readmission, 6 for aspiration and pneumonia. None of the 14 who had Nissen fundoplication via a mini-laparotomy had reflux-related complications requiring further admission at follow-up.

Bonamico *et al.* (2001) found coeliac disease had a prevalence of 4.6% in 1202 people with DS with decreased height and weight percentiles in the coeliac group. Diarrhoea, vomiting, failure to thrive, anorexia, constipation and abdominal distension, lower haemoglobin and serum irons were more frequent. Diagnosis was made an average of 3.8 years from initiation of symptoms. While 69% had classic presentation, 11% had atypical symptoms and 20% had a silent form of coeliac disease. Book *et al.* (2001) found 10.3% of 97 children with DS were positive to serum IgA-anti-endomysial antibody testing. They found that only bloating symptoms were significantly more frequent in those with coeliac disease. Based on these observations it is recommended that children with DS be screened for coeliac disease.

Cornelia de Lange syndrome (CdLS)

Luzzani *et al.* (2003) investigated the incidence of GORD in a series of 43 people with CdLS; GORD was evident in 28/43 (65%). There was a strong correlation between the degree of the oesophageal damage and the behavioural phenotype. Hyperactivity was most frequently associated with the condition (85%). Behavioural symptoms and their evolution during treatment could be used as major signs of oesophageal damage in CdLS. Hall *et al.* (2008) compared 54 people with ID and CdLS and 46 controls with ID alone, matched for degree of ID, mobility and age. The study looked at the presence and severity of health problems within the last month; 71% of the CdLS group compared to 31.8% of the control group had a GI problem sometime in their life ($p < 0.01$), while 44.2% compared to 15.9% had a GI problem in the previous month ($p < 0.01$).

Cerebral palsy

From the initial case series by Cadman *et al.* (1978) the strong association between GORD and people with cerebral palsy has been demonstrated. In particular the high prevalence with spasticity and kyphoscoliosis was noted. A large population study by Bohmer and Klinkenberg-Knol (2002) further highlighted the same strong associations with immobility and swallowing difficulties associated with the condition thought to contribute to the development of the problem.

Pervasive developmental disorder (PDD)

In a review of 118 people with ID Galli-Carminati *et al.* (2006) compared 75 people with ID and no PDD (47 men and 28 women) with a second group of 43 people with ID with PDD (30 men, 13 women). The prevalence of GI disorders was 48.8% in the group with PDD compared to 8.0% in the group without PDD. In the group with PDD, 11.6% had oesophagitis, 13.9% gastritis/duodenitis, 16.3% heartburn and 25.6% had dyspepsia contrasting with none in the control group. The effect was further enhanced in those with more severe degrees of ID.

Diagnosis and treatment

Constipation

In a double-blind, placebo-controlled trial of treatment of dietary fibre glucamannan in 20 children with brain damage and chronic constipation (10 in each group), Staiano *et al.* (2000) showed a significant increase in stool frequency in the treatment group compared to placebo ($p < 0.01$). There was a significant decrease in pain on defaecation, laxative and suppository usage with no effect on motility or colonic transit times. Migeon-Duballet *et al.* (2006) evaluated the tolerability of polyethylene glycol 3350 plus electrolytes (Movicol) in 54/66 residents with severe intellectual and physical disability at a specialist unit. The results indicated an increase in stool numbers with diarrhoea increased and no change in body weight. There was a greater than 50% reduction in cost of laxatives.

Gastro-oesophageal reflux disease (GORD)

Diagnosis

Gossler *et al.* (2007) investigated the link between GORD and behaviour in a prospective study of 19 inpatients with neurological impairment suspected for GORD. All 19 children had repeated pH monitoring and 18 had additional repeated endoscopic investigations with histological examination. A reflux index as a measure of the severity of GORD was significantly higher in the children with auto-aggressive behaviour or agitation than without these behaviours. No association with behaviour and histological findings could be demonstrated. Swender *et al.* (2006) used a case-control design to compare 30 individuals with hand-mouthing behaviour with 30 matched controls using pH testing or endoscopy.

Gastro-oesophageal reflux disease was found in 60% of the hand-mouthing group compared to 23.3% of the controls.

Treatment

Brueton et al. (1990) compared the effect of cisopride on GORD in 6 children with cerebral palsy (3 with athetoid) and 1 with DS with 15 controls and found that the children with neurological disorders did not benefit as much from cisapride as the control group. Cheung et al. (2001) reviewed nine children with ID and a history of GORD and showed that vomiting and pneumonia were reduced significantly by 1.0–2.3 mg/kg of omeprazole. Bohmer and Klinkenberg-Knol (2002) treated 126 people with ID and oesophagitis with 40 mg omeprazole a day for three months followed by 20 mg a day for six months. Endoscopy showed healing in 111 patients (88.1%) with a healing dose of 40 mg omeprazole a day and a maintenance dose of 20 mg a day. Upon dose reduction 13 patients relapsed but all rehealed when the dose was increased back up to 40 mg a day. Two patients with grade II GORD needed a dose of 60 mg a day but did not relapse on 40 mg a day. One person developed skin rash as a side effect.

Campanozzi et al. (2007) reviewed the impact of malnutrition on GI disorders in 21 children with cerebral palsy and severe ID. Gastro-oesophageal reflux disease was present in 14 and 9 had chronic constipation. Four of the 9 children who completed the trial of nutritional treatments improved while the remaining 5 had persistent reflux.

Wales et al. (2002) compared outcomes in 111 neurologically impaired children of fundoplication via laparotomy and gastrostomy (FG, n = 63) with image-guided gastrojejunal tube (GJ, n = 48). The GJ group were more likely to continue anti-reflux medication (p < 0.05), had a trend to have bowel obstruction or intussusception (20.8% vs. 7.9%) and had more problems with repair or adjustment of the tube. In the FG group, 9 (14.3%) individuals had wrap failure with 7 (11.1%) requiring further surgery. Complications from aspiration pneumonia were 31.3% in the GJ group and 36.5% in the FG group. One of 6 deaths in the GJ group and 5 of 11 deaths in the FG group were GORD-related. Cheung et al. (2006) compared the results of open Nissen fundoplication (ONF) on 9 children with severe neurological impairment to those of 11 with laparoscopic fundoplication (LF). There was no difference in incidence of pneumonia, while reflux was significantly reduced by both procedures with a 30% recurrence. Weight increased from an average of 17.4 kg at baseline to 22.8 kg at follow-up. There were two recurrences from ONF and four from LF. Four patients died, two on each side unrelated to surgery or treatment. Neither procedure seemed to have significant changes in rates of pneumonia before or after the operation.

Wilkinson et al. (1981) reviewed surgical and medical treatment in 31 children with severe intellectual and physical disability. Eight (26%) had complete or partial response to medical treatment involving posture, antacid, thickened food and H2 antagonist. Fourteen of those who failed to respond had a Nissen fundoplication with good therapeutic response in 12 and 2 post-operative deaths. The nine without surgery had continuing morbidity from emesis (88%), anaemia (44%) and pulmonary disease (33%) with two (22%) dying. A Cochrane review by Vernon-Roberts and Sullivan (2007) considered fundoplication surgery versus anti-reflux medications for gastro-oesophageal reflux in children with neurological impairment. The review concluded from 55 references that there remains considerable uncertainty regarding the optimal treatment when faced with the decision of who is to undergo gastrostomy insertion. This further emphasised the need for robust scientific evidence in order to provide data on the comparable risks or benefits of the two interventions where mortality rates are so high.

Helicobacter pylori

Wallace *et al.* (2004) reported on reviews of 168 people with ID over 17 years of age, 117 of whom were shown to be infected by *H. pylori*. Of the 96 (82%) who were given standard treatment (omeprazole 20 mg bd, amoxicillin 1 g bd, clarithromycin 500 mg bd, if allergic to amoxicillin this was replaced by metronidazole 400 mg bd), eradication occurred in 61% 31% reported side effects. There were differences in the level of behaviour as measured by the maladaptive behaviour scale (ABS) before or after treatment (Nihira *et al.* 1974) suggesting that maladaptive behaviours may be risk factors for, rather than consequences of, *H. pylori* infection.

Rumination

After a functional relationship between caloric intake and rumination was established by Rast *et al.* (1985) in an experiment that looked at the effect of caloric level on the frequency of rumination they were able to demonstrate a 15% to 43% decrease in rumination compared to baseline with higher caloric intake.

Conclusion

Given the prevalence of GI problems in people with ID there are surprisingly few studies. The studies led by Bohmer (Bohmer and Klinkenberg-Knol, 2002; Bohmer *et al.*, 1997, 2001) and Wallace (Wallace *et al.*, 2002, 2003, 2004) highlight the value of high-quality studies specific to this population with respect to the diagnosis and treatment of GORD and *H. pylori*. The high frequency within the population with ID and within those with PDD and cerebral palsy further emphasises the need to consider this diagnosis in the context of behaviour change or altered blood pathology. The high rates of *H. pylori* infection support the case for regular screening. Vulnerabilities to GI disorders within those with cerebral palsy, PDD, CdLS and DS have been reviewed. While constipation seems to be a perennial problem in this population, there is little research on specific treatment for this group.

References

Beange, H., McElduff, A. and Baker, W. (1995). Medical disorders of adults with mental retardation: a population study. *Am J Ment Retard*, 99, 595–604.

Bohmer, C. J., Klinkenberg-Knol, E. C., Kuipers, E. J. *et al.* (1997). The prevalence of Helicobacter pylori infection among inhabitants and healthy employees of institutes for the intellectually disabled. *Am J Gastroenterol*, 92, 1000–4.

Bohmer, C. J., Taminiau, J. A., Klinkenberg-Knol, E. C. *et al.* (2001). The prevalence of constipation in institutionalized people with intellectual disability. *J Intellect Disabil Res*, 45, 212–18.

Bohmer, C. J. M. and Klinkenberg-Knol, E. C. (2002). Prevalence, diagnosis and treatment of gastro-oesophageal reflux disease in institutionalised persons with an intellectual disability. *J Intellect Dev Disabil*, 27, 92–105.

Bonamico, M., Mariani, P., Danesi, H. M. *et al.* (2001). Prevalence and clinical picture of celiac disease in Italian down syndrome patients: a multicenter study. *J Pediatr Gastroenterol Nutr*, 33, 139–43.

Book, L., Hart, A., Black, J. *et al.* (2001). Prevalence and clinical characteristics of celiac disease in Downs syndrome in a US study. *Am J Med Genet*, 98, 70–4.

Brueton, M. J., Clarke, G. S. and Sandhu, B. K. (1990). The effects of cisapride on gastro-oesophageal reflux in children with and without neurological disorders. *Dev Med Child Neurol*, 32, 629–32.

Buchin, P. J., Levy, J. S. and Schullinger, J. N. (1986). Down's syndrome and the GI tract. *J Clin Gastroenterol*, 8, 111–14.

Cadman, D., Richards, J. and Feldman, W. (1978). Gastro-oesophageal reflux in severely retarded children. *Dev Med Child Neurol*, 20, 95–8.

Campanozzi, A., Capano, G., Miele, E. *et al.* (2007). Impact of malnutrition on GI disorders and gross motor abilities in children with cerebral palsy. [see comment]. *Brain Dev*, 29, 25–9.

Cheung, K. M., Tse, P. W., Ko, C. H. *et al.* (2001). Clinical efficacy of proton pump inhibitor therapy in neurologically impaired children with gastroesophageal reflux: prospective study. *Hong Kong Med J*, 7, 356–9.

Cheung, K. M., Tse, H. W., Tse, P. W. *et al.* (2006). Nissen fundoplication and gastrostomy in severely neurologically impaired children with gastroesophageal reflux. [see comment]. *Hong Kong Med J*, 12, 282–8.

Galli-Carminati, G., Chauvet, I. and Deriaz, N. (2006). Prevalence of gastrointestinal disorders in adult clients with pervasive developmental disorders. *J Intellect Disabil Res*, 50, 711–18.

Gossler, A., Schalamon, J., Huber-Zeyringer, A. *et al.* (2007). Gastroesophageal reflux and behavior in neurologically impaired children. *J Pediatr Surg*, 42, 1486–90.

Hall, S. S., Arron, K., Sloneem, J. *et al.* (2008). Health and sleep problems in Cornelia de Lange syndrome: a case control study. *J Intellect Disabil Res*, 52, 458–68.

Halpern, L. M., Jolley, S. G. and Johnson, D. G. (1991). Gastroesophageal reflux: a significant association with central nervous system disease in children. *J Pediatr Surg*, 26, 171–3.

Kuruvilla, J. and Trewby, P. N. (1989). Gastro-oesophageal disorders in adults with severe mental impairment. *BMJ*, 299, 95–6.

Luzza, F., Concolino, D., Imeneo, M. *et al.* (2004). High seroprevalence of Helicobacter pylori infection in non-institutionalised children with mental retardation. *Clin Microbiol Infect*, 10, 670–3.

Luzzani, S., Macchini, F., Valade, A. *et al.* (2003). Gastroesophageal reflux and Cornelia de Lange syndrome: typical and atypical symptoms. *Am J Med Genet A*, 119A, 283–7.

Migeon-Duballet, I., Chabin, M., Gautier, A. *et al.* (2006). Long-term efficacy and cost-effectiveness of polyethylene glycol 3350 plus electrolytes in chronic constipation: a retrospective study in a disabled population. *Curr Med Res Opin*, 22, 1227–35.

Morad, M., Nelson, N. P., Merrick, J. *et al.* (2007). Prevalence and risk factors of constipation in adults with intellectual disability in residential care centers in Israel. *Res Dev Disabil*, 28, 580–6.

Nihira, K., Foster, R., Shellhaas, M. *et al.* (1974). *AAMD Adaptive Behaviour Scale* (1974 Revision. edn.). Washington: American Association on Mental Deficiency.

Rast, J., Ellinger-Allen, J. A. and Johnston, J. M. (1985). Dietary management of rumination: four case studies. *Am J Clin Nutr*, 42, 95–101.

Satge, D., Sasco, A. J., Vekemans, M. J. *et al.* (2006). Aspects of digestive tract tumors in Down syndrome: a literature review. *Dig Dis Sci*, 51, 2053–61.

Snyder, J. D. and Goldman, H. (1990). Barrett's esophagus in children and young adults. *Dig Dis Sci*, 35, 1185–9.

Sondheimer, J. M. and Morris, B. A. (1979). Gastroesophageal reflux among severely retarded children. *J Pediatr*, 94, 710–14.

Staiano, A., Cucchiara, S., Del Giudice, E. *et al.* (1991). Disorders of oesophageal motility in children with psychomotor retardation and gastro-oesophageal reflux. *Eur J Pediatr*, 150, 638–41.

Staiano, A., Simeone, D., Del Giudice, E. *et al.* (2000). Effect of the dietary fiber glucomannan on chronic constipation in neurologically impaired children. [see comment]. *J Pediatr*, 136, 41–5.

Sullivan, S. G., Hussain, R., Threlfall, T. *et al.* (2004). The incidence of cancer in people with intellectual disabilities. *Cancer Causes Control*, 15, 1021–5.

Swender, S. L., Matson, J. L., Mayville, S. B. *et al.* (2006). A functional assessment of handmouthing among persons with severe and profound intellectual disability. *J Intellect Dev Disabil*, 31, 95–100.

Swischuk, L. E., Hayden, C. K. Jr. and van Caillie, B. D. (1981). Mega-aeroesophagus in children: a sign of gastroesophageal reflux. *Radiology*, 141, 73–6.

Thompson, L. D., McElhinney, D. B., Jue, K. L. *et al.* (1999). Gastroesophageal reflux after repair of atrioventricular septal defect in infants with trisomy 21: a comparison of medical and surgical therapy. *J Pediatr Surg*, 34, 1359–63.

van Trotsenburg, A. S., Heymans, H. S., Tijssen, J. G. *et al.* (2006). Comorbidity, hospitalization, and medication use and their influence on mental and motor development of young infants with Down syndrome. *Pediatrics*, 118, 1633–9.

Vernon-Roberts, A. and Sullivan, P. B. (2007). Fundoplication versus post-operative medication for gastro-oesophageal reflux in children with neurological impairment undergoing gastrostomy. *Cochrane Database Syst Rev*, (1), CD006151.

Wales, P. W., Diamond, I. R., Dutta, S. *et al.* (2002). Fundoplication and gastrostomy versus image-guided gastrojejunal tube for enteral feeding in neurologically impaired children with gastroesophageal reflux. *J Pediatr Surg*, 37, 407–12.

Wallace, R. A. (2007). Clinical audit of gastrointestinal conditions occurring among adults with Down syndrome attending a specialist clinic. *J Intellect Dev Disabil*, 32, 45–50.

Wallace, R. A., Webb, P. M. and Schluter, P. J. (2002). Environmental, medical, behavioural and disability factors associated with Helicobacter pylori infection in adults with intellectual disability. *J Intellect Disabil Res*, 46, 51–60.

Wallace, R. A., Schluter, P. J., Forgan-Smith, R. *et al.* (2003). Diagnosis of Helicobacter pylori infection in adults with intellectual disability. *J Clin Microbiol*, 41, 4700–4.

Wallace, R. A., Schluter, P. J. and Webb, P. M. (2004). Effects of Helicobacter pylori eradication among adults with intellectual disability. *J Intellect Disabil Res*, 48, 646–54.

Wang, K. Y., Hsieh, K., Heller, T. *et al.* (2007). Carer reports of health status among adults with intellectual/developmental disabilities in Taiwan living at home and in institutions. *J Intellect Disabil Res*, 51, 173–83.

Wilkinson, J. D., Dudgeon, D. L. and Sondheimer, J. M. (1981). A comparison of medical and surgical treatment of gastroesophageal reflux in severely retarded children. *J Pediatr*, 99, 202–5.

Systems disorders

9 Urological and male genital diseases

Stefano Lassi

Introduction

Many of the urological conditions which affect the general population are also prevalent among people with intellectual disability (ID). Incontinence shows a higher prevalence amongst such populations, often due to the presence of physical disabilities and impaired mobility (Rogers, 2002). All the other urogenital problems such as urinary tract infections, nephrolithiasis, nephropathies, prostate difficulties, cancer and urogenital abnormalities seem to be more prevalent among people with ID (Gautheron, 1997; Petterson *et al.*, 2007). Nevertheless this topic appears to have received limited attention within the ID literature.

Method

A search in MEDLINE (1966–2008) was made to identify studies on the association between ID and urological and male genital diseases. A broad search strategy included hand-searching journals, policy and good practice guidance. There was no search of unpublished research findings.

The MeSH terms used were urological diseases, male urogenital diseases, male genital diseases, urinary infection, incontinence, prostate diseases, kidney diseases, bladder diseases, sexual diseases, intellectual disability, intellectual disabilities, mental retardation, learning disabilities, intellectual impairment and developmental disability.

The first search was made in September 2008 and updated in January 2009. The focus was on urological and male genital diseases in children and adults with ID. All abstracts found were read, and potentially relevant articles were inspected in more detail. The only exclusion criterion was no abstract available. There was no restriction as to language.

Results

Results were combined which generated 1586 articles for 'urological disorders' and 518 articles for 'male genital disorders'. The final number of abstracts selected after an evidence-based screening was 57 for 'urological disorders' and 60 for 'male genital disorders' (see Table 9.1).

The abstracts of all articles identified were screened and only those that provided direct research findings and evidence on epidemiology, aetiology, diagnostic tools and treatment were accepted and inspected in more detail. Evidence accepted included

Intellectual Disability and Ill Health: A Review of the Evidence, ed. Jean O'Hara, Jane McCarthy and Nick Bouras. Published by Cambridge University Press. © Cambridge University Press 2010.

Table 9.1. Search results

	Urological disorders	Male genital disorders
Before evidence-based screening	1586	518
After evidence-based screening	57	60

Table 9.2. Summary of research studies, clinical trials and guidelines

Study type	References	Country
Research support articles	Badens *et al.*, 2006	France
	Bockenhauer *et al.*, 2008	UK
	Erdmann *et al.*, 2007	USA
	Patja *et al.*, 2001	Finland
	Petterson *et al.*, 2007	Australia
	Gu *et al.*, 2006	China
	Sullivan *et al.*, 2004	Australia
Guidelines	EBPG, 2002	Europe
Randomised controlled trial	van Haelst *et al.*, 2007	UK
Cross-sectional study	Mandell *et al.*, 2008	USA

high-quality population-based and institutional-based studies with or without comparison control groups, review articles, guidelines, research support studies (see Table 9.2) and also case reports since they represented the majority of articles detected. Of the 103 references identified, 69 were case reports, 24 review articles, 7 research support, 1 guideline and 2 clinical trials.

Discussion

The published prevalence of urinary incontinence in children with ID varies between 23% and 86%, due to bladder dysfunction from overactive detrusor and sphincter dyssynergia (Van Laecke, 2008). Nevertheless incontinence cannot be considered to always occur in people with ID although it may take longer for a person with ID to develop continence (Rogers, 2002; Smith *et al.*, 2000; Stanley, 1996; Taylor *et al.*, 1994). Fetal obstructive uropathy and renal abnormalities have been described in Trisomy syndromes, but the relationship of these abnormalities to Trisomy syndromes remains unclear (Qureshi *et al.*, 2000) including partial Trisomy 7p syndrome (Liang *et al.*, 2005), partial Trisomy 13 (Galán *et al.*, 1989) and partial trisomy for the short arm of chromosome 2 (Sekhon *et al.*, 1978).

Urogenital diseases in people with Down syndrome (Trisomy 21) are not as rare as previously thought (Málaga *et al.*, 2005). These include neurogenic or functional bladder dysfunction, which can lead to upper urinary tract deterioration (Ebert *et al.*, 2008), cryptorchidism (Cassidy *et al.*, 1977; Dada *et al.*, 2006) and testicular microlithiasis (Vachon *et al.*, 2006). There are also case reports concerning people with Trisomy 21 with renal tubular dysgenesis (Jain and Beneck, 2003), idiopathic scrotal lymphoedema (Hashem and Ahmed, 1999), thoracic ectopic kidney (Navarro *et al.*, 2005), posterior urethral valves complicated by severe urinary infections with obstructive symptoms (Culty *et al.*, 2006) and prostatic urethral dilatation with pelvic floor spasticity (Handel *et al.*, 2003).

Genital abnormalities and disorders of pubertal development such as hypogonadism, cryptorchidism, genital hypoplasia and delayed or incomplete gonadal maturation are common in Prader-Willi syndrome (Crinò *et al.*, 2003; Vogels *et al.*, 2008). Menkes' kinky hair disease is a poor prognostic congenital disease with X-linked recessive inheritance, characterised by multiple diverticula of the bladder and other urological abnormalities associated with low serum copper levels (Iuchi *et al.*, 1991; Ryoo and Cho, 2008; Zaffanello and Fanos, 2003). Smith-Lemli-Opitz syndrome is a recessive autosomal genetic disease characterised by male pseudohermaphroditism, attributed to a deficit in 7-dehydrocholesterol reductase. The presence of 7-dehydrocholesterol in the serum of individuals is pathognomonic of the disease and genital abnormalities are present in 50–71% of the studied populations (Angle *et al.*, 1998; Roux *et al.*, 2000). The ATR-X syndrome (Alpha thalassaemia X-linked mental retardation syndrome) affecting males is characterised by genital abnormalities in addition to severe ID and distinct facial dysmorphisms (Badens *et al.*, 2006; Wada *et al.*, 2006). Genitopatellar syndrome is characterised by multicystic kidneys or hydronephrosis in addition to absent patellae, dysmorphic features and ID (Cormier-Daire *et al.*, 2000; Lifchez *et al.*, 2003; Reardon, 2002).

There is a high incidence of kidney abnormalities, genital hypoplasia and cryptorchidism in CHARGE (Coloboma, Heart disease, Atresia of choanae, Retarded mental development and growth, Genital hypoplasia, Ear anomalies and deafness) syndrome (Blake and Prasad, 2006; Davenport *et al.*, 1986; Pagon *et al.*, 1981; Pedersen and Skovby, 2007; Ragan *et al.*, 1999; Tellier *et al.*, 1998). Fraser, WAGR (Wilms tumour, aniridia, genitourinary anomalies, and mental retardation) and Denys-Drash syndromes are characterised by ambiguous genitalia, cryptorchidism or hypospadias and renal agenesis (Braun *et al.*, 2007; Dahan *et al.*, 2007; Jadresic *et al.*, 1990, 1991; Le Caignec *et al.*, 2007; Mahale *et al.*, 2007; Martínez-Frías *et al.*, 1998; Morrison *et al.*, 2008; Prasun *et al.*, 2007; Stefan and Semecký, 1998; van Haelst *et al.*, 2007). Lowe syndrome includes low molecular weight proteinuria and hypercalciuria, ID and proximal tubulopathy (Bockenhauer *et al.*, 2008; Erdmann *et al.*, 2007). Xanthinuria with xanthine lithiasis, urinary infections and acute renal failure are characteristic of Lesch-Nyhan syndrome (Lepercq *et al.*, 1973; Oka *et al.*, 1985; Pela *et al.*, 2008; Rebentisch *et al.*, 2004).

There are review articles about urogenital abnormalities in some genetic syndromes associated with ID and many case reports as summarised in Table 9.3 (Hassink *et al.*, 1996; Pinsky and DiGeorge, 1965; Smith, 1978).

Males with ID are found to have a significantly reduced risk of prostate and urinary tract cancer. Low rates of smoking in those with severe and profound ID might explain such significantly low incidence. However, an excess of testicular cancer is found in men with profound ID, as they are more likely to have genetic abnormalities in the germ cells (Dieckmann, 2007; Hafeez *et al.*, 2007; Kuroda *et al.*, 2007; Patja *et al.*, 2001; Suzuki *et al.*, 2005; Sullivan *et al.*, 2004). There is also some evidence of possible increased rates of gonadal tumours in men with Down syndrome (please refer to Chapter 12 on Neoplasms).

Sexually transmitted diseases are considered an important issue in people with ID (Clark and O'Toole, 2007; Mandell *et al.*, 2008). However, only a case report of a boy with Down syndrome who presented disseminated gonorrhoea due to sexual abuse has been reported (Wiggers and Oudesluys-Murphy, 2006). (Please refer to Chapter 4 on Infectious diseases.)

Table 9.3. Summary of case reports of genetic syndromes and urological abnormalities

Study	Country	Genetic syndrome	Urological abnormalities
Yosunkaya Fenerci et al., 2007	Turkey	Emanuel syndrome	Cryptorchidism
Rajcan-Separovic et al., 2007	USA	Sotos syndrome	Chronic renal failure and polycystic kidney disease
Szczepańska et al., 2007	Poland	Tuberous sclerosis	Male genital abnormalities
Cefle et al., 2002	Turkey	Microdeletion syndrome inv. 2p	Male genital abnormalities
Dastot-Le Moal et al., 2007	France	Mowat-Wilson syndrome	Male genital abnormalities
Turnbull et al., 2006	UK	Malpuech syndrome	Male genital abnormalities
Wakui et al., 2005	USA	Potocki-Shaffer syndrome	Male genital abnormalities
Galasso et al., 2003	Italy	Wolf-Pfeiffer type cardiocranial syndrome	Male genital abnormalities
Wieczorek et al., 2000	Germany	DiGeorge syndrome/ velo-cardio-facial syndrome	Male genital abnormalities
Digilio et al., 1997	Italy	Hirschhorn syndrome	Male genital abnormalities
Holmes et al., 1997	USA	Deletion of 7q21 syndrome	Male genital abnormalities
Tajara et al., 1989	Brazil	D13 ring chromosome syndrome	Male genital abnormalities
Mccandless and Walker, 1976	UK	49,XXXXY syndrome	Male genital abnormalities
Musumeci et al., 2006	Italy	Hennekam syndrome	Lymphoedema of the genitalia
Karaman, 2008	Turkey	Bardet-Biedl syndrome	Hypogonadism and renal dysfunction
Rossi et al., 2007	Italy	Lathosterolosis	Hypogonadism and renal dysfunction
Slavotinek et al., 2002	USA	Bardet-Biedl syndrome	Hypogonadism and renal dysfunction
Green et al., 1989	Canada	Bardet-Biedl syndrome	Hypogonadism and renal dysfunction
Blum et al., 2001	USA	Bannayan-Riley-Ruvacalba syndrome	Lentigines on penis
Buoni et al., 2000	Italy	Inv dup (15) syndrome	Macropenis or hypospadias
Labrune et al., 1994	France	Schinzel-Giedion syndrome	Uni- or bilateral hydronephrosis
Wegenke et al., 1975	Germany	Kallmann syndrome	Hypogonadism, unilateral renal aplasia
Caselli et al., 2008	Italy	Deletion in 7q36.1q36.2	Renal hypoplasia
Sartelet et al., 2008	France	Galloway-Mowat syndrome	Nephrotic syndrome
Gimelli et al., 2007	Italy	Invdup(3)(q22.3qter) marker chromosome	Ambiguous genitalia

(cont.)

Table 9.3. (cont.)

Study	Country	Genetic syndrome	Urological abnormalities
Sugayama et al., 2004	Brazil	Williams-Beuren syndrome	Renal and urinary tract anomalies
Pankau et al., 1996	Germany	Williams-Beuren syndrome	Renal anomalies
Stevenson et al., 2005	USA	Renpenning syndrome	Hypogonadism
Unuigbe et al., 2007	Benin	Townes Brocks syndrome	Urethral meatal stenosis
Greco et al., 2007	USA	Fragile X syndrome	Testicular inclusion formation
Gu et al., 2006	China	Fragile X syndrome	Erectile dysfunction
Liebau et al., 2007	Germany	L1CAM mutation	Duplex kidneys
Schulman et al., 1996	Germany	Williams syndrome	Bladder diverticula and uninhibited detrusor contractions

It is relevant to note that severe ID and/or additional disabilities are considered relative contraindications to kidney transplantation by the European best practice guidelines for renal transplantation (EBPG, 2002).

Conclusion

Urogenital anomalies in children and adults with ID of genetic aetiology are frequent but the literature is mainly based on case reports and review articles. Due to the high incidence of potential abnormalities, it is recommended that people with ID who have specific genetic syndromes should undergo a careful genitourinary assessment, including renal and bladder ultrasound, blood and urinary tests and in some syndromes, cystourethrography screening.

Prostate cancer screening with a prostate specific antigen (PSA) test and digital rectal examination should be considered in all men with ID over the age of 50, as for the general population. Testicular palpation is also recommended in children and adults with ID (Peate and Maloret, 2007). Use of screening tests should be based on the benefits and risks for each person and his ability to tolerate a specific procedure.

Incontinence in children and adults with ID is an underestimated problem in urology. Literature is scarce, often limited to the incidence and urodynamics and seldom focused on treatment and prevention. There is a paucity of evidence-based research for urogenital diseases in people with intellectual disability and more research is necessary to inform clinical practice.

References

Angle, B., Tint, G. S., Yacoub, O. A. and Clark, A. L. (1998). Atypical case of Smith-Lemli-Opitz syndrome: implications for diagnosis. *Am J Med Genet*, 80, 322–6.

Badens, C., Lacoste, C., Philip, N. *et al.* (2006). Mutations in PHD-like domain of the ATRX gene correlate with severe psychomotor impairment and severe urogenital abnormalities in patients with ATRX syndrome. *Clin Genet*, 70, 57–62.

Blake, K. D. and Prasad, C. (2006). CHARGE syndrome. *Orphanet J Rare Dis*, 1, 34.

Blum, R. R., Rahimizadeh, A., Kardon, N., Lebwohl, M. and Wei, H. (2001). Genital lentigines in a 6-year-old boy with a family history of Cowden's disease: clinical and genetic evidence of the linkage between Bannayan-Riley-Ruvacalba syndrome and Cowden's disease. *J Cutan Med Surg*, 5, 228–30.

Bockenhauer, D., Bokenkamp, A., van't Hoff, W. *et al.* (2008). Renal phenotype in Lowe Syndrome: a selective proximal tubular dysfunction. *Clin J Am Soc Nephrol*, 3, 1430–6.

Braun, K. P., May, M., Erler, T. and Hoschke, B. (2007). [Multicystic renal tumor in a patient with WAGR syndrome]. *Urologe A*, 46, 671–4.

Buoni, S., Sorrentino, L., Farnetani, M. A., Pucci, L. and Fois, A. (2000). The syndrome of inv dup (15): clinical, electroencephalographic, and imaging findings. *J Child Neurol*, 15, 380–5.

Caselli, R., Mencarelli, M. A., Papa, F. T. *et al.* (2008). Delineation of the phenotype associated with 7q36.1q36.2 deletion: long QT syndrome, renal hypoplasia and mental retardation. *Am J Med Genet A*, 146A, 1195–9.

Cassidy, S. B., Heller, R. M., Chazen, E. M. and Engel, E. (1977). The chromosome 2 distal short arm trisomy syndrome. *J Pediatr*, 91, 934–8.

Cefle, K., Yildiz, A., Palanduz, S. *et al.* (2002). Chronic renal failure in a patient with Sotos syndrome due to autosomal dominant polycystic kidney disease. *Int J Clin Pract*, 56, 316–8.

Clark, L. I. and O'Toole, M. S. (2007). Intellectual impairment and sexual health: information needs. *Br J Nurs*, 16, 154–6.

Cormier-Daire, V., Chauvet, M. L., Lyonnet, S. *et al.* (2000). Genitopatellar syndrome: a new condition comprising absent patellae, scrotal hypoplasia, renal anomalies, facial dysmorphism, and mental retardation. *J Med Genet*, 37, 520–4.

Crinò, A., Schiaffini, R., Ciampalini, P. *et al.* and Genetic Obesity Study Group of Italian Society of Pediatric Endocrinology and Diabetology (2003). Hypogonadism and pubertal development in Prader-Willi syndrome. *Eur J Pediatr*, 162, 327–33.

Culty, T., Delongchamps, N. B., Dominique, S. *et al.* (2006). Posterior urethral valves in adult with Down syndrome. *Urology*, 67, 424.e1–424.e2.

Dada, R., Kumar, R. and Kucheria, K. (2006). A 2-year-old baby with Downs syndrome, cryptorchidism and testicular tumour. *Eur J Med Genet*, 49, 265–8.

Dahan, K., Kamal, M., Noël, L. H. *et al.* (2007). Small glomeruli in WAGR (Wilms Tumor, Aniridia, Genitourinary Anomalies and Mental Retardation) syndrome. *Am J Kidney Dis*, 49, 793–800.

Dastot-Le Moal, F., Wilson, M., Mowat, D. *et al.* (2007). ZFHX1B mutations in patients with Mowat-Wilson syndrome. *Hum Mutat*, 28, 313–21.

Davenport, S. L., Hefner, M. A. and Mitchell, J. A. (1986). The spectrum of clinical features in CHARGE syndrome. *Clin Genet*, 29, 298–310.

Dieckmann, K. P. (2007). Pre- and paraclinical cooperative trials on testicular cancer. Background and overview of current trials. *Urologe A*, 46, 1180–4.

Digilio, M. C, Marino, B., Borzaga, U., Giannotti, A. and Dallapiccola, B. (1997). Intrafamilial variability of Pfeiffer-type cardiocranial syndrome. *Am J Med Genet*, 73, 480–3.

Ebert, A. K., Brookman-Amissah, S. and Rösch, W. H. (2008). [Urological manifestations of Down syndrome: significance and long-term complications – our own patient cohort with an overview]. *Urologe A*, 47, 337–41.

EBPG, Expert Group on Renal Transplantation. (2002). European best practice guidelines for renal transplantation. Section IV: Long-term management of the transplant recipient. IV.11 Paediatrics (specific problems). *Nephrol Dial Transplant*, 17, 55–8.

Erdmann, K. S., Mao, Y., McCrea, H. J. *et al.* (2007). A role of the Lowe syndrome protein OCRL in early steps of the endocytic pathway. *Dev Cell*, 13, 377–90.

Galán, F., García, R., Aguilar, M. S. and Moya, M. (1989). Partial trisomy 13q22—-qter. A new case. *Ann Genet*, 32, 114–16.

Galasso, C., Arpino, C., Fabbri, F. and Curatolo, P. (2003). Neurologic aspects of 49,XXXXY syndrome. *J Child Neurol*, 18, 501–4.

Gautheron, V. (1997). Urination disorders and neurological disease except for o obvious medullary pathology: perinatal brain lesions with mental handicap. *Arch Pediatr*, 4(Suppl 1), 37s–40s.

Gimelli, G., Giorda, R., Beri, S., Gimelli, S. and Zuffardi, O. (2007). A large analphoid invdup(3)(q22.3qter) marker chromosome characterized by array-CGH in a child with malformations, mental retardation, ambiguous genitalia and Blaschko's lines. *Eur J Med Genet*, 50, 264–73.

Greco, C. M., Soontrapornchai, K., Wirojanan, J. *et al.* (2007). Testicular and pituitary inclusion formation in fragile X associated tremor/ataxia syndrome. *J Urol*, 177, 1434–7.

Green, J. S., Parfrey, P. S., Harnett, J. D. *et al.* (1989). The cardinal manifestations of Bardet-Biedl syndrome, a form of Laurence-Moon-Biedl syndrome. *N Engl J Med*, 321, 1002–9.

Gu, F., Zhang, H. Y., Hu, S. Y. *et al.* (2006). Erectile dysfunction in Fragile X patients. *Asian J Androl*, 8, 483–7.

Hafeez, S., Sharma, R. A., Huddart, R. A., Dearnaley, D. P. and Horwich, A. (2007). Challenges in treating patients with Down's syndrome and testicular cancer with chemotherapy and radiotherapy: The Royal Marsden experience. *Clin Oncol (R Coll Radiol)*, 19, 135–42.

Handel, L. N., Barqawi, A., Checa, G., Furness, P. D. 3rd and Koyle, M. A. (2003). Males with Down's syndrome and nonneurogenic neurogenic bladder. *J Urol*, 169, 646–9.

Hashem, F. K. and Ahmed, S. (1999). Idiopathic scrotal lymphoedema in Down's syndrome. *Aust N Z J Surg*, 69, 75–7.

Hassink, E. A., Rieu, P. N., Hamel, B. C. *et al.* (1996). Additional congenital defects in anorectal malformations. *Eur J Pediatr*, 155, 477–82.

Holmes, S. E., Riazi, M. A., Gong, W. *et al.* (1997). Disruption of the clathrin heavy chain-like gene (CLTCL) associated with features of DGS/VCFS: a balanced (21;22)(p12;q11) translocation. *Hum Mol Genet*, 6, 357–67.

Iuchi, H., Mizunaga, M., Miyata, M. *et al.* (1991). A case of Menkes' kinky hair disease with a renal calculus and diverticula of the bladder. *Nippon Hinyokika Gakkai Zasshi*, 82, 994–7.

Jadresic, L., Leake, J., Gordon, I. *et al.* (1990). Clinicopathologic review of twelve children with nephropathy, Wilms tumor, and genital abnormalities (Drash syndrome). *J Pediatr*, 117, 717–25.

Jadresic, L., Wadey, R. B., Buckle, B. *et al.* (1991). Molecular analysis of chromosome region 11p13 in patients with Drash syndrome. *Hum Genet*, 86, 497–501.

Jain, V. and Beneck, D. (2003). Renal tubular dysgenesis in an hydropic fetus with trisomy 21: a case report with literature review. *Pediatr Dev Pathol*, 6, 568–72.

Karaman, A. (2008). Bardet-Biedl syndrome: a case report. *Dermatol Online J*, 14, 9.

Kuroda, N., Amano, S., Shiotsu, T. *et al.* (2007). Mixed testicular germ cell tumor in an adult with cryptorchidism and Down's syndrome. *APMIS*, 115, 1292–5.

Labrune, P., Lyonnet, S., Zupan, V. *et al.* (1994). Three new cases of the Schinzel-Giedion syndrome and review of the literature. *Am J Med Genet*, 50, 90–3.

Le Caignec, C., Delnatte, C., Vermeesch, J. R. *et al.* (2007). Complete sex reversal in a

WAGR syndrome patient. *Am J Med Genet A*, 143A, 2692–5.

Lepercq, G., Poupinet, S., Steinschneider, R. and Weiler, C. (1973). [Urinary lithiasis revealing Lesch-Nyhan syndrome.] *Nouv Presse Med*, 2, 1571–4.

Liang, D. S, Wu, L. Q., Cai, F. *et al.* (2005). [Phenotype positioning on chromosomes in a patient with the syndrome of partial trisomy 7p21.2–>pter]. *Yi Chuan Xue Bao*, 32, 124–9.

Liebau, M. C., Gal, A., Superti-Furga, A., Omran, H. and Pohl, M. (2007). L1CAM mutation in a boy with hydrocephalus and duplex kidneys. *Pediatr Nephrol*, 22, 1058–61.

Lifchez, C. A., Rhead, W. J., Leuthner, S. R. and Lubinsky, M. S. (2003). Genitopatellar syndrome: expanding the phenotype. *Am J Med Genet A*, 122A, 80–3.

Mahale, A., Poornima, V. and Shrestha, M. (2007). WAGR syndrome–a case report. *Nepal Med Coll J*, 9, 138–40.

Málaga, S., Pardo, R., Málaga, I., Orejas, G. and Fernández-Toral, J. (2005). Renal involvement in Down syndrome. *Pediatr Nephrol*, 20, 614–17.

Mandell, D. S., Eleey, C. C., Cederbaum, J. A. *et al.* (2008). Sexually transmitted infection among adolescents receiving special education services. *J Sch Health*, 78, 382–8.

Martínez-Frías, M. L., Bermejo Sánchez, E., Félix, V. *et al.* (1998). Fraser syndrome: frequency in our environment and clinical-epidemiological aspects of a consecutive series of cases. *An Esp Pediatr*, 48, 634–8.

Mccandless, A. and Walker, S. (1976). D13 ring chromosome syndrome. *Arch Dis Child*, 51(6), 449–53.

Morrison, A. A., Viney, R. L., Saleem, M. A. and Ladomery, M. R. (2008). New insights into the function of the Wilms tumor suppressor gene WT1 in podocytes. *Am J Physiol Renal Physiol*, 295, F12–17.

Musumeci, M. L., Nasca, M. R., De Pasquale, R., Schwartz, R. A. and Micali, G. (2006). Cutaneous manifestations and massive genital involvement in Hennekam syndrome. *Pediatr Dermatol*, 23, 239–42.

Navarro, A., Jiménez, J., Ríos, T. *et al.* (2005). Unusual cause of lung and renal disease in a baby with trisomy 21. *Pediatr Pulmonol*, 40, 173–4.

Oka, T., Utsunomiya, M., Ichikawa, Y. *et al.* (1985). Xanthine calculi in the patient with the Lesch-Nyhan syndrome associated with urinary tract infection. *Urol Int*, 40, 138–40.

Pagon, R. A., Graham, J. M. Jr, Zonana, J. and Yong, S. L. (1981). Coloboma, congenital heart disease, and choanal atresia with multiple anomalies: CHARGE association. *J Pediatr*, 99, 223–7.

Pankau, R., Partsch, C. J., Winter, M., Gosch, A. and Wessel, A. (1996). Incidence and spectrum of renal abnormalities in Williams-Beuren syndrome. *Am J Med Genet*, 63, 301–4.

Patja, K., Eero, P. and Iivanainen, M. (2001). Cancer incidence among people with intellectual disability. *J Intellect Dis Res*, 45, 300–7.

Peate, I. and Maloret, P. (2007). Testicular self-examination: the person with learning difficulties. *Br J Nurs*, 16, 931–5.

Pedersen, A. M. and Skovby, F. (2007). Molecular diagnosis of CHARGE syndrome. *Ugeskr Laeg*, 169, 402–6.

Pela, I., Donati, M. A., Procopio, E. and Fiorini, P. (2008). Lesch-Nyhan syndrome presenting with acute renal failure in a 3-day-old newborn. *Pediatr Nephrol*, 23, 155–8.

Petterson, B., Bourke, J., Leonard, H., Jacoby, P. and Bower, C. (2007). Co-occurrence of birth defects and intellectual disability. *Paediatr Perinat Epidemiol*, 21, 65–75.

Pinsky, L. and DiGeorge, A. M. (1965). A familial syndrome of facial and skeletal anomalies associated with genital abnormality in the male and normal genitals in the female: another cause of male pseudohermaphroditism. *J Pediatr*, 66, 1049–54.

Prasun, P., Pradhan, M. and Goel, H. (2007). Intrafamilial variability in Fraser syndrome. *Prenat Diagn*, 27, 778–82.

Qureshi, F., Jacques, S. M., Feldman, B. *et al.* (2000). Fetal obstructive uropathy in trisomy syndromes. *Fetal Diagn Ther*, 15, 342–7.

Ragan, D. C., Casale, A. J., Rink, R. C., Cain, M. P. and Weaver, D. D. (1999). Genitourinary anomalies in the CHARGE association. *J Urol*, 161, 622–5.

Rajcan-Separovic, E., Harvard, C., Liu, X. *et al.* (2007). Clinical and molecular cytogenetic characterisation of a newly recognised microdeletion syndrome involving 2p15–16.1. *J Med Genet*, 44, 269–76.

Reardon, W. (2002). Genitopatellar syndrome: a recognizable phenotype. *Am J Med Genet*, 111, 313–15.

Rebentisch, G., Stolz, S. and Muche, J. (2004). [Xanthinuria with xanthine lithiasis in a patient with Lesch-Nyhan syndrome under allopurinol therapy.] *Aktuelle Urol*, 35, 215–21.

Rogers, J. (2002). Solving the enigma: toilet training children with learning disabilities. *Br J Nurs*, 11, 958, 960, 962.

Rossi, M., D'Armiento, M., Parisi, I. *et al.* (2007). Clinical phenotype of lathosterolosis. *Am J Med Genet A*, 143A, 2371–81.

Roux, C., Wolf, C., Mulliez, N. *et al.* (2000). Role of cholesterol in embryonic development. *Am J Clin Nutr*, 71, 1270S–9S.

Ryoo, J. W. and Cho, J. M. (2008). Multiple bladder diverticula in Menkes disease. *Pediatr Radiol*, 38, 595.

Sartelet, H., Pietrement, C., Noel, L. H. *et al.* (2008). Collapsing glomerulopathy in Galloway-Mowat syndrome: a case report and review of the literature. *Pathol Res Pract*, 204(6), 401–6. Epub 2008 Feb 13.

Schulman, S. L., Zderic, S. and Kaplan, P. (1996). Increased prevalence of urinary symptoms and voiding dysfunction in Williams syndrome. *J Pediatr*, 129, 466–9.

Sekhon, G. S., Taysi, K. and Rath, R. (1978). Partial trisomy for the short arm of chromosome 2 due to familial balance translocation. *Hum Genet*, 44, 99–103.

Slavotinek, A. M., Searby, C., Al-Gazali, L. *et al.* (2002). Mutation analysis of the MKKS gene in McKusick-Kaufman syndrome and selected Bardet-Biedl syndrome patients. *Hum Genet*, 110, 561–7.

Smith, D. W. (1978). Male genital defects in patterns of malformation. *Birth Defects Orig Artic Ser*, 14, 57–61.

Smith, L., Smith, P. and Lee, S. K. (2000). Behavioural treatment of urinary incontinence and encopresis in children with learning disabilities: transfer of stimulus control. *Dev Med Child Neurol*, 42, 276–9.

Stanley, R. (1996). Treatment of continence in people with learning disabilities: 1. *Br J Nurs*, 5, 364–8.

Stefan, H. and Semecký, V. (1998). Aniridia, gonadoblastoma, Wilms' tumor and deletion 11p13. *Acta Medica (Hradec Kralove)*, 41, 29–33.

Stevenson, R. E, Bennett, C. W., Abidi, F. *et al.* (2005). Renpenning syndrome comes into focus. *Am J Med Genet A*, 134, 415–21.

Sugayama, S. M., Koch, V. H., Furusawa, E. A., Leone, C. and Kim, C. A. (2004). Renal and urinary findings in 20 patients with Williams-Beuren syndrome diagnosed by fluorescence in situ hybridization (FISH). *Rev Hosp Clin Fac Med Sao Paulo*, 59, 266–72.

Sullivan, S. G., Hussain, R., Threlfall, T. and Bittles, A. H. (2004). The incidence of cancer in people with intellectual disabilities. *Cancer Causes Control*, 15, 1021–5.

Suzuki, K., Nishimi, D., Yagishita, T., Takanami, M. and Hiruta, N. (2005). Testicular tumor in Down syndrome. *Int J Urol*, 12, 925–7.

Szczepańska, M., Szprynger, K., Winiarski, G., Glowacki, J. and Zajecki, W. (2007). Renal complication in tuberous sclerosis complex. *Wiad Lek*, 60, 483–8.

Tajara, E. H., Varella-Garcia, M. and Gusson, A. C. (1989). Interstitial long-arm deletion of chromosome 7 and ectrodactyly. *Am J Med Genet*, 32, 192–4.

Taylor, S., Cipani, E. and Clardy, A. (1994). A stimulus control technique for improving the efficacy of an established toilet training program. *J Behav Ther Exp Psychiatry*, 25, 155–60.

Tellier, A. L., Cormier-Daire, V., Abadie, V. *et al.* (1998). CHARGE syndrome: report of 47 cases and review. *Am J Med Genet*, 76, 402–9.

Turnbull, C., Lees, M. and Chitty, L. S. (2006). Prenatal sonographic diagnosis of Malpuech syndrome. *Prenat Diagn*, 26, 1121–3.

Unuigbe, E. I., Azubike, C. A., Okaka, E. I., Osarenkhoe, J. O. and Onuora, V. C. (2007). Twenty-one-year-old male with congenital anomalies, obstructive uropathy and chronic renal failure: is this a case of Townes Brocks syndrome? *Niger J Clin Pract*, 10, 91–4.

Vachon, L., Fareau, G. E., Wilson, M. G. and Chan, L. S. (2006). Testicular microlithiasis in patients with Down syndrome. *J Pediatr*, 149, 233–6.

van Haelst, M. M., Scambler, P. J., Fraser Syndrome Collaboration Group and Hennekam, R. C. (2007). Fraser syndrome: a clinical study of 59 cases and evaluation of diagnostic criteria. *Am J Med Genet A*, 143A, 3194–203.

Van Laecke, E. (2008). Elimination disorders in people with intellectual disability. *J Intellect Disabil Res*, 52, 810.

Vogels, A., Moerman, P., Frijns, J. P. and Bogaert, G. A. (2008). Testicular histology in boys with Prader-Willi syndrome: fertile or infertile? *J Urol*, 180, 1800–4.

Wada, T., Sakakibara, M., Fukushima, Y. and Saitoh, S. (2006). A novel splicing mutation of the ATRX gene in ATR-X syndrome. *Brain Dev*, 28, 322–5.

Wakui, K., Gregato, G., Ballif, B. C. *et al.* (2005). Construction of a natural panel of 11p11.2 deletions and further delineation of the critical region involved in Potocki-Shaffer syndrome. *Eur J Hum Genet*, 13, 528–40.

Wegenke, J. D., Uehling, D. T., Wear, J. B. Jr. *et al.* (1975). Familial Kallmann syndrome with unilateral renal aplasia. *Clin Genet*, 7, 368–81.

Wieczorek, D., Krause, M., Majewski, F. *et al.* (2000). Effect of the size of the deletion and clinical manifestation in Wolf-Hirschhorn syndrome: analysis of 13 patients with a de novo deletion. *Eur J Hum Genet*, 8, 519–26.

Wiggers, M. N. and Oudesluys-Murphy, A. M. (2006). [A child presenting with fever and arthritis due to disseminated gonorrhoea.] *Ned Tijdschr Geneeskd*, 150, 1462–5.

Yosunkaya Fenerci, E., Guven, G. S., Kuru, D. *et al.* (2007). Supernumerary chromosome der(22)t(11;22): Emanuel syndrome associates with novel features. *Genet Couns*, 18, 401–8.

Zaffanello, M. and Fanos, V. (2003). Rare urological abnormalities in 2 cases of Menkes' syndrome. *J Urol*, 170, 1335.

10

Obstetric and gynaecological disorders

Maeve Eogan and Mary Wingfield

Introduction

Increasing numbers of women with intellectual disability (ID) are now living with greater longevity in the community rather than in institutions. This social inclusion, however, is not always matched by awareness of their health requirements (Servais, 2006; Wilkinson and Cerreto, 2008). The reproductive health needs of women with ID should be assessed against current standards of obstetric and gynaecological care and management, notwithstanding the fact that particular adjustments may be mandated by individual requirements, abilities and co-morbidity (Grover, 2002).

This chapter aims to review the literature pertaining to obstetric and gynaecological symptomatology within this population. Relevant topics include the management of menstrual problems, contraceptive and sexual healthcare issues, cervical cancer screening and management of the menopause as well as specific concerns relating to pregnancy and delivery. It will not specifically deal with the legal and ethical issues surrounding the care of women with ID as these are complex and vary from one jurisdiction to another. Similarly, a debate of the reproductive rights of women with ID is beyond the scope of this review.

Method

A number of MEDLINE searches from 1950 to September 2008 were performed using the term intellectual disability in combination with a range of obstetric (pregnancy and labour) and gynaecological disorders (specifically menstrual problems, menopause, contraception and sexual health). A broad Internet search strategy was also performed to include other relevant documents.

All abstracts found were reviewed and articles were excluded if they were not available in English, if they were case reports or if they specifically pertained to legal or forensic issues. Full text articles were obtained and reviewed for further information and cross-referencing from papers obtained from the database search was also performed.

Results

We present this systematic review in a number of separate categories (see Table 10.1). From the gynaecological perspective we present a review of the literature on menstrual problems, contraception and sexual health, cervical cancer screening and menopause, in

Intellectual Disability and Ill Health: A Review of the Evidence, ed. Jean O'Hara, Jane McCarthy and Nick Bouras. Published by Cambridge University Press. © Cambridge University Press 2010.

Table 10.1. Search results

	Menstrual health	Cervical cancer screening	Sexual health	Menopause	Pregnancy and childbirth
Articles identified in search	26	5	20	8	3
Articles included in review	24	5	14	7	3

women with ID. This is then followed by a review of pregnancy and labour in this same population.

Discussion

Menstrual health

As for women in the general population, menstruation and perimenstrual symptoms constitute an ongoing source of change and adaptation for women with ID. Some issues, e.g. menorrhagia, dysmenorrhoea and amenorrhoea, are common to all women. However, their management in women with ID needs to be tailored to suit their cognitive, social and environmental needs. Other issues, e.g. problems with menstrual hygiene or premenstrual behavioural problems, are unique to women with ID.

Menstrual hygiene may pose difficulties for women with ID. This arises because of cognitive impairment, often compounded by coexisting motor disabilities (Servais, 2006; Servais *et al.*, 2002), and it can be a significant problem for caregivers (Wingfield *et al.*, 1994a). Inability to manage pads or tampons and smearing of menstrual blood may occur. Appropriate education and support has been shown to be effective in managing physiological menstrual changes, even in those with severe ID (Elkins *et al.*, 1986; Griffin *et al.*, 1994; Rodgers and Lipscombe, 2005). The benefits of such an approach are clear in Elkins' (1986) study where counselling and education were shown to be a valuable alternative for 16 women with ID originally referred for hysterectomy. Education must also be provided for caregivers in the home, in day facilities and in schools (Atkinson *et al.*, 2003; Burbidge *et al.*, 1996). Respite care may also need to be considered. Management of blood products by carers should not be different to concerns regarding urinary and faecal toilet management (Atkinson *et al.*, 2003). Grover notes that a 'positive attitude' on behalf of the carers, health professionals and educators is also of benefit (Grover, 2002).

Several studies have documented pre- and perimenstrual behavioural problems in women with ID. These women have varying levels of communication skills. Willis (2008) explored attitudes to menstruation and menopause in 15 women, 8 with mild and 7 with moderate ID. The women expressed negative attitudes to their periods, concurring with earlier studies (Rodgers, 2001; Rodgers *et al.* 2006). In women with more severe ID and limited communication skills, discomfort or pain may be expressed as self-abuse or aggression (Elkins *et al.*, 1990; Quint *et al.*, 1999). Behavioural symptoms including increased autistic behaviour, irritability, restlessness and seizures have been described in the premenstrual and menstrual phases of the cycle. These symptoms may be misinterpreted if their cyclical nature is not recognised (Servais, 2006). Non-steroidal anti-inflammatory agents or cyclical oral contraceptives may be effective for dysmenorrhoea and menorrhagia while tranexamic acid may also help with menorrhagia.

In managing problems related to menstruation in women with ID, it is now accepted internationally that the treatment options recommended should be the least restrictive available and always in the woman's best interest (Atkinson *et al.*, 2003; Grover, 2002; Servais, 2006). This contrasts with treatment prior to the 1990s when voluntary and involuntary sterilisation or hysterectomy were widely practised as part of eugenics-based practices designed to eliminate the perceived societal burden of these individuals (Servais, 2006). Education, training and support should be the first line of management. In more resistant cases, menstrual suppression may be necessary. A Scandinavian study showed that 67% of women with ID sought therapeutic amenorrhoea at some stage in their lives (Huovinen, 1993). Reversible pharmacological menstrual suppression may be employed using continuous oral contraceptives, depot medroxyprogesterone acetate or progestin implants (Atkinson *et al.*, 2003; Grover, 2002; Servais, 2006; Wilkinson and Cerreto, 2008; Wingfield *et al.*, 1994a). The choice of drug will depend on expected compliance, hormonal status, other medications and social situation. Most methods provide contraception. Combined oral contraceptives are preferable to depot progestagens if oestrogen deficiency is suspected, while depot medroxyprogesterone or implants are preferable if there are concerns regarding compliance or if the woman is taking anticonvulsants which interfere with the efficacy of oral contraceptives. Monophasic oral contraceptives are preferable to triphasic and should be used for a minimum of three months before assessing efficacy or changing to other options (Atkinson *et al.*, 2003). No studies were found of levonorgestrel intrauterine systems in women with ID but they are likely to be equally effective in menstrual management, though sedation or anaesthesia are likely to be required for insertion and uterine size needs to be normal.

Surgical management, e.g. endometrial ablation or hysterectomy, is not reversible and should be reserved for those women whose problems are resistant to reversible methods of control (Atkinson *et al.*, 2003; Grover, 2002; Servais, 2006; Wilkinson and Cerreto, 2008; Wingfield *et al.*, 1994a,b). Indeed in a cohort study of 107 women with ID attending a gynaecological practice over a 9-year period, only 2 required surgical intervention (Wilkinson and Cerreto, 2008). As in the general population, surgical intervention is indicated in the presence of significant pathology, e.g. fibroids, endometriosis or indeed malignancy.

The incidence of amenorrhoea in women with ID is difficult to determine. They are a heterogeneous group and some may be at risk of primary amenorrhoea and hypo-oestrogenaemia. The age of onset of menopause is earlier in this group, particularly those with Down syndrome or Fragile X syndrome, as discussed below. These women are at increased risk of oestrogen deficiency which predisposes them to osteoporosis, particularly if associated physical disability limits their ability to perform adequate weight-bearing exercise (Aspray *et al.*, 1998; Center *et al.*, 1998; Fisher and Kettl, 2005; Jaffe *et al.*, 2001; Lohiya *et al.*, 2004; Wagemans *et al.*, 1998). Anticonvulsant therapy is an additional risk factor (Jaffe *et al.*, 2005; Schrager, 2006).

It has been shown that primary care physicians tend not to focus on menstrual issues for women with ID (Kopac *et al.*, 1998). Indeed carers will find it easier if the woman has amenorrhoea. However, hormone replacement therapy is medically indicated in any woman under the age of 48 with evidence of hypo-oestrogenaemia. Combined oestrogen and progesterone preparations should be given if the woman has a uterus. As in those without ID, if the woman has had a year of amenorrhoea, a continuous preparation should be used; otherwise cyclical preparations which cause regular withdrawal bleeds should be prescribed.

Cervical cancer screening

There has been debate regarding the need for cervical cancer screening in women with ID (Wilkinson and Cerreto, 2008). Two large studies of women with ID residing in institutional settings found an extremely low incidence of abnormal cervical smears (Jaffe *et al.*, 2002; Quint and Elkins, 1997) (please refer to Chapter 12 on Neoplasms). However, as discussed below, an increasing number of women with ID are known to be sexually active. The need for and frequency of cervical cancer screening should therefore be individualised based on the woman's sexual exposure (Wilkinson and Cerreto, 2008).

For many women with ID, the experience of the gynaecological examination may be frightening and painful. Again, education and counselling can be sufficient to enable adequate examination. This should involve education about what will occur during the examination before the actual appointment, to allow time for questions and mental preparation and familiarisation with the medical facility and personnel and even perhaps instrumentation before the examination visit (Servais, 2006). However, sedation or anaesthesia may be required for some women (Servais, 2006; Wingfield *et al.*, 1994a).

Sexual health

The concept of sexual health in women with ID is sensitive, controversial and ethically challenging. As these women are increasingly being cared for in the community the need to ensure appropriate sexual health care for them is vital. Indeed the 58th World Health Assembly urged member states to include a component to address the needs of those with ID in sexual health policies and programmes (WHO, 2005).

The extent of sexual activity engaged in by women with ID will vary according to the degree of disability and their living environment. Chamberlain *et al.* (1984) reported that 50% of a group of 11- to 23-year-olds with mild ID, 32% of those with moderate and 9% with severe ID had engaged in consensual sexual intercourse. Servais *et al.* (2002) reported figures of 33%, 5% and 0% in these groups. Another study noted that 41% of adults in a French institution had engaged in sexual intercourse at least once (Diederich and Greacen, 1996). Not surprisingly, the rates of sexual activity are higher for those living in the community (McCabe, 1999; McGillivray, 1999; Timmers *et al.*, 1981), up to 82% of women in one study (Timmers *et al.*, 1981). Sadly, in some of these studies, the sexual experiences of some women with ID represent rape and sexual assault. Several studies note a discrepancy between the sexual needs and desires expressed by those with ID and that perceived by their caregivers, with parents and caregivers tending to underestimate the needs of these women (Lesseliers and van Hove, 2002; Pueschel and Scola, 1988).

Sexual activity in women with ID, as in those without disability, puts women at risk of sexually transmitted infections and unplanned pregnancy. Those with Down syndrome may be at increased risk because of immunological impairment and those living in institutions are at increased risk of hepatitis transmission. Immunisation against hepatitis B should be considered (Servais, 2006) (please refer to Chapter 4 on Infectious diseases). Education regarding safe sexual practices is paramount but difficult. It is well documented that people with ID have poor sexual knowledge (Galea *et al.*, 2004; Servais, 2006). They have also been shown to have little or no understanding of how to use a condom correctly or consistently (Gust *et al.*, 2003; McGillivray, 1999).

Contraception for women with ID has been mentioned above in the discussion of menstrual suppression. Options include the oral contraceptive pill, progesterones in the form of depot injections or implants and the Mirena intrauterine system (IUS). Barrier methods are unreliable and these women may not be able to manage them, particularly female barrier methods such as diaphragms. Sterilisation has been widely practised in the past but is now rarely justified, given that the Mirena IUS is equally effective, reversible and may also have menstrual benefits. While these methods of contraception are very efficacious, they do not protect against sexually transmitted infections or sexual abuse and hence should be supported by appropriate sexual health education.

People with ID are prone to sexual abuse, with women with mild ID living in the community being at greatest risk (Diederich and Greacen, 1996). Incest may be an issue, while those living in institutions are most likely to be abused by other residents with ID, both male and female (Servais, 2006). Some of the risk factors for abuse include the passive, obedient and affectionate nature of many individuals with ID, their difficulty in distinguishing between consenting and abusive relationships, concomitant immobility and inability to communicate the abuse to carers (McGillivray, 1999; Murphy and O'Callaghan, 2004; Servais, 2006; Wingfield *et al.*, 1994a).

Menopause

The menopause is said to have occurred when a woman has not menstruated for one year, with the 'climacteric' describing the period of transition associated with hypo-oestrogenism and cessation of menstruation. Markers of the menopause include elevated gonadotrophin levels (follicle-stimulating hormone (FSH) and luteinising hormone (LH) and reduced oestrogen levels). A range of symptoms is associated with the menopause, regardless of presence or absence of ID. These include hot flushes, night sweats, headaches and a range of urogenital symptoms including frequency of urination and vaginal atrophy. In the longer term, hypo-oestrogenism increases both osteoporosis and cardiovascular disease.

With regard to menopause in women with ID, the search strategy identified just seven relevant papers. While there is a large research base surrounding menopause and its affects on the general population, there is scant evidence regarding menopause in women with ID, with most work focusing on age of onset of menopause rather than on other relevant diagnostic or therapeutic parameters.

Women with ID, particularly those with Down syndrome, experience menopause at an earlier age. While the mean age of menopause in the general population is just under 51 years (Meschia *et al.*, 2000), three studies found this to be earlier in women with ID. One study found that 69% (87% of those with Down syndrome) had stopped menstruating by the age of 46 and that all had stopped by the age of 54 (Carr and Hollins, 1995) with another study highlighting that the average age of the menopause for Irish women with Down syndrome (44.7 years) was younger than in the general population (Cosgrave *et al.*, 1999). This study also showed that age of onset of dementia correlated with age of menopause, due to the presumed protective influence of oestrogen on Alzheimer's disease. Schupf *et al.* (1997) calculated an age-adjusted likelihood of menopause as being twice as high in women with Down syndrome when compared with women with other forms of ID. Interestingly, this was not found to be related to thyroid dysfunction.

Osteoporosis is associated with the postmenopausal state, but also with sedentary lifestyle, poor diet, small body size, cigarette smoking and anticonvulsant and long-term steroid therapy. Studies have identified a greater risk of osteoporosis among people with ID

(Jaffe *et al.*, 2001; Wagemans *et al.*, 1998), emphasising a need for targeting early screening and risk factor reduction in this population (Guijarro *et al.*, 2008).

McCarthy (2002) explored menopausal experiences through interviews with 30 women with mild to moderate ID and identified poor knowledge and understanding of the menopause. A more recent interview-based study supported these findings and highlighted the paucity of appropriate information on the menopause (Willis, 2008).

There is no published evidence on the role of hormone replacement therapy (HRT) in women with ID. Recent population studies have raised concerns about the risks of prolonged hormone replacement in the postmenopausal population, specifically in relation to breast cancer and cardiovascular disease. In the short term, HRT reduces menopausal symptoms such as vaginal dryness, mood changes and hot flushes with benefits in terms of osteoporotic fractures, colorectal cancer and possibly Alzheimer's disease being seen in the longer term (Nelson *et al.*, 2002). A recent position statement of the North American Menopause Society supports the initiation of HRT for two specific groups of women, either around the time of menopause to treat menopause-related symptoms or to treat or reduce the risk of certain disorders, such as osteoporosis or fractures in select postmenopausal women; or both (Utian *et al.*, 2008). They conclude that the benefit–risk ratio for menopausal HRT is favourable close to menopause but decreases with ageing and with time. Guidelines for HRT now recommend use of the lowest effective dose and shortest treatment duration consistent with individual treatment goals. Nonetheless, with the identified risks of HRT use, medical debate encourages full discussion of perceived risks and benefits of treatment to ensure that women are making an informed choice. Women with ID are unlikely to be able to make these important decisions without appropriate support; placing further emphasis on the need for appropriate health promotion and education in this area.

Pregnancy and childbirth

Compared with the relative wealth of literature available on contraception for women with ID, our search strategy only yielded three relevant papers focusing on issues surrounding pregnancy and childbirth in this population, with some further papers being identified from the cited references of these papers. The search was repeated using a range of search terms including 'obstetrics', 'pregnancy', 'childbirth' and 'labour' in conjunction with 'intellectual disability'. The search, however, did identify a number of papers on parenting issues for women with ID. Interestingly, these studies conclude that maternal IQ is not systematically correlated with parenting competence (Booth and Booth, 1993; Dowdney and Skuse, 1993; Tymchuk and Feldman, 1991). Further discussion of this, however, falls outside of the remit of this review.

Although the scope of this chapter does not include a discussion of reproductive rights for women with ID, one of the papers identified did discuss fertility and pregnancy in general in this population (Servais, 2006). This paper emphasised that pregnancy seemed to be uncommon in women with ID but that data were rare. It cited a study by Chamberlain *et al.* (1984) which recorded 7 pregnancies among 6 subjects in a total of 87 women with ID living in the community and that only 3 were carried to term. Other studies referenced in that paper showed similar low pregnancy rates, but the authors did acknowledge that several factors (e.g. cultural differences with regard to reproductive rights, living environment and termination of pregnancy) make it difficult to assess pregnancy rates within this population.

Another paper identified was a cohort study focusing on pregnancy and birth outcomes of women with ID (McConnell *et al.*, 2008). This study was prompted by a small cross-sectional study which had looked at developmental progress in young children of mothers with ID (McConnell *et al.*, 2003). A significant number of children in this latter study had been born prematurely and weighed less than 2.5 kg but some concerns regarding recruitment and the retrospective nature of data collection meant that the findings required validation. The cohort study invited all women attending their first antenatal clinic visit within a socio-economically disadvantaged area to participate, with medical records being reviewed post-partum to assess birth outcomes. Over 800 women gave informed consent to participate, of these, 33 had ID and 24 had self-reported 'learning difficulties'. Interestingly, a high prevalence of pre-eclampsia was seen in the women with ID or 'learning difficulties' while rates of other pregnancy complications such as gestational diabetes were similar in affected and unaffected women. Furthermore, low birth weight and neonatal intensive care unit admission were higher in the combined group of ID and 'learning difficulties' when compared with women without ID, although rates of preterm delivery were not significantly different. The findings of this study are interesting, with further research being needed to determine the potential contributory influences of nutrition, maternal weight, smoking, anticonvulsant and other drugs as well as social support, stress and anxiety/depression-related influences.

Conclusion

Women with ID are becoming increasingly integrated into our communities and lives. They have proven and documented sexual, gynaecological and obstetric needs. While many of these needs have been minimised and ignored in the past, it now behoves all carers and medical practitioners to address these issues in a way that makes the interests of the woman with ID paramount. Additionally, there is an enormous need for appropriate educational material for these women and their carers. The cooperation and consent of the woman with disability should be sought before any decisions are made regarding care, regardless of her legal status regarding consent. The decision to induce amenorrhea, suppress fertility or perform gynaecological surgery for non-life-threatening situations in these women requires careful consideration of the legal and ethical aspects of consent.

Ideally, recommendations must be evidence-based, rather than being based on carers' and health providers' general and personal assumptions about women with ID. It is, however, clear from this systematic review that despite the large number of papers referenced, many of these are observational studies and reviews. A robust evidence base for obstetric and gynaecological practice within the ID community is lacking. When issues of informed consent are considered, it is probably not surprising that no relevant randomised controlled trials (level I evidence) were identified by the literature review; even the level II evidence, however, is based on studies involving relatively small numbers. Nonetheless, some well-informed guidelines (Atkinson *et al.*, 2003; Grimes, 1997; Sullivan *et al.*, 2006; Wilkinson et al, 2007) for best practice have been published in recent years, and we welcome ongoing contribution to the literature to optimise the care of this group.

References

Aspray, T. J., Francis, R. M., Thompson, A. *et al.* (1998). Comparison of ultrasound measurements at the heel between adults with mental retardation and control subjects. *Bone*, 22(6), 665–8.

Atkinson, E., Bennett, M. J., Dudley, J. *et al.* (2003). Consensus statement: Menstrual and contraceptive management in women with an intellectual disability. *Aust N Z J Obstet Gynaecol*, 43, 109–10.

Booth, T. and Booth, W. (1993). Parenting with learning difficulties: lessons for practitioners. *Br J Soc Work*, 23, 459–80.

Burbidge, M., Tracy, J. and Butler, J. (1996). *Menstrual Management and Women with Intellectual Disability: a guide for families and carers.* Melbourne: Centre for Developmental Disability. Health Victoria.

Carr, J. and Hollins, S. (1995). Brief report: menopause in women with learning disabilities. *J Intellect Disabil Res*, 39(2), 137–9.

Center, J., Beange, H. and McElduff, A. (1998). People with mental retardation have an increased prevalence of osteoporosis: a population study. *Am J Ment Retard*, 103(1), 19–28.

Chamberlain, A., Rauh, J., Passer, A. *et al.* (1984). Issues in fertility for mentally retarded female adolescents: sexual activity, sexual abuse and contraception. *Pediatrics*, (73), 445–50.

Cosgrave, M. P., Tyrrell, J., McCarron, M., Gill, M. and Lawlor, B. A. (1999). Age at onset of dementia and age of menopause in women with Down's syndrome. *J Intellect Disabil Res*, 43(6), 461–5.

Diederich, N. and Greacen, T. (1996). Enquête sur la sexualité et la prévention du sida chez les adultes handicapés mentaux en lle de France. *Rev Eur Handicap Ment*, 3, 20–32.

Dowdney, L. and Skuse, D. (1993). Parenting provided by adults with mental retardation. *J Child Psychol Psychiatry*, 34, 25–47.

Elkins, T. E., Gafford, L. S., Wilks, C. S. *et al.* (1986). A model clinic approach to the reproductive health concerns of the mentally handicapped. *Obstet Gynecol*, 68, 185–8.

Elkins, T. E., McNeely, S. G., Punch, M. *et al.* (1990). Reproductive health concerns in Down syndrome: a report of eight cases. *J Reprod Med*, 35, 745–50.

Fisher, K. and Kettl, P. (2005). Aging with mental retardation: increasing population of older adults with MR require health interventions and prevention strategies. *Geriatrics*, 60(4), 26–9.

Galea, J., Butler, J., Iacono, T. *et al.* 2004. The assessment of sexual knowledge in people with intellectual disability. *J Intellect Dev Disabil*, 29, 350–65.

Griffin, J., Carlson, G., Taylor, M. and Wilson, J. (1994). Menstrual management and intellectual disability: new perspectives. *Occup Ther Int*, 1, 141–57.

Grimes, D. (ed.) (1997). Reproductive health care for the mentally handicapped. *Contracept Rep*, 8(4), 4–11.

Grover, S. (2002). Menstrual and contraceptive management in women with an intellectual disability. *Med J Aust*, 176, 108–110

Guijarro, M., Valero, C., Paule, B., Gonzalez-Macias, J. and Riancho, J. A. (2008). Bone mass in young adults with Down's syndrome. *J Intellect Disabil Res*, 52, 182–9.

Gust, D. A., Wang, S. A., Grot, J. *et al.* (2003). National survey of sexual behaviour and sexual behaviour policies in facilities for individuals with mental retardation/developmental disabilities. *Ment Retard*, 5, 365–73.

Huovinen, K. J. (1993). Gynecological problems of mentally retarded women. *Acta Obstet Gynecol Scand*, 72, 475–80.

Jaffe, J. S., Timell, A. M. and Gulanski, B. I. (2001). Prevalence of low bone density in women with intellectual disabilities. *J Clin Densitom*, 4(1), 25–9.

Jaffe, J. S., Timell, A. M., Eisenberg, M. S. and Chambers, J. T. (2002). Low prevalence of abnormal cervical cytology in an institutionalized population with intellectual disability. *J Intellect Disabil Res*, 46(Pt 7), 569–74.

Jaffe, J. S., Timell, A. M., Elolia, R. and Thatcher, S. S. (2005). Risk factors for low bone mineral density in individuals residing in a facility for the people with intellectual disability. *J Intellect Disabil Res*, 49(Pt 6), 457–62.

Kopac, C. A., Fritz, J. and Holt, R. A. (1998). Gynecologic and reproductive services for women with developmental disabilities. *Clin Excell Nurs Pract*, 2(2), 88–95.

Lesseliers, J. and Van Hove, G. (2002). Barriers to the development of intimate relationships and the expression of sexuality among people with developmental disabilities: their perceptions. *Res Pract Pers Severe Disabil*, 27, 69–81.

Lohiya, G. S., Tan-Figueroa, L. and Iannucci, A. (2004). Identification of low bone mass in a developmental center: finger bone mineral density measurement in 562 residents. *J Am Med Dir Assoc*, 5(6), 371–6.

McCabe, M. P. (1999). Sexual knowledge, experience and feelings among people with disability. *Sex Disabil*, 17, 157–70.

McCarthy, M. (2002). Going through the menopause: perceptions and experiences of women with learning disability. *J Intellect Dev Disabil*, 27(4), 281–95.

McConnell, D., Llewellyn, G., Mayes, R., Russo, D. and Honey, A. (2003). Developmental profiles of children born to mothers with intellectual disability. *J Intellect Dev Disabil*, 28, 122–34.

McConnell, D., Mayes, R. and Llewellyn, G. (2008). Women with intellectual disability at risk of adverse pregnancy and birth outcomes. *J Intellect Disabil Res*, 52, 529–35.

McGillivray, J. A. (1999). Level of knowledge and risk of contacting HIV/AIDS amongst young adults with mild/moderate intellectual disability. *J Appl Res Intellect Disabil*, 12, 113–26.

Meschia, M., Pansini, F., Modena, A. M. *et al.* (2000). Determinants of age at menopause in Italy: results from a large cross sectional study. ICARUS Study Group, Italian Climacteric Research Group Study. *Maturitas*, 34(2), 119–25.

Murphy, G. H. and O'Callaghan, A. (2004). Capacity of adults with intellectual disabilities to consent to sexual relationships. *Psychol Med*, 34, 1347–57.

Nelson, H. D., Humphrey, L. L., Nygren, P., Teutsch, S. M. and Allan, J. D. (2002). Postmenopausal hormone replacement therapy: scientific review. *JAMA*, 288(7), 872–81.

Pueschel, S. M. and Scola, P. S. (1988). Parents' perception of social and sexual functions in adolescents with Down syndrome. *J Ment Defic Res*, 32, 215–20.

Quint, E. and Elkins, T. (1997). Cervical cytology in women with mental retardation. *Obstet Gynecol*, 89(1), 123–6.

Quint, E. H., Elkins, T. E., Sorg, C. A. *et al.* (1999). The treatment of cyclical behavioral changes in women with mental disabilities. *J Pediatr Adolesc Gynecol*, 12, 139–42.

Rodgers, J. (2001). Pain, shame, blood and doctors: how women with learning difficulties experience menstruation, *Womens Stud Int Forum*, 24(5), 523–39.

Rodgers, J. and Lipscombe, J. (2005). The nature and extent of help given to women with intellectual disabilities to manage menstruation. *J Intellect Dev Disabil*, 30, 45–52.

Rodgers, J., Lipscombe, J. and Santer, M. (2006). Menstrual problems experienced by women with learning disabilities. *J Appl Res Intellect Disabil*, 19(10), 364–73.

Schrager, S. (2006). Epidemiology of osteoporosis in women with cognitive impairment. *Ment Retard*, 44(3), 203–11.

Schupf, N., Zigman, W., Kapell, D. *et al.* (1997). Early menopause in women with Down's syndrome. *J Intellect Disabil Res*, 41, 264–7.

Servais, L. (2006). Sexual health care in persons with intellectual disabilities. *Ment Retard Dev Disabil Res Rev*, 12, 48–56.

Servais, L. and Jacques, D., Leach, R. *et al.* (2002). Contraception of women with intellectual disabilities: prevalence and determinants. *J Intellect Disabil Res*, 46(Pt 2), 108–19.

Sullivan, W. F., Heng, J., Cameron, D. *et al.* (2006). Consensus guidelines for primary care of adults with developmental disabilities. *Can Fam Physician*, 52(11), 1410–18.

Timmers, R. L., DuCharme, P. and Jacob, G. (1981). Sexual knowledge, attitudes and behaviours of developmentally disabled adults living in a normalized apartment setting. *Sex Disabil*, 4, 27–39.

Tymchuk, A. J. and Feldman, M. A. (1991). Parents with mental retardation and their children: review of research relevant to professional practice. *Can Psychol*, 32, 486–96.

Utian, W. H., Archer, D. F., Bachmann, G. A. *et al.* (2008). Estrogen and progestogen use in postmenopausal women: July 2008 position statement of The North American Menopause Society. *Menopause*, 15, 584–602.

Wagemans, A. M., Fiolet, J. F., van der Linden, E. S. and Menheere, P. P. (1998). Osteoporosis and intellectual disability: is there any relation? *J Intellect Disabil Res*, 42(Pt5), 370–4.

WHO (2005). Disability, including prevention, management and rehabilitation. Available from: www.who.int/gb/ebwha/pdf_files/WHA58/WHA58_23-en.pdf.

Wilkinson, J., Culpepper, L. and Cerreto, M. C. (2007). Primary care screening tests for adults with intellectual disabilities. *J Am Board Fam Med*, 20(4), 399–407. Available from: www.mass.gov/Eeohhs2/docs/dmr/health_screening_brochure.pdf.

Wilkinson, J. E. and Cerreto, M. C. (2008). Primary care for women with intellectual disabilities. *J Am Board Fam Med*, 21(3), 215–22.

Willis, D. S. (2008). A decade on: what have we learnt about supporting women with intellectual disabilities through the menopause. *J Intellect Disabil*, 12(1), 9–23.

Wingfield, M., Healy, D. L. and Nicholson, A. (1994a). Gynaecological care for women with intellectual disability. *Med J Aust*, 160, 536–8.

Wingfield, M., McClure, N., Mamers, P. M. *et al.* (1994b). Sexual health: the intellectually disabled: menstrual management and gynaecological care. *Med J Aust*, 160, 533–6.

Metabolic and endocrine diseases

Joav Merrick and Mohammed Morad

Introduction

Metabolic disease

The term *'inborn error of metabolism'* was coined by a British physician, Archibald Garrod (1857–1936), in the early twentieth century. Metabolism is carried out by enzymes and if a genetic abnormality affects the function of an enzyme or causes it to be deficient or missing altogether, various disorders can occur. Inborn errors of metabolism can be divided into three major pathophysiological diagnostic groups:

- Disorders that disrupt the synthesis or catabolism of complex molecules with symptoms that are permanent, progressive, independent of intercurrent events and not related to food intake. These include lysosomal disorders, peroxisomal disorders and disorders of intracellular transport and processing.
- Disorders that lead to an acute or progressive accumulation of toxic compounds as a result of metabolic block. These include disorders of amino acid metabolism (phenylketonuria (PKU), homocystinuria, maple syrup urine disease), organic acidurias, congenital urea cycle defects and sugar intolerances (galactosaemia).
- Disorders with symptoms due to a deficiency of energy production or utilisation within the liver, myocardium, muscle or brain. These include congenital lactic acidaemias, fatty acid oxidation defects, gluconeogenesis defects and mitochondrial respiratory chain disorders.

The mechanisms for brain damage resulting in intellectual disability (ID) are not well understood and relatively few metabolic conditions cause ID in isolation (Kahler and Fahey, 2003).

Endocrine disease

The study of endocrinology began in China; by the year 200 BC they had isolated sex and pituitary hormones from human urine and were using them for medicinal purposes. The word endocrinology comes from Greek, endon meaning 'within' and krino 'to separate'. It is a branch of medicine dealing with disorders of the endocrine system and its specific chemical mediators, called hormones.

People with ID often have associated endocrine problems (Botero and Fleischman, 2006; McElduff, 2002) and sometimes the endocrine disease can be the cause of the ID. People with ID may have (Botero and Fleischman, 2006):

Intellectual Disability and Ill Health: A Review of the Evidence, ed. Jean O'Hara, Jane McCarthy and Nick Bouras. Published by Cambridge University Press. © Cambridge University Press 2010.

Table 11.1. Search results for metabolic disease

Before evidence-based screening	9593
After evidence-based screening	557

- their disability caused by endocrinopathies
- endocrine conditions associated with chromosomal and non-chromosomal syndromes
- other abnormalities of growth and development
- endocrine manifestations caused by medications taken
- endocrine disease as in the general population.

Method

Metabolic disease

A search in MEDLINE (1967–2008) was made to find studies on the association between ID and metabolic disease. A broad search strategy also included Google Scholar, Elsevier, Eric, Ovid and Springer. The MeSH terms used were mental retardation, intellectual disability, mental handicap, chronic disease and metabolic disease. The first search was made in July 2008 and updated in August 2008.

Endocrine disease

A search in MEDLINE (1967–2008) was made to find studies on the association between ID and endocrine disease. A search strategy included MeSH terms mental retardation and endocrine disease together with a hand search of journals and other material relevant to the topic of ID.

Results

Metabolic disease

The Google Scholar search for metabolic disease and mental retardation found 45 papers, while for metabolic disease and intellectual disability only 2 papers. The MEDLINE/PubMed search for metabolic disease and mental retardation yielded 480 papers, while metabolic disease and intellectual disability resulted in 30 papers. All abstracts were read and relevant articles inspected in more detail and used for this chapter. The search results are shown in Table 11.1.

Endocrine disease

A Google Scholar search for endocrine disease and mental retardation found eight articles, while there were no papers for endocrine disease and intellectual disability. The MEDLINE/PubMed search for endocrine disease and mental retardation produced 256 articles, while endocrine disease and intellectual disability found 29 articles. All relevant abstracts were read and relevant articles inspected in more detail and used for this review. The search results are shown in Table 11.2.

Table 11.2. Search results for endocrine disease

Before evidence-based screening	5114
After evidence-based screening	293

Discussion

Metabolic disease

Prevalence and screening

Metabolic disorders are a heterogeneous group of genetic conditions mostly occurring in childhood and individually rare, but collectively numerous resulting in substantial morbidity and mortality.

One study from the UK looked at the 1999–2003 period and found the overall birth prevalence at 1 in 784 live births (95% CI 619–970) (Sanderson *et al.*, 2006). Of a total of 396 new cases the most frequent diagnoses were mitochondrial disorders (1 in 4929; 95% CI 2776–8953), lysosomal storage disorders (1 in 5175; 95% CI 2874–9551), amino acid disorders excluding PKU (1 in 5354; 95% CI 2943–9990) and organic acid disorders (1 in 7962; 95% CI 3837–17 301). Most of the diagnoses (72%) were made by the age of 15 years and a third by the age of 1 year. Another study from Luxembourg looked at all school children with ID in special school and residential care centres for people with ID and found that 1% showed metabolic abnormality (Kutter and Metz, 1968).

A classic example of how neonatal screening has progressed is PKU. Phenylketonuria was discovered in 1934, when a Norwegian mother brought her son and daughter, who had ID, to Professor Ivar Asbjørn Følling (1888–1973) at the University of Oslo School of Medicine for a consultation (Guttler, 1984). In 1947, Jervis (1947) showed that usually the administration of phenylalanine to normal humans led to a prompt rise in blood tyrosine, whereas no increase in blood tyrosine could be detected in individuals with PKU, indicating both the normal pathway of phenylalanine metabolism and the metabolic error in PKU. Several years later this inborn error of the amino acid metabolism, caused by the deficiency of the liver enzyme phenylalanine hydroxylase (PAH), changed to become a preventable form of ID, when Bickel *et al.* (1954) published the results of dietary treatment. The work of Jervis (1947) and Bickel *et al.* (1954) was the incentive that led to the large field of investigations into the inborn errors of metabolism that became the basis for the understanding of a range of causes of ID and the possibility for treatment and prevention.

Several further studies stressed the importance of diet for people with PKU and a drive started to develop a diagnostic method to measure phenylalanine in the blood. Guthrie and Susi (1963) developed a bacterial 'inhibition assay' that facilitated a sensitive, specific, inexpensive and fast method for the determination of blood phenylalanine.

From 1964 to 1973 different types of PKU were found and worldwide (Guttler, 1984), neonatal screening started, resulting in early treatment and prevention of ID with more screening for other diseases added. In Israel, neonatal screening started in 1963. Whilst there was agreement that treatment with a phenylalanine-restricted diet must start as soon as possible (in the first two weeks of life), there was not universal agreement on when to stop. In recent years we have come to understand the need for a 'diet for life' (Merrick *et al.*, 2001). A study from the UK traced people with PKU who were born before screening began and so were never treated, but were still alive (Murphy *et al.*, 2008). They found no significant differences between those who had or had not tried the phenylalanine–restricted diet. Further study is therefore required to examine the effect of trying the low-phenylalanine diet for people with untreated PKU.

Tandem mass spectrometry is now being used as an analytical method for neonatal screening. The method can determine the content of amino acids and acylcarnitines in neonatal screening samples in one integrated analysis. This allows detection of more than 20 inherited disorders of amino acid, fatty acid and organic acid metabolism.

Metabolic disorders

Inborn errors of metabolism are inherited defects in human metabolism. To improve the prognosis for metabolic diseases, early recognition is necessary. Many infants with metabolic diseases can be diagnosed with routine biochemical tests and metabolic screening of urine. For some metabolic diseases, an early diagnosis will lead to specific treatment and improved prognosis, for others to genetic counselling and prenatal diagnosis.

Metabolic disorders can present with a great assortment of signs and symptoms that mimic non-genetic disorders. Common presenting symptoms are acute neonatal symptoms, failure to thrive, central nervous system (CNS) symptoms such as developmental delay, movement or psychiatric disorder or cerebral palsy, sudden infant death syndrome (SIDS), episodic illness (anorexia, vomiting, lethargy, coma), cardiomyopathy, muscular (hypotonic, weakness, cramps), gastrointestinal (anorexia, vomiting, diarrhoea, malabsorption), liver disease, ophthalmic abnormalities, Reye's syndrome-like illness, dysmorphic features or metabolic manifestations (acidosis, hypoglycaemia).

Acute symptoms in the neonatal period can be very non-specific such as respiratory distress, hypotonia, poor sucking reflex, vomiting, diarrhoea, dehydration, lethargy and seizures, which can be just the same symptoms as in infection. Children or babies with metabolic disorders of accumulation can show deterioration after a normal initial period that can last hours or weeks.

Another type of late-onset symptoms is seen with metabolic disorders of toxic accumulation or energy production, where the child has a symptom-free period for a year or more, some extending into late childhood, adolescence or even adulthood. Symptoms may be triggered by a viral infection, fever or diarrhoea, which result in the body reverting to the breakdown of stored protein within the cells and tissue. The child can improve despite missed or prolonged diagnosis and therefore without intervention. General or chronic gastrointestinal, neurological and muscular complaints may also eventually lead to diagnosis.

Lysosomal storage disorders

Lysosomal storage diseases are a heterogeneous group of disorders (over 40 known today) with a progressive accumulation of undegraded catabolites (Kahler and Fahey, 2003). Due to the deficiency, catabolites will be stored in the reticuloendothelial and nervous system with CNS damage resulting in ID. The lysosomal storage diseases are classified by the nature of the primary stored material involved into lipid storage disorders, mainly sphingolipidoses (including Gaucher's and Niemann-Pick diseases), gangliosidosis (like Tay-Sachs disease), leukodystrophies, mucopolysaccharidoses, glycoprotein storage disorders and mucolipidoses.

Treatment is symptomatic for this group of metabolic diseases. Bone marrow transplantation and enzyme replacement therapy have been tried with some success, but it is hoped that gene therapy (introducing the gene for a missing enzyme product in to the blood, liver or other cells) may offer cures in the future (Kahler and Fahey, 2003).

Phenylketonuria

Phenylketonuria (PKU) as discussed above, is a metabolic disease causing ID, where universal screening, early detection and early diet treatment has resulted in the prevention of ID. In the early days of diet treatment the idea was that the diet should only be implemented while the brain was still developing. However, with children and especially female children growing up and entering the fertile age, it was found that their offspring became affected with ID (Kahler and Fahey, 2003). A 'diet for life' is now recommended for every child diagnosed with PKU (Merrick *et al.*, 2001).

Mitochondrial disorders

Research on mitochondrial and metabolic medical conditions (called mitochondrial cytopathies) has taken a rapid development since the first case was diagnosed in 1959 (Shoffner, 2006). A mitochondrion is part of every cell in the body that contains genetic material and is responsible for processing oxygen and converting substances into energy for essential cell functions. Mitochondria produce energy in the form of adenosine triphosphate (ATP), which is then transported to the cytoplasm of a cell for use in numerous cell functions. Mitochondrial disorders now include more than 40 different identified diseases that have different genetic features (more than several hundred phenotypes). In all these diseases, the mitochondria are unable to completely burn food and oxygen in order to generate energy and the incompletely burned food accumulates inside the body.

Mitochondrial diseases might affect the cells of the brain, nerves (including nerves to the stomach and intestines), muscles, kidneys, heart, liver, eyes, ears or pancreas. In some individuals, only one organ is affected, while in other patients all the organs are involved. Depending on how severe the mitochondrial disorder is, the illness can range in severity from mild to fatal.

Symptoms are not specific and include delayed growth, loss of muscle coordination and muscle weakness, visual and/or hearing problems, developmental delays, ID, heart, liver or kidney disease, gastrointestinal disorders, respiratory disorders, diabetes, seizures and dementia. In adults, many diseases of ageing have been found to have defects of mitochondrial function, such as Type 2 diabetes, Parkinson's disease, atherosclerotic heart disease, stroke, Alzheimer's disease and cancer.

Endocrine disease

Primary congenital hypothyroidism occurs in approximately 1 of every 3000–4000 newborns in the United States (US Preventive Services Task Force, 2008). Neonatal screening, which originated from Quebec in 1971, and implemented together with PKU screening at birth results in early diagnosis and treatment, which prevent neurological, motor and growth deficits, including irreversible ID. In the Centers for Disease Control and Prevention studies of birth cohorts in Atlanta from 1981 to 1995, 216 children tested positive for metabolic and endocrine disorders at neonatal screening and only nine children showed developmental disability (speech and language impairment) (Braun *et al.*, 2003).

Several large studies of adults with ID aged 40 years and older in New York State (1371 persons), Israel (2282 persons) and Taiwan (1128 persons) showed that the Israeli cohort had increased odds of dermatological, endocrine, gastrointestinal and infectious diseases/conditions compared with the New York State cohort (Janicki *et al.*, 2002; Merrick *et al.*, 2004, Wang *et al.*, 2007). Of these, endocrine and infectious diseases, as well as musculoskeletal and respiratory diseases, were two to three times more likely in males than females in the Israeli cohort when compared to the New York cohort, but in the Israeli cohort diabetes was at a lower frequency than the general Israeli population. The Taiwan study showed much lower frequencies of all conditions compared to New York and Israel, with the exception of neurological conditions. Endocrine disorders were found with increased ageing in people with Down syndrome and in the total cohort of all three studies 32% showed endocrine problems.

In studies with smaller sample sizes, of people referred for genetic evaluation, a 9% prevalence of metabolic and endocrine disorders was found (Maves *et al.*, 2007).

Disability caused by endocrinopathies

The main two entities are congenital hypothyroidism and neonatal hypoglycaemia, which should be diagnosed in the early neonatal period and treated to prevent ID.

Screening implemented in the 1970s has been able to detect congenital hypothyroidism more accurately (US Preventive Services Task Force, 2008). Congenital hypothyroidism seems to be a sporadic and not hereditary disease (Gruters *et al.*, 2003).

Glucose is the major energy source for the fetus and neonate, since the newborn brain depends upon glucose, but at birth glucose regulatory mechanisms are not always functioning well. The infant is therefore susceptible to hypoglycaemia, when glucose demands are increased. Severe or prolonged hypoglycaemia may result in long-term neurological damage and ID. Symptoms are non-specific and monitoring is important to prevent hypoglycaemia in the neonatal period, especially in premature infants (Botero and Fleischman, 2006).

Endocrine conditions associated with chromosomal and non-chromosomal syndromes

There are several syndromes with an endocrine component that the clinician should be aware of and anticipate, but only the most common in clinical practice are mentioned below.

Down syndrome (DS) is associated with several endocrinological and autoimmune manifestations, the most prominent being hypothyroidism, but also diabetes mellitus, chronic lymphocytic thyroiditis, Graves' disease and short stature (Botero and Fleischman, 2006). Regular thyroid function tests should therefore be carried out in people with DS all through their life. Prasher and Gomez (2007) investigated annual thyroid function tests in 200 adults with DS over a 10-year period and concluded that routine screening for adults with DS who are euthyroid can be reduced to every 5 years rather than to current usual practice of every 1–2 years.

Turner syndrome, Klinefelter syndrome, Prader-Willi syndrome, Noonan syndrome and Williams syndrome all have related endocrine disorders requiring regular screening (Botero and Fleischman, 2006; Höybye, 2004).

Other abnormalities of growth and development

Intrauterine growth retardation can have long-term complications for development and health with increased prevalence of essential hypertension, impaired glucose tolerance, Type 2 diabetes, polycystic ovary syndrome, ischaemic heart disease, hypertriglyceridaemia and low high-density lipoprotein on top of the increased risk for seizures and developmental disability (Botero and Fleischman, 2006; Vining, 2008).

Precocious puberty has also been described in association with ID (Botero and Fleischman, 2006; Raphaelson *et al.*, 1983; Vining, 2008) and can coexist with any CNS abnormality causing ID. Each case of the development of secondary sexual characteristics before age 8–9 years should include a careful examination, clinical and laboratory investigations.

Mills *et al.* (2007) found that children with autistic spectrum disorder had significantly elevated levels of growth-related hormones.

Endocrine manifestations caused by medication

In the last national survey of over 6000 people with ID living in residential care centres in Israel it was found that nearly 80% received medication every day (30% received antiepileptic drugs and 51% received psychotropic medications) (Morad *et al.*, 2007). Many of the medications used had thyroid-stimulating hormone suppression, thyroid suppression, effects on thyroid binding proteins, inactivation of vitamin D, osteoporosis, diabetes, obesity, galactorrhoea and growth retardation (Botero and Fleischman, 2006).

Obesity

Obesity is a common problem in people with ID, due to the fact that there is often habitual overeating and decreased daily activities. There are also several syndromes with ID associated with obesity, e.g. DS (Merrick and Kandel, 2008) and Prader-Will syndrome (Höybye, 2004). Prevention programmes and physical activity should be part of interventions.

Diabetes

As obesity and sedentary lifestyle are common in people with ID, it would be expected to find a higher prevalence of diabetes. In a large cohort study of adults with ID in Israel diabetes was found with increasing age, decreased as ID became severe, but with a lower prevalence than the general Israeli population (Merrick *et al.*, 2004). Regular screening should be conducted.

Conclusion

Recent scientific and medical advances in early screening for metabolic and endocrine diseases have contributed in the detection and treatment of some of these diseases and the prevention of ID associated with them. There is a great need for evidence-based research including gene therapy to provide effective treatments.

Several studies have shown that endocrine problems are common in people with ID as in the general population, but also as part of several syndromes and conditions seen in this population. People with ID should therefore have a comprehensive assessment of their endocrine function and be part of screening procedures as in the general population.

References

Bickel, H., Gerrard, J. and Hickmans, E. M. (1954). The influence of phenylalanine intake on the chemistry and behavior of a phenylketonuria child. *Acta Paediatr Scand*, 43, 64–77.

Botero, D. and Fleischman, A. (2006). Endocrinology. In *Medical Care for Children and Adults with Developmental Disabilities*, ed. I. L. Rubin and A. C. Crocker. Baltimore: Paul Brookes, pp. 387–98.

Braun, K. V. N. , Yeargin-Allscop, M., Schendel, D. and Fernhoff, P. (2003). Long-term developmental outcomes of children identified through a newborn screening program with a metabolic and endocrine disorder: a population-based approach. *J Pediatr*, 143, 236–42.

Gruters, A., Biebermann, H. and Krude, H. (2003). Neonatal thyroid disorders. *Horm Res*, 59(Suppl 1), 24–9.

Guthrie, R. and Susi, A. (1963). A simple phenylalanine method for detecting phenylketonuria in populations of newborn infants. *Pediatrics*, 32, 338–43.

Guttler, F. (1984). Phenylketonuria: 50 years since Folling's discovery and still expanding our clinical and biochemical knowledge. *Acta Paediatr Scand*, 73, 705–16.

Höybye, C. (2004). Endocrine and metabolic aspects of adult Prader-Willi syndrome with special emphasis on the effect of growth hormone treatment. *Growth Horm IGF Res*, 15, 1–15.

Janicki, M. P., Davidson, P. W., Henderson, C. M. *et al.* (2002). Health characteristics and health services utilization in older adults with intellectual disability living in community residences. *J Intellect Disabil Res*, 47(4), 287–98.

Jervis, G. A. (1947). Studies on phenylpyruvic oligophrenia. The position of the metabolic error. *J Biol Chem*, 169, 651–6.

Kahler, S. G. and Fahey, M. C. (2003). Metabolic disorders and mental retardation. *Am J Med Genet C Semin Med Genet*, 117C, 31–41.

Kutter, D. and Metz, H. (1968). [The frequency of some oligophrenias due to metabolic disease in the grand-duchy of Luxembourg.] *Schweiz Arch Neurol Neurochir Psychiatr*, 101, 369–82.

Maves, S. N., Williams, M. S., Williams, J. L., Levonian, P. J. and Josephson, K. D. (2007). Analysis of 88 adult patients referred for genetic evaluation. *Am J Med Genet C Semin Med Genet*, 145C, 232–40.

McElduff, A. (2002). Endocrinological issues. In *Physical Health of Adults with Intellectual Disabilities*, ed. V. P. Prasher and M. P. Janicki. Oxford: Blackwell, pp. 160–80.

Merrick, J. and Kandel, I. (2008). Down syndrome and obesity. *Int J Child Health Hum Dev*, 1(4), 437–40.

Merrick, J., Aspler, S. and Schwarz, G. (2001). Should adults with phenylketonuria have treatment? *Ment Retard*, 39(3), 216–17.

Merrick, J., Davidson, P. W., Morad, M. *et al.* (2004). Older adults with intellectual disability in residential care centers in Israel: health status and service utilization. *Am J Ment Retard*, 109(5), 413–20.

Mills, J. L., Hediger, M. L., Molloy, C. A. *et al.* (2007). Eleveated levels of growth-related hormones in autism and autism spectrum disorder. *Clin Endocrinol*, 67, 230–7.

Morad, M., Kandel, I. and Merrick, J. (2007). National survey 2001 on medical services for persons with intellectual disability in residential care in Israel. *Int J Disabil Hum Dev*, 6(3), 317–22.

Murphy, G. H., Johnson, S. M., Amos, A. *et al.* (2008). Adults with untreated phenylketonuria: out of sight, out of mind. *Br J Psychiatry*, 193(6), 501–2.

Prasher, V. and Gomez, G. (2007). Natural history of thyroid function in adults with Down syndrome–10-year follow-up study. *J Intellect Disabil Res*, 51(4), 312–17.

Raphaelson, M. I., Stevens, J. C., Elders, J., Comite, F. and Theodore, W. H. (1983). Familial spastic paraplegia, mental retardation, and precocious puberty. *Arch Neurol*, 40(13), 809–10.

Sanderson, S., Green, A., Preece, M. A. and Burton, H. (2006). The incidence of inherited metabolic disorders in the West Midlands, UK. *Arch Dis Child*, 91(11), 896–9.

Shoffner, J. M. (2006). Mitochondrial disorders. In *Medical Care for Children and Adults with Developmental Disabilities*, ed. I. L. Rubin and A. C. Crocker. Baltimore: Paul Brookes, pp. 130–7.

US Preventive Services Task Force (2008). Screening for congenital hypothyroidism (CH): U.S. Preventive Services Task Force reaffirmation recommendation statement.

Ann Fam Med, 6(2), 166. Available from: http://www.annfammed.org/cgi/content/full/6/2/166-a/DC1.

Vining, E. P. (2008). You've come a long way, baby: or have you? *Epilepsy Curr*, 8(5), 118–19.

Wang, K. Y., Hsieh, K., Heller, T., Davidson, P. W. and Janicki, M. P. (2007). Carer reports of health status among adults with intellectual/developmental disabilities in Taiwan living at home and in institutions. *J Intellect Disabil Res*, 51(3), 173–83.

Neoplasms

Simon Bonell

Introduction

There has been interest in the study of neoplasms in people with intellectual disability (ID) for many years. Early interest focused on leukaemia in Down syndrome (DS) (Krivit and Good, 1957) and on people with ID living in institutions (Jancar and Jancar, 1977). It is important that this area of health care is understood to ensure that public health measures are suitably directed and that clinical suspicion and early diagnosis are improved (Turner and Moss, 1996).

This chapter reviews the evidence on the incidence of neoplasms in people with ID. There will be little discussion of aetiology, screening, diagnosis or treatment. As the focus is on the ID population as a whole, it is beyond the scope of this chapter to review rare genetic syndromes that are associated with malignancy, although there will be some mention of more common conditions (e.g. DS).

Method

A MEDLINE search was performed (1950–2008) to find co-morbidity or incidence studies on ID and neoplasms. The MeSH terms used were mental retardation, neoplasms and co-morbidity or incidence.

Free text searches were also performed using MEDLINE, PsycINFO and CINAHL databases, using the search terms 'mental AND retardation' OR 'intellectual AND disability' OR 'learning AND disability' AND 'cancer' OR 'neoplasm' OR 'tumour'. Additional references were identified from reference lists of retrieved papers. The initial search took place in July 2008 and was updated in October 2008.

Results

A total of 1156 papers were found (please refer to Table 12.1). No exclusion was made by language. All abstracts were read and the papers studied in more detail if deemed to be relevant. High-quality cohort studies with or without control groups were included.

Discussion

Mortality

Historically, the incidence of neoplasms (cancers) in people with ID has been measured through studying populations in institutions. These studies are often limited to mortality

Intellectual Disability and Ill Health: A Review of the Evidence, ed. Jean O'Hara, Jane McCarthy and Nick Bouras. Published by Cambridge University Press. © Cambridge University Press 2010.

Table 12.1. Summary of search results

Articles identified in the search	1156
Articles included in the review	32

surveys. Often there is no control group and data may be lacking about the institutionalised population making it impossible to compare the rates with an age-matched general population. Information is often based upon death certificates and medical notes and thus does not take into account treated malignancies. Although these studies can show the proportions of deaths from different cancers and trends over time, the hospital population is constantly changing, especially given the move away from institutionalisation. Any changes over time should be interpreted with caution.

Probably the most influential institutional study of cancer deaths, is that on the Stoke Park Group of hospitals in Bristol (UK) (please refer to Table 12.2). Jancar and Jancar (1977) carried out their study after noticing that the proportion of deaths from cancer had doubled from 1936 to 1975 within their group of hospitals. This 40-year review was updated (Jancar, 1990) and completed with a 60-year review (Cooke, 1997). There were dramatic changes in the population being studied over this time period. The original population of 1690 patients declined to 293 by 1995. Over the study period there was a marked increase in life-expectancy, most striking in the residents with DS, whose life-expectancy increased by 40 years in a 50-year period (Carter and Jancar, 1983). There was also a decrease in the average IQ score, as more able people were discharged to the community. Data relied on death records, and rates of post-mortem studies had dropped to only 3 out of 29 cancer cases between 1986 and 1995.

As these studies lacked a control group the data could not be compared to the general population but the proportion of people with ID dying from cancers was noted to be lower than expected. The incidence of cancer was noted to increase during the first five decades, as the life expectancy increased. The average age of death due to cancer also increased. The pattern of cancers that occurred was also noted to be different from the general population. The high proportion of gastrointestinal (GI) cancer deaths was reanalysed by Duff *et al.* (2001), who confirmed that this was due to increased rates of stomach cancers, possibly due to increased rates of *Helicobacter pylori* infection (please refer to Chapter 4 on Infectious diseases and Chapter 8 on Digestive system diseases).

A number of mortality studies were identified that were not primarily investigating cancer rates thus highlighting the limited reliability of this method (e.g. Chaney and Eyman, 2000). McLoughlin (1988) published mortality data from the Prudhoe hospital, Northumberland, UK. Between 1983 and 1987 the proportion of deaths recorded on death certificates due to cancer was 10.7%. The hospital population comprised 50.7% with severe ID who also had significantly shorter life expectancy. O'Brien *et al.* (1991) studied mortality in a large institution in the USA. Over the study period (1974–85), there were 19 deaths with cancer, oesophageal and digestive system cancers being the most frequent. Again, there was a decline over the study period in the proportion of deaths from cancer. They noted that tobacco use was positively associated with IQ although there were no cases of lung cancer. However, tobacco use was significantly related to death by cancer, particularly of the oesophagus and digestive system.

Table 12.2. Cancer rates in the ID population: selected mortality papers

Paper	Country	Time period	Sample	Significant findings
Jancar and Jancar, 1977	UK	1936–75	Stoke Park Hospitals – population of 1690 patients. 1125 deaths over the study period. 48% had post-mortems. Cause of death from death certificate and medical records	Lower cancer rate in ID population than general population and cancer accounted for lower proportion of deaths. High proportion of carcinoma of the GI tract (58%)
Jancar, 1990	UK	1976–85	Stoke Park Hospitals – population declined over the study period from 1240 to 1051. There were 302 deaths	Increased proportion of deaths for all types of cancer and age of death from carcinoma when compared to previous 40 years. GI tract accounted for 58% of cancer deaths
Cooke, 1997	UK	1986–95	Stoke Park Hospitals – population fell from 828 in 1986 to 293 in 1995. 213 deaths over the study period	13.6% of deaths due to cancer versus 26% in general population. Incidence of cancer declined from the previous decade. 55% of cancers were from GI tract
O'Brien et al., 1991	USA	1974–85	Institutional facility with 1000 beds. 165 deaths occurred during the study period. Information on cause of death was from medical and nursing records and autopsy reports	11.5% of deaths due to cancer. Tobacco use was positively associated with cancer and significantly with IQ. GI tract were most prevalent tumours. No cases of lung cancer recorded
Durvasula et al., 2002	Australia	1989–99	693 people with ID identified by contact with services. 40 deaths occurred during the study period and information was obtained from death certificates, medical notes and post-mortems	A total of 7 cancer deaths were recorded – all in over 40-year-olds. 17.5% of all deaths were due to cancer compared with 38.7% in the general population. Men had significantly more stomach and brain cancers, women more colorectal cancers and leukaemia occurred more frequently in both men and women with ID

GI, gastrointestinal.

No prospective studies were identified that looked particularly at cancer incidence in the ID population. Evenhuis (1997) carried out a ten-year prospective longitudinal study exploring medical conditions, including cancer, in an elderly institutional ID population (average age 70) in the Netherlands. Out of the 77 subjects, 16 had a current or previous diagnosis of cancer. The small numbers did not allow for comparison with the general population but Evenhuis noted a high rate of oesophageal cancer (two cases) and one of the small intestine. A further prospective study was carried out by Hollins et al. (1998) to look at mortality rates in two London districts. They found that malignancy was the third most common cause of death in their population, with similar rates to the general population. They note the low rates of post-mortem examination and the unreliability of death certification.

Durvasula et al. (2002) carried out a population-based study into mortality in the ID population in the Lower North Shore area of Sidney, Australia (please refer to Table 12.2). It is noticeable that all cancer deaths (seven) occurred in the over 40s. Of all deaths, 17.5% were from cancer as compared to 38.7% in the general population in that area.

Table 12.3. Incidence papers of cancers in the ID population

Paper	Country	Time period studied	Sample and method	Significant findings
Patja et al., 2001	Finland	1967–97	2173 people with ID identified in a survey in 1962; diagnosis by neuropsychological testing. Names linked to national cancer register and compared with age-matched rates for general population	Overall cancer rate lower than general population (ns); no difference in overall cancer rates by level of ID. Mild/moderate ID had lower rates of prostate and urinary tract cancers (SIR 0.2 for both). Severe/profound ID had lower lung cancer (no cases) and increased gall bladder (SIR 10.3), testicular (SIR 9.9) and central nervous system (SIR 3.5) cancers
Sullivan et al., 2003	Australia	1982–2000	2370 women with ID aged over 25 from the Disability Services Commission of Western Australia. Linked with the mandatory cancer registry	Lower rate of breast cancer in ID than general population over total study period. Lower rate of breast cancer in all age groups (ns). Lower uptake of screening services (34.7% vs 54.6% in general population)
Sullivan et al., 2004	Australia	1982–2001	9409 people with ID from the Disability Services Commission. Linked to the mandatory cancer registry	No difference with overall cancer rates in general population. High rates of leukaemia, increased rates of stomach and brain cancers in men and colorectal cancers in women

ns, not significant; SIR, standardised incidence ratio.

Incidence

More robust data regarding the incidence of cancers in the ID population has been provided by recent data linkage studies (please refer to Table 12.3). These rely on the quality of national databases for people with ID and with cancer. Databases of people with ID can come from people accessing services or from cytogenetic laboratory testing. They have the advantages of being cohort studies, thus allowing comparisons with age-matched controls and giving incidence ratios.

Patja et al. (2001) was the first study of its kind. Using a Finnish register that had identified ID cases in a survey in 1962, 2173 people with ID made up the cohort. Diagnosis of ID was by neuropsychological testing. A national personal identity number was introduced in 1967 which allowed for the names from this cohort to be linked to the national cancer register between 1967 and 1997. The age range for the cohort was from 7 to 69. Overall, there were slightly fewer cancers in the ID population as compared to the age-matched general population, but this did not reach significance. Of interest, overall cancer incidence did not vary by level of ID. However, significant differences were noted in the age at which cancers occurred as compared to the general population and in the cancer profile depending on the level of ID. There was a higher risk of cancer in the 15 to 29 year age range than the general population and a lower risk in men with ID over 60.

A similar study design was employed in Western Australia (Sullivan et al., 2004). Cases of ID were identified through the Disability Services Commission, which covers 70% of the ID population. In this study, 9409 individuals were identified and were linked to the mandatory cancer registry service (WA cancer registry) between 1982 and 2001. When compared to the age-matched general population there were no differences in overall cancer rates. This did not hold in the 0–4 year age group, in which seven times more cancers occurred in the ID group than the general population. An earlier study by Sullivan *et al.* (2003) had found a reduced rate of breast cancer overall, but this was postulated to be due to the overall reduced life expectancy among people with ID. A low rate of uptake of breast screening services was noted, particularly associated with the level of ID, the presence of physical disability, urban residence and being unmarried.

Various studies have been carried out looking at specific malignancies. Bohmer *et al.* (1997) compared the age-related incidence of oesophageal cancer in an institution-based ID population in the Netherlands with that in the general population. Data were obtained from the Netherlands Cancer Registry. The standardised incidence ratio (SIR) was found to be almost three times higher in the ID population as compared to the general population.

Jaffe *et al.*'s (2002) study of abnormal cervical cytology in an institutionalised ID population in the USA found that 151 women had a total of 229 Papanicolau smears over a two-year period as part of routine cancer screening. The slides were rescreened for the study and three were found to be abnormal. The rate of cervical dysplasia was 0.32%, compared with 1.5–6% in the general population. They postulate that this may be due to a lower risk factor profile including lower rates of sexually transmitted diseases, smoking and average age.

Down syndrome

Numerous studies have confirmed the increased rates of leukaemia in DS since the first large study in 1957 (Krivit and Good, 1957). Studies are plentiful due to the prevalence and easy recognition of DS, the high incidence of leukaemia in this group and the availability of registers for people with DS. A review of cancers in DS is provided by Satge *et al.* (1998) with discussion of the 20-fold excess of leukaemia and relatively uncommon occurrence of solid tumours in general. However, they note that lymphomas, gonadal and extragonadal germ cell tumours and possibly retinoblastomas, pancreatic and bone tumours are in excess.

Of note is the increased rate of leukaemia in younger age groups. Baird and Sadovnick (1988) found a relative risk of 7.4 for leukaemia in the 1–9 year age group. Mili *et al.* (1993a) found an SIR of 50.8 for leukaemia in children with DS in Atlanta and an SIR of 32.1 in Iowa (Mili *et al.* (1993b), although numbers were small leading to wide confidence intervals. Hasle *et al.* (2000) carried out a large study using information from the Danish Cytogenetic Register (please refer to Table 12.4). Diagnosis of DS was from cytogenetic laboratories and gave a sample of 2814 individuals with DS from 1968. These individuals were linked to the Danish Cancer Register. Overall, there was no significant difference between those with DS and the age- and sex-matched general population for cancer rates. However, there were significant differences for specific cancers and in different age groups. The SIR for leukaemia was 17.6 in all age groups, and was 54 in the 0–4 year age group. They also found a decreased SIR for solid tumours (0.5 in all age groups). Notably there were no cases of breast cancer (7.3 cases expected).

Boker and Merrick (2002) carried out a population-based study on people with DS in Israel between 1948 and 1995. They identified 2635 people with DS; either from the Israel DS register which started in 1978 or from people receiving institutional care prior to this. This is likely to have introduced bias, as it did not include people raised by families. Information on

Table 12.4. Selected papers investigating the incidence of cancers in Down syndrome

Paper	Country	Time period studied	Sample and method	Significant findings
Hasle *et al.*, 2000	Denmark	1968–95	Cohort of 2814 cases from the Danish cytogenetic register. Linked to Danish Cancer Registry. Number of expected cases calculated for age- and sex-matched general population and SIRs calculated	Slightly increased rates of cancers overall (SIR 1.2 (ns)). Leukaemia accounted for 60% of malignant disease, with a significantly higher number occurring than expected in the general population (SIR 17.6). Highest risk in first 4 years, gradually reducing. No cases of leukaemia were identified in over 30-year-olds. Significantly reduced incidence of solid tumours (SIR 0.5). SIR significantly lower for solid tumours in females than in males
Hill *et al.*, 2003	Sweden and Denmark	1965–93	4872 individuals with DS identified from hospital discharge records and linked to the cancer registry of each respective country	Overall there was an increased incidence of cancers in the DS group (SIR 1.7). SIR for leukaemia was 19.5. SIR for solid tumours was 0.8 (ns). Raised incidence of liver cancer (SIR 6.0), testis cancer (SIR 3.7) and male genital cancers based on 3 cases of penile cancer (SIR 45.5)
Goldacre *et al.*, 2004	UK	1963–2001	A cohort of 1453 people with DS identified from hospital discharge records was compared to a cohort of over 460 000 people admitted with other conditions. Linked with data on treatment for cancers and death certification	Overall 2.7 times increased rate of all cancers in DS group compared to reference group. 18.9 times increased rate of leukaemia in DS group. Significantly increased rate of cancer of the testis (12 times above reference group)
Patja *et al.*, 2006	Finland	1978–2002	Cases identified between 1978 and 1986 for the Finnish registry of people with ID; identified from providers. 3581 people with confirmed DS identified. Followed up for cancer occurrence via linkage with the Finnish Cancer Registry	Overall risk of cancer very similar to general population. Leukaemia accounted for 38% of all cancers, and rates were significantly increased as compared to the general population (SIR 10.5). Highest risk in 0–9 year age range (SIR 32.5) and a higher risk in women than men with DS. Significantly reduced incidence of solid tumours. SIR for testicular cancer raised at 4.8
Sullivan *et al.*, 2007	Australia	1982–2001	1298 people with DS identified from the Disability Services Commission of Western Australia (based on people accessing services). Linked to the State Cancer Registry	Overall, no significant difference in numbers of cancers. Leukaemia accounted for 62% of all cancer, occurring with an SIR of 8.4. Highest in the 0–4 year age group (SIR 61.6). Reduced risk of solid tumours (SIR 0.44) overall, although not for women alone

DS, Down syndrome; ns, not significant; SIR, standardised incidence ratio.

cancer came from the cancer registry. A raised SIR of 25.2 was found for leukaemia in those from the register group and a slight excess of gastric cancer in males, based on two cases.

Hill *et al.* (2003) used Swedish and Danish hospital discharge diagnoses to identify a DS cohort of 4872. This methodology has its limitations, as cases identified through hospital admission may have an increased risk of mortality or cancer. They attempted to minimise this by excluding cancer diagnoses made within 12 months of first hospital admission (i.e. entry into the study). The DS cohort was followed up until death, emigration or the end of the study (1993) and linked to the cancer registries. The risk of leukaemia was found to be increased 20-fold in people with DS as compared to the age-matched general population and there was a modest increase in liver and testes cancers. Three penile cancers also led to an increased risk of genital cancers.

A similar hospital admissions study by Goldacre *et al.* (2004) in the UK found an overall increased risk of cancer in the DS cohort, with leukaemia being over 18 times more common. They also note an increased risk of testicular cancer, although this was based on three cases. The authors discuss the weaknesses of their sampling method including the absence of cytogenetic data and lack of follow-up of those who left the area. Likewise, Patja *et al.*'s (2006) Finnish study found an SIR of over 10 for leukaemia but also an increased SIR for testicular cancer of 4.8. This had been reported previously by Dieckmann *et al.* (1997).

Sullivan *et al.* (2007) found similar data for an Australian population. Overall, there were no differences in the cancer incidence rates but in the 0–4 year age group individuals with DS were over 60 times more likely to develop leukaemia than the general population. Sullivan also found a similarly decreased SIR of 0.44 for solid tumours.

Population studies into other causes of ID are few. A Danish study used the national cytogenetic register to identify cases of Fragile X syndrome and linked them to the cancer register (Schultz-Pedersen *et al.*, 2001). Of 223 people identified with Fragile X syndrome, 4 cancers occurred between 1943 and 1996. The age-matched SIR, at 0.28, was significantly reduced. The authors suggest that genetic factors may play a part, as might reduced exposure to environmental risk factors. Diagnostic failure may also be significant.

Conclusion

Early studies of populations in institutions suggested that the risk of cancer in ID was lower than the general population. However, this has not been replicated by population registry studies which suggest that overall there is an equal incidence of cancer rates between people with ID and the general age-matched population.

However, people with ID have a different profile of cancers compared to the general population. In institutionalised cohorts high rates of stomach and oesophageal cancers have been found, possibly related to the high rates of *Helicobacter pylori* infection. They have also been shown to have lower rates of cervical cancer. Wider population studies also suggest a different profile of cancers in ID than the general population but further large high-quality studies are required before firm conclusions can be drawn.

It is well established that there is an increased incidence of leukaemia in DS and there is some evidence of increased rates of testicular cancers and lower rates of solid tumours. Satge *et al.* (2006) provides a review of this area with some discussion of the possible underlying genetic basis that is beyond the scope of this chapter.

There have been reports of a higher incidence of cancer in mild to moderate ID than severe to profound ID. This has also been used to explain the apparent reduction in cancer incidence in populations in institutions. However, this could be confounded by the reduced life expectancy among people with more severe ID (Hogg *et al.* 2001) and was not found by Patja *et al.* (2001) who controlled for age.

As the life expectancy of people with ID continues to rise it is likely that the overall incidence of cancer will also rise. The increase in community access over recent decades has also changed the risk factor exposure in this population, including alcohol and tobacco consumption and increasing obesity (Turner and Moss, 1996), and is thus likely to have an influence on cancer rates.

References

Baird, P. A. and Sadovnick, A. D. (1988). Causes of death to age 30 in Down syndrome. *Am J Hum Genet*, 43, 239–48.

Bohmer, C. J., Klinkenberg-Knol, E. C., Niezen-de Boer, R. C. and Meuwissen, S. G. (1997). The age-related incidences of oesophageal carcinoma in intellectually disabled individuals in institutes in The Netherlands. *Eur J Gastroenterol Hepatol*, 9(6), 589–92.

Boker, L. K. and Merrick, J. (2002). Cancer incidence in persons with Down syndrome in Israel. *Downs Syndr Res Pract*, 8(1), 31–6.

Carter, G. and Jancar, J. (1983). Mortality in the mentally handicapped: a 50 year survey at the Stoke Park group of hospitals (1930–1980). *J Ment Defic Res*, 27, 143–56.

Chaney, R. and Eyman, R. (2000). Patterns in mortality over 60 years among persons with mental retardation in a residential facility. *Ment Retard*, 38(3), 289–93.

Cooke, L. B. (1997). Cancer and learning disability. *J Intellect Disabil Res*, 41, 312–16.

Dieckmann, K. P., Rube, C. and Henke, R. P. (1997). Association of Down's syndrome and testicular cancer. *J Urol*, 157, 1701–4.

Duff, M., Scheepers, M., Cooper, M., Hoghton, M. and Baddeley, P. (2001). *Helicobacter pylori*: has the killer escaped from the institution? A possible cause of increased stomach cancer in a population with intellectual disability. *J Intellect Disabil Res*, 45, 219–25.

Durvasula, S., Beange, H. and Baker, W. (2002). Mortality of people with intellectual disability in northern Sydney. *J Intellect Dev Disabil*, 27(4), 255–64.

Evenhuis, H. M. (1997). Medical aspects of ageing in a population with intellectual disability: III. Mobility, internal conditions and cancer. *J Intellect Disabil Res*, 41, 8–18.

Goldacre, M. J., Wotton, C. J., Seagroatt, V. and Yeates, D. (2004). Cancers and immune related diseases associated with Down's syndrome: a record linkage study. *Arch Dis Child*, 89, 1014–17.

Hasle, H., Clemmensen, I. H. and Mikkelsen, M. (2000). Risks of leukaemia and solid tumours in individuals with Down's syndrome. *Lancet*, 355(9199), 165–9.

Hill, D. A., Gridley, G., Cnattingius, S. *et al.* (2003). Mortality and cancer incidence among individuals with Down syndrome. *Arch Intern Med*, 163, 705–11.

Hogg, J., Northfield, J. and Turnbull, J. (2001). *Cancer and People with Learning Disabilities*. Worcestershire, UK: BILD publications, p. 33.

Hollins, S., Attard, M. T., von Fraunhofer, N., McGuigan, S. and Sedgwick, P. (1998). Mortality in people with learning disability: risks, causes, and death certification findings in London. *Dev Med Child Neurol*, 40, 50–6.

Jaffe, J. S., Timell, A. M., Eisenberg, M. S. and Chambers, J. T. (2002). Low prevalence of abnormal cervical cytology in an institutionalized population with intellectual disability. *J Intellect Disabil Res*, 46(7), 569–74.

Jancar, J. (1990). Cancer and mental handicap. *Br J Psychiatry*, 156, 531–3.

Jancar, M. P. and Jancar, J. (1977). Cancer and mental retardation. *Bristol Med Chir J*, 92, 3–7.

Krivit, W. and Good, R. A. (1957). Simultaneous occurrence of mongolism and leukemia; report of a nationwide survey. *Am J Dis Child*, 94(3), 289–93.

McLoughlin, I. J. (1988). A study of mortality experiences in a mental-handicap hospital. *Br J Psychiatry*, 153, 645–9.

Mili, F., Khoury, M. J., Flanders, W. D. and Greenberg, R. S. (1993a). Risk of childhood cancer for infants with birth defects. I. A record-linkage study, Atlanta, Georgia, 1968–1988. *Am J Epidemiol*, 137(6), 629–38.

Mili, F., Lynch, C. F., Khoury, M. J., Flanders, W. D. and Edmonds, L. D. (1993b). Risk of childhood cancer for infants with birth defects. II. A record-linkage study, Iowa, 1983–1989. *Am J Epidemiol*, 137(6), 639–44.

O'Brien, K. F., Tate, K. and Saharia, E. S. (1991). Mortality in a large southeastern facility for persons with mental retardation. *Am J Ment Retard*, 95, 397–403.

Patja, K., Pukkala, E. and Iivanainen, M. (2001). Cancer incidence among people with intellectual disability. *J Intellect Disabil Res*, 45, 300–7.

Patja, K., Pukkala, E., Sund, R., Iivanainen, M. and Kaski, M. (2006). Cancer incidence of persons with Down syndrome in Finland: a population-based study. *Int J Cancer*, 118, 1769–72.

Satge, D., Sommelet, D., Geneix, A. *et al.* (1998). A tumor profile in Down syndrome. *Am J Med Genet*, 78, 207–16.

Satge, D., Sasco, A., Vekemans, M. J. J. *et al.* (2006). Aspects of digestive tract tumors in Down syndrome: A literature review. *Dig Dis Sci*, 51(11), 2053–61.

Schultz-Pedersen, S., Hasle, H., Olsen, J. H. and Friedrich, U. (2001). Evidence of decreased risk of cancer in individuals with fragile X. *Am J Med Genet*, 103(3), 226–30.

Sullivan, S. G., Glasson, E. J., Hussain, R. *et al.* (2003). Breast cancer and the uptake of mammography screening services by women with intellectual disabilities. *Prev Med*, 37(5), 507–12.

Sullivan, S. G., Hussain, R., Threlfall, T. and Bittles, A. H. (2004). The incidence of cancer in people with intellectual disabilities. *Cancer Causes Control*, 15, 1021–5.

Sullivan, S. G., Hussain, R., Glasson, E. J. and Bittles, A. H. (2007). The profile and incidence of cancer in Down syndrome. *J Intellect Disabil Res*, 51, 228–31.

Turner, S. and Moss, S. (1996). The health needs of adults with learning disabilities and the health of the nation strategy. *J Intellect Disabil Res*, 40, 438–50.

Systems disorders

Otorhinolaryngological disorders

Vishwa Radhakrishnan

Introduction

People with intellectual disability (ID) constitute approximately 2% of the population. They die prematurely and often have a number of unrecognised or poorly managed medical conditions as well as inadequate health promotion and disease prevention (Lennox *et al.*, 2007). If satisfactory health care is to be achieved for people with ID, medical needs must be monitored, regular specialist reassessments offered, access to specialist services facilitated and reports clearly explained to carers (Kerr *et al.*, 2003). This chapter focuses on the evidence related to the association between otorhinolaryngological (ENT) disorders and ID.

Method

A search in MEDLINE was made to find studies related to otorhinolaryngological disorders in people with ID. The MeSH terms used were 'mental retardation' and 'otorhinolaryngologic diseases'. A broad search strategy included AMED, BNI, CINAHL, EMBASE, MEDLINE, HEALTH BUSINESS ELITE, HMIC and PsycINFO databases. Search terms used were otorhinolaryngolog* OR otorhinolog* OR otolaryng* OR otolog* OR rhinolog* OR laryngolog*, hearing AND impairment, intellectual AND disability OR learning AND disability OR developmental AND disability OR mental AND retardation. The first search was made in November 2008 and updated in January 2009. All abstracts found were read, and potentially relevant articles were inspected in more detail. No exclusion criteria or restrictions (language or country of origin) were used.

Results

The search results are shown in Table 13.1.

Discussion

Hearing impairment

Recognition and management of hearing impairment can lead to significant improvement in the quality of life of people with ID (Lavis *et al.*, 1997). Hearing impairment in people with ID is anything from 40 to 100 times above the rate in the general population (Carvill, 2001) but testing people with ID for hearing impairment can be difficult (Wilson and Haire, 1990). People with ID are unlikely to be assessed for sensory impairments due to staff attributing

Intellectual Disability and Ill Health: A Review of the Evidence, ed. Jean O'Hara, Jane McCarthy and Nick Bouras. Published by Cambridge University Press. © Cambridge University Press 2010.

Table 13.1. Search results

Search method	Before screening	After screening
MEDLINE	1649	189
Broader search	1121	23

lower levels of functioning to the person's ID (Lavis *et al.*, 1997; Yeates, 1995) and are unlikely to receive aids to hearing (Yeates, 1995). Rates of hearing impairment were also shown to be different for testing (38.9%) and questionnaire (9.4%) in a study by Lavis *et al.* (1997).

In a longitudinal observation study of the hearing and speech development of 110 children with Down syndrome (DS) between 1982 and 1991, otitis media with effusion was detected in 34 (63%) of the 54 children with moderate hearing loss (Harigai, 1994). Active treatment led to significant improvement in hearing in 26 children. They used hearing aids for individuals with prolonged otitis media and those with a hearing loss greater than 50 dB in both ears. This led to improvement in their social interaction and speech development. In another study, 12 882 children were screened and further audiological examination of 151 children with ID was conducted, with a randomly selected control group of 101 children without ID (Karjalainen *et al.*, 1983). Tympanograms were obtained from 206 children (81.7%) and 30.9% of ears were classed as abnormal in the case of children with ID, but in only 17.8% of children without ID. An aetiological study on 122 deaf pupils (57 aged < 20 years, 65 aged > 20 years) found that apart from having hearing impairment with thresholds of > 60 dB, all the participants had ID with a non-verbal IQ of 40–80 (Admiraal and Huygen, 1999). The cause of hearing impairment was acquired in 48%, inherited in 17%, chromosomal in 4% and unknown in 30%. Male predominance among the hearing-impaired pupils was higher.

A prospective cohort study of 1602 people with ID reported high prevalence and incidence of hearing impairment, which was even more pronounced in people with DS than in people with ID resulting from other causes (Lantman-de Valk *et al.*, 1997). In a cross-sectional population-based study on the prevalence of hearing loss in 1598 adults with ID, DS and age were confirmed to be risk factors (Meuwese-Jongejeugd *et al.*, 2006). The age-related increase in prevalence in persons with DS appears to occur approximately three decades earlier, and in persons with ID by other causes approximately one decade earlier, than in the general population. Hearing loss occurs in almost one in three adults with ID, which is two times higher than the prevalence of 16–17% in the general population. Timehin and Timehin (2004) studied a community population of adults with ID to determine the prevalence of hearing impairment, problem behaviours and their access to audiology. They report a prevalence rate of 9.2% for hearing impairment; 70% had been seen by audiology services at some time in their life but only 24% had ongoing assessments and hearing-aid maintenance. Problem behaviours were also reported in 62% of their sample with 34% exhibiting self-injurious behaviour.

More recently, Hild *et al.* (2008) screened 552 athletes with ID during the German Special Olympics Summer Games 2006 and found the prevalence of hearing impairment to be considerably higher than in the general population. The proportion of undetected hearing impairment is large, even among people with only mild and moderate ID.

Dysphagia

Patients with ID and neurological disabilities associated with swallowing difficulties are vulnerable to dehydration and undernutrition (Kennedy *et al.*, 1997). Sano *et al.* (2007) studied 57 patients with severe motor dysfunction and ID suspected of having dysphagia and found that severe dysphagia such as retention of solid food in the pharynx could only be detected on videofluoroscopic examination of swallowing. In a study done by Samuels and Chadwick (2006), speech and language therapists working with adults with ID and dysphagia gathered data from case notes, clinical assessment and videofluoroscopic assessment reports. Speed of eating, cramming food and premature loss of the bolus into the pharynx were identified as significant predictors of asphyxiation risk in this population. Rogers *et al.* (1994) examined the feeding skills and health of 73 adults with severe developmental disabilities who aspirated between 1986 and 1990. Sixty individuals had profound ID (82%) and 48 had cerebral palsy (66%). Mealtime respiratory distress (65%) or chronic lung disease (55%), however, were significantly associated with aspiration. (Please refer to Chapter 7 on Respiratory diseases.)

Sheppard (1991) recommends a dysphagia management protocol for people with ID, which includes screening to identify individuals at risk, diagnostic evaluation of dysphagia, daily management to promote optimal mealtime function and dysphagia therapy to improve underlying neuromotor competency and eating skills.

Down syndrome and otorhinolaryngological disorders

Accurate knowledge of the pathophysiology underlying ENT disorders (facial dysmorphism, ear abnormalities, upper airway abnormalities and immunodeficiency) allow an understanding of the reasons for the development of upper airway obstruction, obstructive sleep apnoea syndrome, subglottic stenosis, deafness, speech delay and ENT infections that occur frequently in people with DS. Early screening and specific treatment may allow some of the long-term sequelae to be avoided, or at least their prognosis to be improved (Venail *et al.*, 2004). Shott *et al.* (2001) conducted a five-year longitudinal study following the otolaryngological problems seen in 48 children with DS. After treatment of easily reversible hearing loss from chronic otitis media, with either medical treatment or surgical treatment with PETs (pressure equalisation tubes), 98% of the children had normal hearing levels. Zarate *et al.* (2001) studied the prevalence and presentation of oesophageal motor dysfunction in 58 people with DS and 38 controls. The most frequent symptoms in people with DS were dysphagia for liquids and solids, vomiting/regurgitation and chest pain. Oesophageal motor disorders, particularly achalasia, are frequent in people with DS.

In their study, Chen *et al.* (2006) investigated peripheral nasal pathology as a contributor to olfactory impairment in 20 individuals with DS and 16 without DS. Those with DS were impaired on olfactory threshold and odour identification. They suggest that olfactory deficits in DS appear to be secondary to central, rather than rhinological, pathology. Price *et al.* (2004) compared the efficacy of adenoidectomy in 27 children with DS and 53 age- and sex-matched control patients by reviewing medical records between January 1978 and September 1997. After adenoidectomy, more controls than patients with DS had improvement in symptoms, including nasal obstruction, snoring, mouth breathing and middle ear disease. Individuals with DS were 7.7 times more likely to have chronic ear drainage after adenoidectomy.

Dahle and McCollister (1986) designed a study to determine the prevalence of otological disorders in children with DS compared to children with other causes of ID. The results indicated that children with DS had a significantly higher prevalence of hearing impairment and otological disorders. Libb *et al.* (1985) investigated the relationship between hearing disorder and performance on intelligence tests among 28 children and young adults with DS. They found that the performance on intelligence tests by individuals with abnormal tympanograms was inferior to that of individuals with normal tympanograms. Evenhuis *et al.* (1992) assessed the hearing function of 35 institutionalised persons with DS, age 35 to 62 years, and reported hearing losses of 20 dB to over 90 dB in 56 of their ears. They suggest that hearing loss should be considered and excluded as a contributing factor in social and mental deterioration in middle-age persons with DS. Laczkowska-Przybylska and Szyfter (1999) examined 61 patients with DS and diagnosed otitis media in 19 patients. Conductive hearing impairment after otitis media was observed.

Sheehan and Hans (2006) evaluated the indications, surgical techniques and postoperative problems seen in children with DS fitted with bone-anchored hearing aids (BAHA) in the United Kingdom and Ireland. They conclude that BAHA is a valuable method of hearing amplification in children with DS and should be considered not as a primary method of amplification, but in the overall management of individuals with DS after conventional hearing aids and/or ventilation tubes have been considered or failed.

Other syndromes

Roberts *et al.* (2005) conducted a study to determine whether 23 young males with Fragile X syndrome (FRAX) displayed atypical auditory brainstem responses compared to typically developing males when conductive and sensorineural hearing losses are ruled out. They had normal hearing sensitivity and middle ear function and scored similarly to the typically developing children on the measures of auditory brainstem pathway integrity. Auditory brainstem responses in young males with FRAX were within normal limits. Hagerman *et al.* (1987) evaluated records of 30 prepubertal boys with FRAX retrospectively to document the incidence of recurrent otitis media by physician records. The number of documented otitis media infections in the first five years of life was significantly more than those of the normal male siblings and of unrelated, cytogenetically normal controls. They also highlight that males with FRAX are at high risk for recurrent ear disease.

People with Williams syndrome (WS) experience debilitating symptoms such as hyperacusis and phonophobia. The mothers of 49 children with WS completed a Hyperacusis Screening Questionnaire and those children with reported hyperacusis and sufficient developmental capacity underwent comprehensive audiological and brainstem auditory-evoked response testing (Gothelf *et al.*, 2006). Compared to a control group, the results indicate that hyperacusis in WS is associated with a high-frequency hearing loss resembling the configuration of noise-induced hearing loss. According to the authors, the hyperacusis and hearing loss in WS may stem from a deficiency in the acoustic reflex resulting from auditory nerve dysfunction. Klein *et al.* (1990) also used parental questionnaires to determine the prevalence of hyperacusis and otitis media in individuals with WS. Prevalence rates of 95% for hyperacusis and 61% for otitis media were found, both significantly higher than in the general population. Levitin *et al.* (2005) collected data from parents of people with WS (n = 118) and comparison groups of people with DS, autistic spectrum disorder and controls.

The findings revealed four phenomenologically separate auditory abnormalities, all of which were significantly more prevalent in WS than the three comparison groups.

In a cross-sectional study, Pillion *et al.* (2003) examined the auditory status of 81 females with Rett syndrome (RS) using auditory brainstem response testing and measures of acoustic admittance. They found bilateral hearing loss in 16 (19.8%) of the participants and unilateral hearing loss in 13 (16%). The prevalence of hearing loss was increased in older RS participants and in those with seizures requiring the use of anticonvulsants. Morton *et al.* (1997) studied the feeding abilities in 20 individuals with RS aged $1\frac{1}{2}$ to 33 years by history and clinical assessment during a meal, followed by videofluoroscopy of feeding. All were shown to have reduced movements of the mid and posterior tongue, with premature spill over of food and liquid from the mouth into the pharynx. They also showed delayed pharyngeal swallow, but otherwise pharyngeal problems were minimal.

Cornelia de Lange syndrome (CdLS) is characterised by multiple congenital malformations and ID. Sataloff *et al.* (1990) examined 45 patients with CdLS; almost all had hearing loss and most had impaired language development. Other otolaryngological abnormalities identified were external auditory canal stenosis and cleft palate. Sakai *et al.* (2002) examined the auditory brainstem-evoked responses of 13 children with CdLS to evaluate hearing and the utility of hearing aids in hearing-impaired individuals. They suggest that the fitting of hearing aids and early consistent training have a significant effect on auditory development in CdLS children. Marchisio *et al.* (2008) investigated 50 children (aged 1–18 years) with CdLS for the prevalence of otitis media with effusion and/or hearing loss and its impact on the children's performance. The findings indicate that otitis media with effusion and/or hearing loss is an important feature of children with CdLS and may negatively affect their performance.

Other otorhinolaryngological conditions

A major sequelae of impacted cerumen (earwax) is conductive hearing loss, which can be deleterious to linguistic, social and intellectual development, particularly for individuals with ID. The longitudinal incidence (over a 12-year period) of excessive or impacted cerumen and related conductive hearing loss of 117 adults with ID was examined by Crandell and Roeser (1993). Results indicated a considerably higher incidence of excessive cerumen and cerumen impaction with associated conductive hearing loss in adults with ID (28%) than in the general adult population (2% to 6%). Brister *et al.* (1986) determined the incidence of occlusion of the external auditory canal due to impacted cerumen for 44 individuals with ID in comparison with 44 people without ID. Results confirmed that adolescents with ID have a significantly higher incidence of occlusion of the external auditory canal due to impacted cerumen than do adolescents without ID.

Diagnosis, therapy and prevention

Primary care physicians should be aware of the necessity of screening for sensory impairments. It is also important that the primary care physician plays a more active role in the detection of age-related sensory loss in older adults with ID and the assessment of younger adults whose sensory functions have never or incompletely been evaluated. Whilst annual sensory screening is not deemed necessary, annual otoscopy to detect impacted earwax or unidentified middle ear infection, as well as checks of the proper use of glasses and hearing aids, are suggested (Evenhuis *et al.*, 1997). Training carers and staff to recognise possible signs of a sensory impairment is valuable. This should be followed by accurate assessment by specialist services (Yeates, 1991). Kunst *et al.* (2007) assess the impact and the subjective benefit of BAHA through a case-control study of 22 individuals with conductive or mixed hearing loss. The use of BAHA proved beneficial in most of those with hearing impairment and moderate ID. Benham-Dunster and Dunster (1985) assessed residents with moderate (n = 61) and profound (n = 103) ID in a large institution using three audiometric procedures: behavioural observation audiometry (BOA, both speech and tonal), acoustic reflex measures and brainstem auditory-evoked responses audiometry to compare the three methods to determine whether a battery of tests might provide a more accurate assessment. Results indicated that a battery of tests was beneficial. Lennox *et al.* (2007) conducted a cluster randomised controlled trial with matched pairs. The participants were 453 adults with ID (34 clusters). The intervention was a health assessment programme to enhance interactions between the adult with ID, their carer and their primary care physician. Following the intervention there was a 30-fold increase in hearing testing. The intervention increased detection of new disease by 1.6 times. Most adults with mild or moderate ID can be assessed with methods that are normally used by primary care physicians. People who are unable to tolerate these methods should be referred for screening with specialised methods (Evenhuis *et al.*, 1997).

Evenhuis (1996) recommend structured cooperation of an audiological physician, ENT surgeon, audiological scientist, specialised speech and hearing therapist and hearing aid technician (e.g. by cooperation of district audiological centres and centres for people with ID). They highlight the need to encourage referral by primary care physicians, paediatricians and ENT specialists.

Conclusion

More studies examining the impact of otorhinolaryngological disorders on the health of people with intellectual disability are needed, as the majority tend to focus on people with DS. There is a need for studies evaluating the effect of early interventions for otorhinolaryngological conditions on social interaction, communication, behaviour and quality of life of people with ID. Research to develop training programmes for carers and professionals working closely with this population would enable better identification of need. Studies on care pathways to streamline the diagnosis, management and follow-up of people with ID with otorhinolaryngological disorders will be hugely beneficial to both individuals and organisations.

References

Admiraal, R. J. and Huygen, P. L. (1999). Causes of hearing impairment in deaf pupils with a mental handicap. *Int J Pediatr Otorhinolaryngol*, 51(2), 101–8.

Benham-Dunster, R. A. and Dunster, J. R. (1985). Hearing loss in the developmentally handicapped: a comparison of three audiometric procedures. *J Aud Res*, 25(3), 175–90.

Brister, F., Fullwood, H. L., Ripp, T. and Blodgett, C. (1986). Incidence of occlusion due to impacted cerumen among mentally retarded adolescents. *Am J Ment Defic*, 91(3), 302–4.

Carvill, S. (2001). Sensory impairments, intellectual disability and psychiatry. *J Intellect Disabil Res*, 45(Pt 6), 467–83.

Chen, M. A., Lander, T. R. and Murphy, C. (2006). Nasal health in Down syndrome: a cross-sectional study. *Otolaryngol Head Neck Surg*, 134(5), 741–5.

Crandell, C. C. and Roeser, R. J. (1993). Incidence of excessive/impacted cerumen in individuals with mental retardation: a longitudinal investigation. *Am J Ment Retard*, 97, 568–74.

Dahle, A. J. and McCollister, F. P. (1986). Hearing and otologic disorders in children with Down syndrome. *Am J Ment Defic*, 90(6), 636–42.

Evenhuis, H. M. (1996). Dutch consensus on diagnosis and treatment of hearing impairment in children and adults with intellectual disability. *J Intellect Disabil Res*, 40(5), 451–6.

Evenhuis, H. M., van Zanten, G. A., Brocaar, M. P. and Roerdinkholder, W. H. (1992). Hearing loss in middle-age persons with Down syndrome. *Am J Ment Retard*, 97(1), 47–56.

Evenhuis, H. M., Mul, M., Lemaire, E. K. and de Wijs, J. P. (1997). Diagnosis of sensory impairment in people with intellectual disability in general practice. *J Intellect Disabil Res*, 41(Pt 5), 422–9.

Gothelf, D., Farber, N., Raveh, E., Apter, A. and Attias, J. (2006). Hyperacusis in Williams syndrome: characteristics and associated neuroaudiologic abnormalities. *Neurology*, 66(3), 390–5.

Hagerman, R. J., Altshul-Stark, D. and McBogg, P. (1987). Recurrent otitis media in the fragile X syndrome. *Am J Dis Child*, 141(2), 184–7.

Harigai, S. (1994). Longitudinal studies in hearing-impaired children with Down's syndrome. *Nippon Jibiinkoka Gakkai Kaiho*, 97(12), 2208–18.

Hild, U., Hey, C., Baumann, U. *et al.* (2008). High prevalence of hearing disorders at the Special Olympics indicate need to screen persons with intellectual disability. *J Intellect Disabil Res*, 52(Pt 6), 520–8.

Karjalainen, S., Kaariainen, R. and Vohlonen, I. (1983). Ear disease and hearing sensitivity in mentally retarded children. *Int J Pediatr Otorhinolaryngol*, 5(3), 235–41.

Kennedy, M., McCombie, L., Dawes, P., McConnell, K. N. and Dunnigan, M. G. (1997). Nutritional support for patients with intellectual disability and nutrition/dysphagia disorders in community care. *J Intellect Disabil Res*, 41(Pt 5), 430–6.

Kerr, A. M., McCulloch, D., Oliver, K. *et al.* (2003). Medical needs of people with intellectual disability require regular reassessment, and the provision of client- and carer-held reports. *J Intellect Disabil Res*, 47(2), 134–45.

Klein, A. J., Armstrong, B. L., Greer, M. K. and Brown, F. R. III. (1990). Hyperacusis and otitis media in individuals with Williams syndrome. *J Speech Hear Disord*, 55(2), 339–44.

Kunst, S. J., Hol, M. K., Cremers, C. W. and Mylanus, E. A. (2007). Bone-anchored hearing aid in patients with moderate mental ID: impact and benefit assessment. *Otol Neurotol*, 28(6), 793–7.

Laczkowska-Przybylska, J. and Szyfter, W. (1999). Otitis media in patients with Down's syndrome. *Otolaryngol Pol*, 53(1), 83–6.

Lantman-de Valk, H. M., Van Den Akker, M., Maaskant, M. A. *et al.* (1997). Prevalence and incidence of health problems in people with intellectual disability. *J Intellect Disabil Res*, 41(1), 42–51.

Lavis, D., Cullen, P. and Roy, A. (1997). Identification of hearing impairment in people with a learning disability: from questionnaire to testing. *Br J Learn Disabil*, 25(3), 100–5.

Lennox, N., Bain, C., Rey-Conde, T. *et al.* (2007). Effects of a comprehensive health assessment programme for Australian adults with intellectual disability: a cluster randomized trial. *Int J Epidemiol*, 36(1), 139–46.

Levitin, D. J., Cole, K., Lincoln, A. and Bellugi, U. (2005). Aversion, awareness, and attraction: investigating claims of hyperacusis in the Williams syndrome phenotype. *J Child Psychol Psychiatry*, 46(5), 514–23.

Libb, J. W., Dahle, A., Smith, K., McCollister, F. P. and McLain, C. (1985). Hearing disorder and cognitive function of individuals with Down syndrome. *Am J Ment Defic*, 90(3), 353–6.

Marchisio, P., Selicorni, A., Pignataro, L. *et al.* (2008). Otitis media with effusion and hearing loss in children with Cornelia de Lange syndrome. *Am J Med Genet A*, 146A(4), 426–32.

Meuwese-Jongejeugd, A., Vink, M., van Zanten, B. *et al.* (2006). Prevalence of hearing loss in 1598 adults with an intellectual disability: cross-sectional population based study. *Int J Audiol*, 45(11), 660–9.

Morton, R. E., Bonas, R., Minford, J., Kerr, A. and Ellis, R. E. (1997). Feeding ability in Rett syndrome. *Dev Med Child Neurol*, 39(5), 331–5.

Pillion, J. P., Rawool, V. W., Bibat, G. and Naidu, S. (2003). Prevalence of hearing loss in Rett syndrome. *Dev Med Child Neurol*, 45(5), 338–43.

Price, D. L., Orvidas, L. J., Weaver, A. L. and Farmer, S. A. (2004). Efficacy of adenoidectomy in the treatment of nasal and middle ear symptoms in children with Down syndrome. *Int J Pediatr Otorhinolaryngol*, 68(1), 7–13.

Roberts, J., Hennon, E. A, Anderson, K. *et al.* (2005). Auditory brainstem responses in young males with fragile X syndrome. *J Speech Lang Hear Res*, 48(2), 494–500.

Rogers, B., Stratton, P., Msall, M. *et al.* (1994). Long-term morbidity and management strategies of tracheal aspiration in adults with severe developmental disabilities. *Am J Ment Retard*, 98(4), 490–8.

Sakai, Y., Watanabe, T. and Kaga, K. (2002). Auditory brainstem responses and usefulness of hearing aids in hearing impaired children with Cornelia de Lange syndrome. *Int J Pediatr Otorhinolaryngol*, 66(1), 63–9.

Samuels, R. and Chadwick, D. D. (2006). Predictors of asphyxiation risk in adults with intellectual disabilities and dysphagia. *J Intellect Disabil Res*, 50(Pt 5), 362–70.

Sano, N., Morimoto, T., Yano, Y. *et al.* (2007). [Dysphagia and videofluoroscopic examination of swallowing in patients with severe motor and intellectual disabilities, and the results of dysphagia rehabilitation for these patients.] *No To Hattatsu*, 39(4), 275–8.

Sataloff, R. T., Spiegel, J. R., Hawkshaw, M., Epstein, J. M. and Jackson, L. (1990). Cornelia de Lange syndrome. Otolaryngologic manifestations. *Arch Otolaryngol Head Neck Surg*, 116(9), 1044–6.

Sheehan, P. Z. and Hans, P. S. (2006). UK and Ireland experience of bone anchored hearing aids (BAHA) in individuals with Down syndrome. *Int J Pediatr Otorhinolaryngol*, 70(6), 981–6.

Sheppard, J. J. (1991). Managing dysphagia in mentally retarded adults. *Dysphagia*, 6(2), 83–7.

Shott, S. R, Joseph, A. and Heithaus, D. (2001). Hearing loss in children with Down syndrome. *Int J Pediatr Otorhinolaryngol*, 61(3), 199–205.

Timehin, C. and Timehin, E. (2004). Prevalence of hearing impairment in a community population of adults with learning disability: access to audiology and impact on behaviour. *Br J Learn Disabil*, 32(3), 128–32.

Venail, F., Gardiner, Q. and Mondain, M. (2004). ENT and speech disorders in children with

Down's syndrome: an overview of pathophysiology, clinical features, treatments, and current management. *Clin Pediatr (Phila)*, 43(9), 783–91.

Wilson, D. N. and Haire, A. (1990). Health care screening for people with mental handicap living in the community. *BMJ*, 301(6765), 1379–81.

Yeates, S. (1991). Hearing loss in adults with learning disabilities. *BMJ*, 303, 427–30.

Yeates, S. (1995). The incidence and importance of hearing loss in people with learning disabilities. *Br J Learn Disabil*, 23(2), 79–84.

Zarate, N., Mearin, F., Hidalgo, A. and Malagelada, J. R. (2001). Prospective evaluation of esophageal motor dysfunction in Down's syndrome. *Am J Gastroenterol*, 96(6), 1718–24.

14

Eye diseases and visual impairment

J. Margaret Woodhouse

Introduction

This chapter will evaluate the evidence for eye and visual abnormalities amongst people with intellectual disability (ID). The conditions included are those which affect sight to some degree, and therefore will have an impact on daily living skills. There are no eye conditions unique to people with ID; all occur in the general population and the question posed is whether the prevalence is higher amongst our study population than amongst the general population.

Method

An advanced PubMed search of the MEDLINE database was conducted and additional peer-reviewed published studies known to the author, but not included on MEDLINE, were accessed. There was no search of unpublished research findings.

The search period was from 1970 to the present using the following MeSH terms: (intellectual disability/disabilities OR learning disability/disabilities OR mental retardation) AND (vision OR visual impairment OR eye diseases OR refractive errors).

The initial search was conducted in September 2008 and updated in November 2008. The abstracts of all articles identified were screened and only those that provided direct research findings and evidence on prevalence were accepted. Additional exclusion criteria were studies limited to: a clinical population, participants selected for suspected visual problems, infants, data collection by questionnaire, techniques for evaluating/diagnosing defects, only one specific subject condition such as motor disability, literature review, audit of healthcare outcomes and economic costing of health care.

Results

The initial search yielded 6048 articles. After screening, a selection of 32 articles were included in the review. (Please refer to Table 14.1.)

All but two of the studies suffer from a lack of controls. In addition, evaluation of the evidence is complex because of a lack of consistency of assessment techniques, variations in definitions of defects and in many cases absence of definitions of defects. In the discussion, separate inclusion criteria for the studies will be described for each topic.

Intellectual Disability and Ill Health: A Review of the Evidence, ed. Jean O'Hara, Jane McCarthy and Nick Bouras. Published by Cambridge University Press. © Cambridge University Press 2010.

Table 14.1. Search results

	MEDLINE and hand-search results
Before evidence-based screening	6048
After evidence-based screening	32

Discussion

Refractive errors

Amongst the general population, refractive errors (long sight, short sight and astigmatism) are not generally considered visual defects, because of the ready availability of optical correction by spectacles and contact lenses, at least in the developed world. However, if such errors are neglected amongst people with ID then the resulting poor vision forms an unnecessary visual impairment. The topic is, therefore, an important one in this context.

The criteria for describing refractive error as hypermetropia (long sight) or myopia (short sight) vary amongst studies and can be somewhat arbitrary. For prevalence studies, refractive error should be described for one eye of each participant only, as there is usually a strong association between the refractive status of the two eyes of an individual (the exception to this, a difference between the two eyes is called anisometropia). Inclusion criteria for this topic are: criteria for classifying refractive error type, description of which eye was used in the analysis, and unselected participants assessed for refractive error.

Six papers fulfilled the above criteria. Only one study used a (non-random) control group, so it may be considered the most valuable on this topic (Akinci et al., 2008). The researchers examined 724 children with ID (age 1–17 years) and 151 children with 'no known neurological or medical disorders related to ocular functioning' (age 3–15 years), attending an assessment clinic in Turkey. The authors raise the issue of the control group not being a 'visually normal population', since participants were attendees at a clinic. However, if anything, refractive errors would be more prevalent than amongst a true control group and any differences are therefore minimised rather than exaggerated. The inclusion of very young children in the study group may potentially confound the results, as refractive errors can change rapidly in early infancy (Saunders, 1995). However, the mean and standard deviation of the study group was given as 9.3 ± 3.0 years, and we may, therefore, conclude that the numbers of very young children were limited and their contribution probably minimal.

Akinci et al. (2008) reported a prevalence of refractive errors (including anisometropia) of 82% amongst children with ID, compared to 39% amongst controls. They also showed a tendency for refractive errors to increase with the severity of ID. Intelligence quotient scores were used to categorise participants into groups with mild, moderate and severe ID. Astigmatism and anisometropia were significantly more common amongst individuals with severe as opposed to mild ID, and hypermetropia more common amongst those with mild than moderate ID.

Of the other five studies selected on this topic, two compared their data with those published by Sorsby et al. (1960) (Woodhouse et al., 2000, 2003). These 'control' data were collected from 1017 young men aged 17–27 entering National Service (plus 16 cases selected from those rejected from the army; since the British Army had limits on refractive errors permitted in recruits). They are not, therefore, randomly selected data or representative of

Table 14.2. The prevalence of uncorrected refractive errors and inadequate spectacles amongst people with ID

Study	Location	Population	Uncorrected errors	Inadequately corrected errors
Haire *et al.* (1991)	UK	75 people aged 15 years and over attending a day centre	13% required a correction and had no previous spectacles	1.3% wore an inadequate correction
Haugen *et al.* (1995)	Norway	183 people aged 15 years and over resident in an institution	70% required a correction and had no previous spectacles	18.9% of 37 people wearing glasses had inadequate correction
Woodhouse *et al.* (2000)	UK	154 people over 19 years old attending day centres	79% of all those with a significant refractive error (including presbyopia) did not have adequate spectacles	17% of 46 people with spectacles wore inadequate correction
van Splunder *et al.* (2004)	Netherlands	1106 people aged 18 years and over using ID services	49% of 670 people with refractive errors had no spectacles	6.3% of 343 people with spectacles had inadequate correction

Note that 'population' describes the number successfully completing testing for this attribute.

the age range of participants with ID. However, they are the most widely used control data for refractive errors.

Overall, it is apparent that the prevalence of myopia and astigmatism amongst people with ID (2.9–13.5% and 19–39.2% respectively) is higher than amongst controls (3.7% and 7.5% respectively) (Block *et al.*, 1997; Jacobson, 1988; Karadag *et al.*, 2007; Woodhouse *et al.*, 2000, 2003).

Correction of refractive errors

Of more relevance to healthcare needs than prevalence rates for refractive errors is a consideration of how often these errors are corrected, as they are in the general population, with spectacles or contact lenses. Papers were examined with the following inclusion criteria: reports of corrected, inadequately corrected and uncorrected refracted errors at presentation. There are no evidence-based guidelines for the clinical significance of refractive errors in terms of prescribing spectacles, and most researchers use clinical judgement in determining whether spectacles should be prescribed. Only one study describes the criteria for how much the measured refractive error must differ from the spectacle prescription in order to identify an inadequate correction (Woodhouse *et al.*, 2000).

Table 14.2 shows the prevalence of uncorrected and inadequately corrected refractive errors reported by four studies. The variation in prevalence of uncorrected errors (particularly the relatively low prevalence reported by Haire *et al.* (1991)) may reflect variations in service provision in different areas.

Amongst the general population, most people expect to wear spectacles for near tasks in middle-age. The condition in which near focus fails is presbyopia and is a normal consequence of ageing. Although all people with ID will encounter presbyopia, few studies consider problems with near focusing. Woodhouse *et al.* (2000) reported that 43% of individuals with ID of pre-presbyopic age had difficulty with near focusing, with no specific optical correction, and 85% of those of presbyopic age had no appropriate spectacles. van Splunder *et al.* (2004) reported that 56% of their participants with presbyopia had no spectacles for near tasks.

It is quite clear then, that people with ID have greater need for spectacle correction than do members of the general population, and yet are much less likely to have that correction. Woodhouse *et al.* (2000) showed that the more severe the ID, the less likely that refractive errors would be corrected. Uncorrected refractive errors reduce visual abilities and have an impact on daily living skills. Two of the studies reported improvements in visual acuity (van Splunder *et al.*, 2004) and improvement in daily living abilities and general interest in activities (Jacobson, 1988) when refractive errors were corrected. Future healthcare planning must address this prevalence of unnecessary visual deficit as a matter of some urgency.

Vision and visual impairment

Many studies report poor scores of visual acuity (detail vision) at examination amongst people with ID. To address this topic, the following inclusion criteria were used: evidence that ability-appropriate acuity tests were employed, criteria for reduced visual acuity were described and a description was given of whether acuity was recorded with present spectacles if worn. Nine papers fulfilled the above criteria, of which four presented data for individuals with particular levels of disability. (Note that studies of Special Olympics athletes, such as Block *et al.* (1997) and Woodhouse *et al.*, 2003, while not selecting for levels of ID, may over-represent mild and moderate ID.)

The nine studies use different criteria for poor vision, and the details are shown in Table 14.3. Note that 'normal' visual acuity for adults is usually taken to be 6/9 (0.67 or 20/15) or better and the World Health Organization uses visual acuity of poorer than 6/18 (0.3 or 20/60) as a definition of visual impairment. As Table 14.3 shows, below-normal visual acuity in the habitual state is extremely common amongst people with ID, and there is good evidence that the more severe the ID, the more likely acuity is to be reduced.

Uncorrected refractive errors are common amongst people with ID, so at least some of the poor vision reported in the above studies is unnecessary. Warburg (2001) estimated that amongst 837 individuals assessed in Denmark, 37% of cases of visual impairment (acuity poorer than 6/18) were due purely to uncorrected refractive errors. Using the same criteria, Evenhuis *et al.* (2001) in the Netherlands, reported a prevalence of visual impairment of 23% of their 611 participants after correction with spectacles. In their study of 135 UK Special Olympics athletes, Woodhouse *et al.* (2003) reported that 42.2% had reduced acuity (poorer than 6/9.5) when refractive errors were fully corrected.

Strabismus

Strabismus, or squint, is a misalignment of one eye during binocular viewing that has prevalence in the general population of 2–4% (Sorsby *et al.*, 1960). This condition disrupts binocular depth perception, and can result in poor vision in one eye. Not all studies report strabismus, presumably not considering the condition to constitute a visual defect. Inclusion criterion was simply reporting the prevalence of strabismus in the study group.

Ten papers provide data, two of which make use of a control group. Tuppurainen (1983) examined 149 children, aged 9–10 years, identified from a birth cohort in Finland as having ID by psychological testing, and 100 control children randomly selected from the same cohort. Strabismus was noted in 25.5% of children with ID and 4.0% of controls. Akinci *et al.*

Table 14.3. Visual acuity findings amongst people with ID (all are presenting acuities, that is, in the subjects' habitual state..

Study	Location	Population	Visual acuity findings
Jacobson (1988)	Sweden	219 people over 20 years old and resident in an institution	Poorer than 6/60 = 24.2%
Haire et al. (1991)	UK	61 people aged 16 and over attending a day centre	Poorer than 6/18 = 28%
Block et al. (1997)	USA	905 athletes aged 9 and over from 70 countries entering Special Olympics World Games	Poorer than 6/12 = 26.7%
Woodhouse et al. (2003)	UK	486 UK athletes aged 9* and over attending Special Olympics UK Summer Games	Poorer than 6/9.5 = 58.2%
Warburg (2001)	Denmark	594* people aged 20 and over, resettled from institutions to community homes	Poorer than 6/18 = 15.7%
Woodhouse et al. (2000)	UK	143 people over 19 years old and attending day centres	Poorer than 6/10 = 62.6% Poorer than 6/19 Mild/Moderate ID = 21% Severe/Profound ID = 37%
McCulloch et al. (1996)	UK	56 people 20 years old and over resident in an institution	Poorer than 6/24 Mild ID = 12% Severe ID = 42% Profound ID = 100%
Kwok et al. (1996)	Hong Kong	260 young people aged 3–25 educated in special school, all with 'severe mental deficiency'	Poorer than 6/60 = 25%
Van Den Broek et al. (2006)	Netherlands	76 people, ages not given, resident in a care facility, all with 'severe/profound multiple impairments'	Poorer than 6/18 = 92%

Note that 'population' describes the number successfully completing testing for visual acuity. * Number excludes those unable to perform an optotype (picture) test.

(2008) in a study in Turkey, reported strabismus amongst 14% of 724 children with ID (age 1–17 years) and amongst 1.3% of 151 control children aged 3–15 years.

Prevalence in the remaining eight studies ranged from 18.5% to 44.1% (Aitchison et al., 1990; Karadag et al., 2007; Levy, 1984; McCulloch et al., 1996; van Splunder et al., 2004; Woodhouse et al., 2000, 2003; Woodruff et al., 1980). McCulloch et al. (1996) showed that prevalence increased with the severity of ID; 25% of subjects with mild ID had strabismus, whereas 60% of subjects with profound ID had the condition.

Cataract

Establishing the prevalence of cataract in any population is problematic for two reasons. Firstly, the prevalence increases markedly with age, and most studies of the general population examine only older individuals. For example, a UK study of men aged 63 and over being followed for cardiovascular disease reported an overall prevalence of 28% with some degree of lens opacification (Stocks et al., 2002). In a study in Denmark, Buch et al. (2001) estimated the prevalence of visual impairment due to cataract amongst 1000 people aged 65 years and over to be 1%. Secondly, few studies of people with ID define criteria for reporting the condition. Cataract is opacification of the lens within the eye. The condition can range from small discrete congenital opacities with no visual consequences, through general age-related cloudiness with minimal visual impact, to dense sight-obscuring opacification. Cataract is treated by surgical extraction (removal of the lens) and currently, replacement by an implant. If an implant is not used, the eye is termed aphakic. Therefore in cataract prevalence studies, cases of implants and aphakia might rightfully be included since they indicate treated cataract. Inclusion criteria for this topic were: age of subjects with reported cataract/aphakia/implant and definition of cataract.

Only two papers fulfilled the above criteria. Woodhouse *et al.* (2003) in their UK study of Special Olympics athletes distinguished between 'lens opacities' (not visually limiting) and 'cataract' (visually limiting), based on the examiner's judgement. Of 494 individuals with ID, 7.5% had lens opacities, 4.9% had cataract and 0.8% had interocular lens implant. The 24 people with cataract were aged 12 to 54 years, with only 2 over the age of 50 years. The 4 individuals with implants were aged 30, 34, 34 and 58 years.

van Splunder *et al.* (2004) defined lens opacities as any opacity visible in the lens in a person with good vision, and cataract as any opacity in a person classified as visually impaired (acuity poorer than 6/18). Among 1416 individuals in the Netherlands, 18.1% had lens opacities, 6.1% had cataract associated with visual impairment and an additional 4.9% had previous cataract surgery. In a comprehensive evaluation of the influence of age in comparison to published figures for the general population, the authors showed that people with ID are at increased risk of developing lens opacities 'at a relatively young age'. van Splunder *et al.* (2004) concluded that 'people with Down syndrome seem to have a forward shift of approximately 40 years and other people with ID of approximately 20 years'.

One additional study contributes to this topic because of the inclusion of a control group (Tuppurainen, 1983). Although the definition of cataract is not given, the individuals' ages are 9–10 years, which excludes lens changes due to normal ageing. Their study group of 149 children with ID showed a prevalence of cataract or aphakia of 2%, whereas none of the 100 children in the control group had cataract.

Other ocular abnormalities

There are many ocular anomalies of which people with ID are at risk. For example, in their study of 494 UK Special Olympics athletes, Woodhouse *et al.* (2003) reported 28 separate abnormalities, excluding lens opacities. Here we consider only the most common sight-impairing conditions. Inclusion criterion was prevalence of named ocular anomalies (e.g. 'keratoconus' rather than 'corneal abnormality').

Table 14.4 shows the findings of the seven studies that fulfilled the above criterion. Many of the studies constituted screening and did not include full ophthalmological examination, so it is reasonable to presume that early or borderline conditions were missed. The nature of the studies would, therefore, underestimate the total number of ocular abnormalities. Keratoconus, a progressive distortion of the cornea, has an onset around adolescence, and therefore studies that include young children would underestimate the prevalence of this condition. Amongst adults, the prevalence of keratoconus in the general population is estimated to be 0.05% (Rabinowitz, 1998). Nystagmus has an overall prevalence of 0.05% to 0.01%, according to the UK charity Nystagmus Network, but this figure will probably include people with ID. Since optic nerve anomalies such as optic atrophy and optic nerve hypoplasia are associated

Table 14.4. Named sight-impairing ocular abnormalities and overall prevalence of all anomalies amongst individuals with ID

Study	Location	Population	Keratoconus	Nystagmus	Optic nerve abnormality	Overall prevalence of ocular anomalies
Tuppurainen (1983)	Finland	149 children aged 9–10* years selected from birth cohort	None reported	10.7%	5.4%	Not reported
Levy (1984)	Canada	298 people aged 20–40 years in a training/working environment	2.0%	6.4%	0.7%	49% (includes cataract and strabismus)
Jacobson (1988)	Sweden	228 people over 20 years old and resident in an institution	11.4%	0.9%	7.9%	59.2% (includes cataract)
Woodhouse et al. (2000)	UK	154 people over 19 years old and attending day centres	3.2%	3.9%	1.9%	22.08% (includes cataract)
Warburg (2001)	Denmark	837 people aged 20 years and over, resettled from institutions to community homes	2.2%	1.4%	5.0%	24% (includes cataract and high myopia)
Karadag et al. (2007)	Turkey	180 people aged 9–50* years attending a rehabilitation centre	0.6%	2.4%	1.2%	75.3% (includes cataract and strabismus)
Akinci et al. (2008)	Turkey	724 children aged 1–17* years attending a psychiatric clinic for initial evaluation	None reported	5.2%	0.27%	77% (includes refractive errors and strabismus)

Note that 'population' describes the number successfully completing testing for this attribute. * Inclusion of children may underestimate the prevalence of keratoconus compared to an adult population.

with visual impairment, studies of prevalence will be limited to studies of impairment and figures for the general population are difficult to estimate.

Cerebral visual impairment

Cerebral (or cortical) visual impairment is visual loss or visual disturbance attributed to brain injury or brain maldevelopment. The condition can range from mild difficulties with visual perceptual skills through to total blindness. Under screening conditions, it is seldom reported as the diagnosis is usually a process of elimination and requires full ophthalmological (and possibly neurological) examination. In studies of people with ID, the term is used to describe cases of visual impairment in which there is no obvious ocular defect. Only two studies report cerebral visual impairment. Warburg (2001) estimated that amongst 837 individuals with ID in Denmark, 6.1% had cerebral visual impairment. Kwok *et al.* (1996) studied 260 young people aged 3–25 years in Hong Kong. All had 'severe mental deficiency' and included 51 (19.6%) with cerebral visual impairment.

Conclusion

This chapter has restricted evaluation to the most rigorous studies of eye and vision disorders amongst people with ID. Exclusion and inclusion criteria have been strict, and, as a result, the total number of papers is small. The consequence is that data are reliable. The papers present results from a number of different locations worldwide and for a wide age range; the latter can make comparisons difficult. What has emerged is that people with ID are much more likely than members of the general population in the developed world to have unnecessary visual impairment because of uncorrected refractive errors. There is also evidence that this unnecessary impairment is more pronounced amongst people with more severe ID. This review shows that treatable impairment due to cataract is also more common, leading to the inevitable conclusion that people with ID are not accessing the same standard or frequency of eye care as the rest of the population. In addition, sight-impairing defects such as keratoconus, nystagmus and optic nerve anomalies have a higher prevalence. Overall, a large proportion of this vulnerable group has a level of sight that is markedly poorer than normal. The implications for primary eye care provision, ophthalmological treatment and rehabilitation services are obvious. This population is under-served and needs urgent attention to allow each and every person with ID to access quality eye care and visual rehabilitation.

References

Aitchison, C., Easty, D. L. and Jancar, J. (1990). Eye abnormalities in the mentally handicapped. *J Ment Defic Res*, 34, 41–8.

Akinci, A., Oner, O., Bozkurt, O. H. *et al.* (2008). Refractive errors and ocular findings in children with intellectual disability: a controlled study. *J AAPOS*, 12, 477–81.

Block, S. S., Beckerman, S. A. and Berman, P. E. (1997). Vision profile of the athletes of the 1995 Special Olympics World Summer Games. *J Am Optom Assoc*, 68, 699–708.

Buch, H., Vinding, T. and Nielson, N. V. (2001). Prevalence and causes of visual impairment according to World Health Organization and United States criteria in an aged, urban Scandinavian population: the Copenhagen City eye study. *Ophthalmology*, 108, 2347–57.

Evenhuis, H. M., Theunissen, M., Denkers, I., Verschuure, H. and Kemme, H. (2001). Prevalence of visual and hearing impairment in a dutch institutionalized population with intellectual disability. *J Intellec Disabil Res*, 45, 457–64.

Haire, A. R., Vernon, S. A. and Rubinstein, M. P. (1991). Levels of visual impairment in a day centre for people with a mental handicap. *J R Soc Med*, 84, 542–4.

Haugen, O. H., Aasved, H. and Bertelsen, T. (1995). Refractive state and correction of refractive errors among mentally retarded adults in a central institution. *Acta Ophthalmol Scand*, 73, 129–32.

Jacobson, L. (1988). Ophthalmology in mentally retarded adults. A clinical survey. *Acta Ophthalmol (Copenh)*, 66, 457–62.

Karadag, R., Yagci, R., Erdurmus, M. *et al.* (2007). Ocular findings in individuals with intellectual disability. *Can J Ophthalmol*, 42, 703–6.

Kwok, S. K., Ho, P. C., Chan, A. K., Gandhi, S. R. and Lam, D. S. (1996). Ocular defects in children and adolescents with severe mental deficiency. *J Intellect Disabil Res*, 40(4), 330–5.

Levy, B. (1984). Incidence of oculo-visual anomalies in an adult population of mentally retarded persons. *Am J Optom Physiol Opt*, 61, 324–6.

McCulloch, D. L., Sludden, P. A., McKeown, K. and Kerr, A. (1996). Vision care requirements among intellectually disabled adults: a residence-based pilot study. *J Intellect Disabil Res*, 40(2), 140–50.

Rabinowitz, Y. S. (1998). Keratoconus. *Surv Ophthalmol*, 42, 297–319.

Saunders, K. J. (1995). Early refractive development in humans. *Surv Ophthalmol*, 40, 207–16.

Sorsby, A., Sheridan, M., Leary, G. A. and Benjamin, B. (1960). Vision, visual acuity and ocular refraction of young men. *Br Med J*, 1, 1394–8.

Stocks, N. P., Patel, R., Sparrow, J. and Davey-Smith, G. (2002). Prevalence of cataract in the Speedwell Cardiovascular Study: a cross-sectional survey of men aged 65–83. *Eye*, 16, 275–80.

Tuppurainen, K. (1983). Ocular findings among mentally retarded children in Finland. *Acta Ophthalmol (Copenh)*, 61, 634–44.

Van Den Broek, E. G., Janssen, C. G., Van Ramshorst, T. and Deen, L. (2006). Visual impairments in people with severe and profound multiple disabilities: an inventory of visual functioning. *J Intellect Disabil Res*, 50, 470–5.

van Splunder, J., Stilma, J. S., Bernsen, R. M. and Evenhuis, H. M. (2004). Prevalence of ocular diagnoses found on screening 1539 adults with intellectual disabilities. *Ophthalmology*, 111, 1457–63.

Warburg, M. (2001). Visual impairment in adult people with moderate, severe, and profound intellectual disability. *Acta Ophthalmol Scand*, 79, 450–4.

Woodhouse, J. M., Griffiths, C. and Gedling, A. (2000). The prevalence of ocular defects and the provision of eye care in adults with learning disabilities living in the community. *Ophthalmic Physiol Opt*, 20, 79–89.

Woodhouse, J. M., Adler, P. M. and Duignan, A. (2003). Ocular and visual defects amongst people with intellectual disabilities participating in Special Olympics. *Ophthalmic Physiol Opt*, 23, 221–32.

Woodruff, M. E., Cleary, T. E. and Bader, D. (1980). The prevalence of refractive and ocular anomalies among 1242 institutionalized mentally retarded persons. *Am J Optom Physiol Opt*, 57, 70–84.

Systems disorders

Dentition and oral health diseases

Stefano Fedele and Crispian Scully

Introduction

Intellectual disability (ID) has been often associated with poor oral health (Dougall and Fiske, 2008; Stanfield *et al.*, 2003), but controversy exists as to whether or not this is related to a real increase in prevalence of oral diseases with respect to the general population (Dougall and Fiske, 2008). Oral health is often linked to systemic disease, and issues relevant to prevalence and management of oral diseases in individuals with ID appear to be similar to those of systemic diseases. This chapter attempts to review the available evidence regarding ID and oral health.

People with ID are known to experience poorer general health, have unmet health needs and have a lower uptake of screening services (The Royal College of Surgeons of England and British Society of Disability and Oral Health, 2001). Interestingly, ID has been often associated with poverty (in the UK about 39% of children with disability were reported to live below the official poverty level) (Emerson and Hatton, 2007) and the exposure to this economic disadvantage has been suggested to account for the health inequalities experienced by people with ID.

Oral health is reported to be significantly impaired in individuals with ID (Gallagher and Fiske, 2007; Kerr *et al.*, 1996). Systemic disease associated with ID and related chronic medical therapies have the potential to increase the risk of oral and dental diseases (e.g. dental caries and oral candidosis caused by drug-induced xerostomia). However, significant disparities in oral health care and outcomes are well known to exist in individuals with and without disability (Tiller *et al.*, 2001). In the UK it is unlawful for oral healthcare providers to treat people with disability less favourably and it is recognised that they should have equal access to oral healthcare services and equitable oral health outcomes (in terms of function, comfort, appearance and social interaction) (Dougall and Fiske, 2008). Nevertheless, as a consequence of deinstitutionalisation, people with ID currently rely on community and general dental practitioners who might not be experienced in and might lack the required skills for the challenging management of these individuals (Dougall and Fiske, 2008; Stanfield *et al.*, 2003).

Oral health in people with ID is an important issue. Oral diseases, as a group, represent a significant burden on the general population worldwide, but an even larger health problem in underprivileged groups, including individuals with disability, in both developing and developed countries (Petersen *et al.*, 2005). Whilst a few oral conditions are life-threatening (e.g. oral cancer and potentially malignant conditions), the vast majority of diseases affecting the soft and hard tissues of the oral cavity (e.g. dental caries, periodontitis, edentulism) are

Intellectual Disability and Ill Health: A Review of the Evidence, ed. Jean O'Hara, Jane McCarthy and Nick Bouras. Published by Cambridge University Press. © Cambridge University Press 2010.

chronic but can result in continuous pain and suffering, and can reduce the overall quality of life (Mignogna and Fedele, 2006). Oral diseases are also known to potentially alter individual psychosocial well-being, because of interference with fundamental activities, such as speaking, smiling, swallowing, kissing and conveying feelings and emotions through facial expressions (Mignogna and Fedele, 2006; Petersen *et al.*, 2005). Moreover, there is a strong correlation between chronic oral diseases and the four major chronic diseases (cardiovascular diseases, cancer, chronic respiratory diseases and diabetes), due to common risk factors (dietary factors, lack of exercise, tobacco and alcohol misuse) and possibly because of a potential pathogenetic association (at least between chronic oral infections and both diabetes and cardiovascular diseases) (Elter *et al.*, 2003; Mignogna and Fedele, 2006; Petersen *et al.*, 2005). The impact of all these aspects on the oral, general and psychological health of individuals with ID can be significant. For example, pain caused by dental diseases is known to have the potential to exacerbate pre-existing psychiatric disorders (McCall, 1991). The aim of this chapter is to critically review current evidence regarding the prevalence of oral and dental diseases in individuals with ID.

Method

A review on oral diseases and ID is restricted by the fact that little high-quality research has been done and differing terminologies and definitions have been used to indicate ID. Moreover, as ID can be part of a more generalised medical disorder, a portion of research and publications falls under the name of a specific medical condition or syndrome rather than ID (e.g. Down syndrome).

A search in MEDLINE was made to find studies on the association between ID and both prevalence of dental and oral diseases and provision of dental treatment. A broad search strategy included (i) electronic searching of PubMed database (1966–2008), (ii) hand searching the main dentistry and ID journals, (iii) checking references of included studies and reviews and (iv) clinical guidelines such as those developed by The Royal College of Surgeons of England Faculty of Dental Surgery and those from the British Society of Disability and Oral Health. The MeSH terms used were 'intellectual disability', 'learning disability', 'mental retardation', 'developmental disability' and 'oral health', 'dentistry' and 'dental'. The first search was made in May 2008 and updated in July 2008. The focus was on studies regarding epidemiology of oral and dental disease in individuals with ID. The title and abstract of each article resulting from the different search strategies were examined separately by the two authors. When at least one author considered the article relevant, it progressed in the review process and was included in a digital archive prepared using dedicated software. Full reports were obtained for all relevant studies. No restriction as to language was applied.

Results

The number of references/hits was 23 for 'learning disability AND dentistry', 21 for 'intellectual disability AND dentistry', 32 for 'learning disability AND dental', 26 for 'intellectual disability AND dental', 8 for 'learning disability AND oral health', 14 for 'intellectual disability AND oral health', 148 for 'developmental disabilities and dental', 1045 for 'mental retardation AND dental', giving a total of 1317. After abstract reading, 127 were found to be relevant to oral dental disease and intellectual disability. Among these 127 papers, 23 were specifically focused on epidemiology of oral diseases. (Please refer to Table 15.1.) Evidence included

Table 15.1. Search results for ID and epidemiology of oral diseases

References before abstract reading and before evidence-based screening	1317
References after abstract reading and before evidence-based screening	127
References after evidence-based screening	23

high-quality population-based studies with a control group, population-based studies and longitudinal studies.

Discussion

There is controversial evidence whether or not individuals with ID experience more oral diseases than the general population. Certainly, many studies from the UK and abroad have consistently found that people with ID have more untreated dental decay, more extractions, worse oral hygiene levels and more gum inflammation and periodontal disease than the general population (Francis *et al.*, 1991; Gizani *et al.*, 1997; Nunn, 1987; Shyma *et al.*, 2000). Long-term longitudinal studies also showed that the incidence of tooth loss due to periodontal disease is higher among individuals with ID compared to the general population (Gabre *et al.*, 1999). However, many other studies have found similar prevalence estimates of decayed, missing and filled teeth among individuals with ID compared to those in the general population, even though these studies included individuals living in all types of environments and with varying levels of ID (Cumella *et al.*, 2000; Nowak, 1984; Tesini, 1981; Whyman *et al.*, 1995). Indeed the major difference between these two groups of studies relies on the characteristics of the population studied. Research including individuals with ID as a single group usually found no increased prevalence of oral and dental disease with respect to the general population. Studies differentiating individuals on the basis of degree of disability (mild versus moderate) and social environment (institution versus community or own home and socio-economic deprivation of the area where they live) usually did find significant differences with respect to the general population and also within different subgroups of individuals with disability. For example, a study researching the oral health of participants at the 2005 Glasgow Special Olympics (SO), showed that SO participants with ID had relatively good dental health (in terms of fewer fillings and untreated decay) compared with the general population studied in the 1998 UK Adult Dental Health Survey (ADHS) (Turner *et al.*, 2008). However, it was highlighted that SO participants are hardly representative of most people with ID as they are younger and have less severe disability, and thus are likely to be healthier, better supported and integrated (Reid *et al.*, 2003; Turner *et al.*, 2008). A low incidence of dental caries was observed in another longitudinal study on a population of individuals with ID provided with preventive dental care and optimal fluoride concentration in drinking water (Gabre *et al.*, 2001). In general, within the group of individuals with ID, the prevalence and incidence of dental caries among those living in institutions or in richer areas is low compared to individuals living in community, among relatives or in poorer areas (Pezzementi and Fisher, 2005; Rodríguez Vázquez *et al.*, 2002).

Smaller studies showed that ID is observed in about 46% of children with cleft palate (Broder *et al.*, 1998) and that congenital insensitivity to pain, leading to self-mutilation of oral tissues and progression of untreated dental caries, can be associated with ID in the context of hereditary sensory and autonomic neuropathies (Butler *et al.*, 2006).

When the type of oral health care provided rather than the prevalence of oral disease is studied, significant disparities are evident between individuals with and without ID. People with ID living in community settings are less likely to have received dental treatment and, even when treatment is offered, it is more likely to result in tooth extractions rather than more conservative treatments such as restorations, crowns and bridges (Tiller *et al.*, 2001).

Conclusion

Overall, individuals with ID as a group seem not to have an increased prevalence of oral and dental disease with respect to the general population but they are less likely to receive appropriate and conservative dental treatment. Individuals with severe ID and those living in the community or in deprived areas have an increased prevalence of oral disease with respect to the general population, individuals with mild ID or those living in less deprived areas. Some subgroups of individuals with mild ID and high levels of care and assistance can even have better oral health than the general population.

However, there are no definitive data regarding the association between ID and oral diseases. Results of studies should be considered with caution as (i) the population of individuals with ID is non-homogeneous (ii) subgroups of individuals can present co-morbid medical disorders that have the potential to increase the risk of oral diseases and (iii) the socio-economic environment surrounding people with ID can affect their risk of oral disease and their access to oral health care.

Further research should investigate the prevalence of oral disease with respect to variables such as different degree of disability, age, co-morbid disorders and socio-economic environments.

References

Broder, H. L., Richman, L. C. and Matheson, P. B. (1998). Learning disability, school achievement, and grade retention among children with cleft: a two-center study. *Cleft Palate Craniofac J*, 35, 127–31.

Butler, J., Fleming, P. and Webb, D. (2006). Congenital insensitivity to pain–review and report of a case with dental implications. *Oral Surg Oral Med Oral Pathol Oral Radiol Endod*, 101, 58–62.

Cumella, S., Ransford, N., Lyons, J. and Burnham, H. (2000). Needs for oral care among people with intellectual disability not in contact with community dental services. *J Intellect Disabil Res*, 44, 45–52.

Dougall, A. and Fiske, J. (2008). Access to special care dentistry, part 1. Access. *Br Dent J*, 204, 605–16.

Elter, J. R., Offenbacher, S., Toole, J. F. and Beck, J. D. (2003). Relationship of periodontal disease and edentulism to stroke/TIA. *J Dent Res*, 82, 998–1001.

Emerson, E. and Hatton, C. (2007). Poverty socio-economic position, social capital and the health of children and adolescents with intellectual disabilities in Britain: a replication. *J Intellect Disabil Res*, 51, 866–74.

Francis, J. R., Stevenson, D. R. and Palmer, J. D. (1991). Dental health and dental care requirements for young handicapped adults in Wessex. *Community Dent Health*, 8, 131–7.

Gabre, P., Martinsson, T. and Gahnberg, L. (1999). Incidence of, and reasons for, tooth mortality among mentally retarded adults during a 10-year period. *Acta Odontol Scand*, 57, 55–61.

Gabre, P., Martinsson, T. and Gahnberg, L. (2001). Longitudinal study of dental caries, tooth mortality and interproximal bone loss in adults with intellectual disability. *Eur J Oral Sci*, 109, 20–6.

Gallagher, J. E. and Fiske, J. (2007). Special care dentistry: a professional challenge. *Br Dent J*, 202, 619–29.

Gizani, S., Declerck, D., Vinckier, F. *et al.* (1997). Oral health condition of 12-year-old handicapped children in Flanders (Belgium). *Community Dent Oral Epidemiol*, 25, 352–7.

Kerr, M., Richards, D. and Glover, G. (1996). Primary care for people with a learning disability – a group practice survey. *J Appl Res Intellect Disabil*, 9, 347–52.

McCall, W. V. (1991). Exacerbation of mental illness by dental disease. *Psychosomatics*, 32, 114–15.

Mignogna, M. D. and Fedele, S. (2006). The neglected global burden of chronic oral diseases. *J Dent Res*, 85, 390–91.

Nowak, A. J. (1984). Dental disease in handicapped persons. *Spec Care Dentist*, 4, 66–9.

Nunn, J. H. (1987). The dental health of mentally and physically handicapped children: a review of the literature. *Community Dent Health*, 4, 157–68.

Petersen, P. E., Bourgeois, D., Ogawa, H., Estupinan-Day, S. and Ndiaye, C. (2005). The global burden of oral diseases and risks to oral health. *Bull WHO*, 83, 661–9.

Pezzementi, M. L. and Fisher, M. A. (2005). Oral health status of people with intellectual disabilities in the southeastern United States. *J Am Dent Assoc*, 136, 903–12.

Reid, B., Chenette, R. and Macek, M. (2003). Prevalence and predictors of untreated caries and oral pain among Special Olympics athletes. *Spec Care Dentist*, 23, 139–42.

Rodríguez Vázquez, C., Garcillan, R., Rioboo, R. and Bratos, E. (2002). Prevalence of dental caries in an adult population with mental disabilities in Spain. *Spec Care Dentist*, 22, 65–9.

The Royal College of Surgeons of England and British Society of Disability and Oral Health (2001). *Clinical Guidelines and Integrated Care Pathways for the Oral Health Care of People with Learning Disabilities*. Available from: http://www.bsdh.org.uk/guidelines.html (accessed on 15 September 2008).

Shyma, M., Al-Mutawa Honkala, S., Sugathan, T. and Honkala, E. (2000). Oral hygiene and periodontal conditions in special needs children and young adults in Kuwait. *J Disabil Oral Health*, 1, 13–19.

Stanfield, M., Scully, C., Davison, M. F. and Porter, S. R. (2003). The oral health of clients with learning disability: changes following relocation from hospital to community. *Br Dent J*, 194, 271–7.

Tesini, D. A. (1981). An annotated review of the literature of dental caries and periodontal disease in mentally retarded individuals. *Spec Care Dentist*, 1, 75–87.

Tiller, S., Wilson, K. I. and Gallagher, J. E. (2001). The dental health and dental service use of adults with learning disabilities. *Community Dent Health*, 18, 167–71.

Turner, S., Sweeney, M., Kennedy, C. and Macpherson, L. (2008). The oral health of people with intellectual disability participating in the UK Special Olympics. *J Intellect Disabil Res*, 52, 29–36.

Whyman, R. A., Treasure, E. T., Brown, R. H. and MacFadyen, E. E. (1995). The oral health of long-term residents of a hospital for the intellectually handicapped and psychiatrically ill. *N Z Dent J*, 91, 49–56.

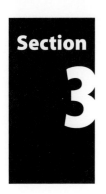

Section 3

Disorders of the nervous system and neurodevelopment

16 Mental illness

Stephen Ruedrich

Introduction

The medical or psychiatric evaluation of persons with intellectual disability (ID) is often complicated by issues of assessment itself. Individuals with ID have limited ability to characterise problems or cooperate with standard physical examination. However, if clinicians can obtain standardised assessments, diagnosis of most medical/physical illness is substantively similar to that of individuals without ID (US Public Health Service, 2001).

The presence of ID affects both the individual's ability to participate in assessment and the form of the psychiatric/behavioural disorder(s) itself (Sturmey, 2007). In the central nervous system, ID and psychiatric/behavioural disorders are co-occurring and interdependent (Harris, 2006). The presence and type of psychiatric disorder(s) seen are dependent on, and influenced by, the aetiology of ID, as well as the developmental level and life experience of the person (Tsakanikos *et al.*, 2007).

The prevalence of psychiatric illnesses in people with ID also depends on age and gender, diagnostic strategy employed, experience of the examiner, setting and any current treatment already in place (Sturmey, 2007). Ideally, attempts to characterise psychiatric disorders in persons with ID should utilise a recognised diagnostic classification system and standardised assessments and should be population-based; include all ages, genders and levels of severity; be over multiple observations (O'Hara, 2007).

Diagnostic systems in psychiatry

Most reports of psychiatric disorders in people with ID have utilised the two mainstream diagnostic systems available: the Diagnostic and Statistical Manual of Mental Disorders (DSM) or International Classification of Diseases (ICD); current versions are the DSM-IV and DSM-IV-TR and the ICD-10 (APA, 1994; WHO, 1992). Neither system is universally applicable to individuals with ID, particularly those with limited communication abilities and/or more severe ID (Fletcher *et al.*, 2007). Two additional diagnostic manuals have been recently proffered to address this difficulty: the Diagnostic Criteria for Psychiatric Disorders for use with Adults with Learning Disabilities/Mental Retardation (DC-LD) (RCP, 2001) and the Diagnostic Manual for Intellectual Disabilities (DM-ID) (Fletcher *et al.*, 2007). The DC-LD is intended to be utilised for adults, as a companion to the ICD-10. It has undergone significant field testing (52 field investigators; over 700 patients), demonstrating acceptable validity and reliability (Cooper *et al.*, 2003). The DM-ID is not yet field tested, although an initial clinician survey (63 clinicians, 845 patients) reported significant satisfaction (Fletcher *et al.*, 2009).

Intellectual Disability and Ill Health: A Review of the Evidence, ed. Jean O'Hara, Jane McCarthy and Nick Bouras. Published by Cambridge University Press. © Cambridge University Press 2010.

Table 16.1. Search results

Database	Number of references	With evidence-based medicine screen
PubMed/MEDLINE	731	51
CINAHL	713	6
PsycFIRST	190	14
PBHSC	193	14

Concepts of co-morbidity (dual diagnosis)

Individuals with ID appear susceptible to the entire range of mental illnesses (Harris, 2006). Behavioural or emotional difficulties seen in people with ID were previously attributed to the ID itself, characterised as 'diagnostic overshadowing' (Reiss *et al.*, 1982). The contemporary concept of 'dual diagnosis' (co-occurring psychiatric disorder and ID) is attributed to Meno-lascino (Schroeder *et al.*, 1998). Three theoretical constructs have been posited to explain dual diagnosis (Harris, 2006):

1. Psychiatric illness and ID arise from the same underlying neurobiological substrate.
2. Individuals with ID are specifically vulnerable to developing psychiatric disorder(s), surrounding stressful life circumstances and compromised coping capacity.
3. Severe social and environmental deprivation can sometimes result in both ID and psychiatric illness.

Most scholars combine the first two explanations, arguing that dual diagnosis combines neurobiological predisposition, stressful life events and limited coping skills, resulting in specific co-morbidities (Cowley *et al.*, 2004).

Method

The electronic databases PubMed, CINAHL, PsycFIRST, and Psychology and Behavioural Health Sciences Collection (PBHSC) were searched, along with selective hand searches of psychiatric and ID journals.

Electronic searches employed the specialised MeSH terms and keywords: intellectual disabilities, mental retardation, learning disabilities, mental disorders/illness, psychiatric disorders/illness, behavioural disorders, dual diagnosis/epidemiology, diagnostic systems, DSM-IV, ICD-10, DC-LD.

Initial searches were conducted in summer 2008. Abstracts were screened, relevant abstracts read and potentially relevant articles inspected in more detail. Reports in English or with English abstracts were included.

Results

The total number of references found was 1827; reduced to 85 by applying an evidence-based medicine screen (please refer to Table 16.1). The types of references identified were: population-based studies, some with comparison controls; large non-controlled case series, reviews and book chapters.

Discussion

Prevalence studies

Prevalence reports can be categorised into five sometimes-overlapping groups:

1. Large population studies
2. Large institutional or community-based samples
3. Reviews of people with ID referred for psychiatric evaluation
4. Reviews of specific psychiatric disorders
5. Reviews of co-morbidity of specific psychiatric disorders with a specific ID aetiology.

Population studies

The most classic population study was from the Isle of Wight, UK in the 1960–70s; children aged 9–11 with ID were much more likely to have psychiatric disorders, compared to their peers (Rutter *et al.*, 1976). Borthwick-Duffy and Eyman (1990) reported 10% of 78 000 persons in California with ID had a dual diagnosis; Stromme and Diseth (2000) found that 37% of 30 000 Norwegian children with ID had co-morbid psychiatric illness, utilising ICD-10. In an Australian sample, 23% of 42 000 adults with ID had ICD-10 psychotic, depressive or anxiety disorders (White *et al.*, 2005).

Large institutional and community-based samples

Many studies focus specifically on individuals with ID, in either hospital or community settings. Lund (1985) reported that 27% of 302 Danish adults with ID manifested psychiatric disorder. The prevalence of co-morbid psychiatric illness was 15% of 1273 institutionalised adults in Virginia, USA (Crews *et al.*, 1994). Finally, Cooper *et al.* (2007a) examined over 1000 adults with ID utilising the DC-LD, ICD-10 and DSM-IV-TR. Point prevalence of psychiatric disorder was 35.2% for the DC-LD, 16.6% for ICD-10 and 15.7% for DSM-IV-TR.

Reviews of people with ID referred for psychiatric evaluation

Not surprisingly, prevalence of co-morbidity in referred individuals is even higher, ranging from 68% of adults (using the DSM-III); 90% of individuals with severe/profound ID (DSM-III-R), to 60% of young adults (using ICD-10) (Eaton and Menolascino, 1982; King *et al.*, 1994; Kishore *et al.*, 2004). Using ICD-10, Bouras *et al.* (2003) found 53% of 752 adults referred to a specialist mental health service over 18 years had psychiatric illness.

Reviews of specific psychiatric disorders

Multiple studies focus on specific psychiatric disorders in persons with ID, often seen in specialised diagnostic/treatment settings.

Attention deficit hyperactivity disorder (ADHD)

Fox and Wade (1998) reported that 15% of adults with severe/profound ID had co-morbid ADHD, using DSM-IV criteria. Hastings *et al.* (2005) found 60% of children with ID had ADHD, compared to only 2.7% of their siblings without ID. Tonge (2007) followed 500 children with ID over a 14-year period, reporting symptoms of ADHD decreased from 32% to 14%, perhaps reflecting a maturational effect. Seager and O'Brien's (2003) review of over 200 studies concluded that rates were substantially higher than in the general population, especially among those with severe ID. (Please refer to Chapter 17 on Neurodevelopmental disorders.)

Mood disorders

Mood disorders have been widely studied. Richards *et al.* (2001) found a fourfold greater risk of affective disorder among those with ID, by age 40. Tonge (2007) reported stable rates of depression (9%) in Australian children with ID over a 14-year period. Masi *et al.* (1999) estimated 20% of adolescents with ID could have dysthymic disorder. Cooper *et al.* (2007b) described point prevalence for depression of 3.8%, 0.6% for mania and 1.0% for bipolar illness in remission. Stavrakaki and Lunsky (2007) concluded that mood disorders are common, and more frequent than previously considered.

Psychotic disorders

Reports describing psychotic disorders in ID span 100 years. Conventional wisdom holds that schizophrenia can be reliably diagnosed in individuals with mild ID, but is problematic with more severe ID (Clarke, 2007). Melville (2003) noted that little research has addressed the validity or reliability of ICD-10 non-affective psychotic disorders in ID. White *et al.* (2005) found 1.3% of persons with ID had psychotic disorders. Cooper *et al.* (2007b) found 2.6%, using the ICD-10. Prevalence utilising the DC-LD was higher at 3.8%. In two large Australian cohorts, Morgan *et al.* (2008) reported that 3.7–5.2% of people with ID had co-morbid schizophrenia.

Eating disorders

Gravestock (2003) reviewed eating disorders (ED) in ID, noting few controlled or population studies. Most reports are descriptions of abnormal eating behaviours (AEB) in specific ID syndromes (e.g. hyperphagia in Prader-Willi syndrome). The DC-LD has broadened the diagnosis of ED beyond anorexia, bulimia and pica (in ICD-10 and DSM-IV), to include other AEB often seen in ID. Ali (2001) reported pica in 9–25% of individuals with ID in institutional settings, and Cooper *et al.* (2007b) found 2% in > 1000 community-based individuals.

Substance misuse

Traditionally, substance misuse has been under-reported in ID (McGillicuddy, 2006). Burgard *et al.* (2000) found that adults with ID are just as likely as their peers without ID to abuse alcohol, but not other drugs. Taggart *et al.* (2006) reported that 75% of substance abusers with ID had primarily alcohol-related problems. Hassiotis *et al.* (2008) reported prevalent substance misuse among community-living individuals with borderline intellectual functioning, compared to their peers in the general population.

Anxiety disorders

Stavrakaki and Mintsioulis (1997) reported that most of the referred adults with ID and anxiety disorders had experienced a major life event or trauma in the preceding six months, and Sequeira *et al.* (2003) reported that 35% of 54 adults with ID who had suffered sexual abuse met criteria for post-traumatic stress disorder (PTSD). Tonge (2007) reported that longitudinal anxiety prevalence rates for boys remained near 8%; but in girls increased to 20%. Cooper *et al.* (2007b) reported anxiety disorder prevalence at 2.8%, but Bailey and Andrews (2003) concluded that true prevalence estimates await more systematic research.

Obsessive-compulsive disorders (OCD)

Bodfish *et al.* (1995) reported that 40% of adults with severe/profound ID had compulsions, but Cooper *et al.* (2007b) found only a 0.2% prevalence of OCD in a community sample. The overlap between OCD and autism may create difficulty in determining true prevalence rates (Bailey and Andrews, 2003).

Dementia

Dementia is associated with ageing in people with Down syndrome (DS), but Cooper (1997) found 21% of elderly persons with other causes of ID also had dementia. However, Zigman *et al.* (2004), in New York State, found that rates of dementia in individuals with ID (excluding DS) no different from persons without ID. Strydom *et al.* (2007) screened 222 adults with ID above age 60 (none with DS) with DSM-IV, ICD-10 and DC-LD. All yielded similar rates of dementia (9.9–12.2%), with Alzheimer's subtype the most common (8.6%). (Please refer to Chapter 19 on Neurodegenerative diseases.)

Personality disorders (PD)

The diagnosis of PD in people with ID is controversial. Reported prevalence varies widely (1–22%); over time, setting and diagnostic assessment utilised (Cooper *et al.*, 2007b; Lindsay, 2007). Alexander and Cooray (2003) noted the lack of accurate evidence-based prevalence data, and argued that PD diagnosis in people with severe ID may not be possible.

Behaviour disorders

Behavioural disorders are common in people with ID, but difficult to quantify. Cooper *et al.* (2007a) found 22.5% of a large sample demonstrated problem behaviour. The ICD-10 allows for coding of behavioural problems across a variety of other categories (WHO, 1992). The DC-LD provides diagnostic criteria for 12 separate problem behaviours, and/or associates problem behaviour with pervasive developmental disorders, psychiatric illness, personality disorders and medical conditions (RCP, 2001). In a cross-sectional sample of 214 adults with ID, Hemmings *et al.* (2006) reported problem behaviours in more than 10%, and noted that self-injurious and aggressive behavioural problems were associated with affective type symptoms.

Reviews of co-morbidity of specific psychiatric disorders with a specific ID aetiology (behavioural phenotypes)

Newer studies focus on psychiatric disorders in persons with ID of known aetiology. 'Behavioural phenotype' has been defined as 'the heightened probability or likelihood that people with a given syndrome will exhibit certain behavioural or developmental sequel relative to those without the syndrome' (Hodapp and Dykens, 2007).

Down syndrome (DS)

Most widely studied is the behavioural phenotype associated with DS. Utilising ICD-10 criteria, 10% of children and adults with DS have co-morbid autism (Pary and DesNoyers-Hurley, 2002). However, children with DS have fewer serious behavioural problems than age- and ID-matched peers (Dykens, 2007). In adults with DS, depression is common (6–11%) (Dykens, 2007); and bipolar illness uncommon (Craddock and Owen, 1994). The early onset of degenerative dementia Alzheimer's disease may develop as much as 30 years earlier than in the general population (Holland *et al.*, 1998). Using ICD-10, Mantry *et al.* (2008) reported point prevalence in DS for any psychiatric disorder of 11.3% (19% with DC-LD), making psychiatric illness less prevalent in DS compared to other ID aetiologies.

Prader-Willi syndrome (PWS)

Children and adults with PWS demonstrate frequent tantrums, impulsivity, stubbornness and skin-picking relative to peers with ID (Dykens, 2000; Hiraiwa *et al.*, 2007). Adults are susceptible to mood disorders and psychosis (Dykens, 2000). Clarke *et al.* (2002) found 24–49% of adults with PWS demonstrated ritualistic behaviour.

Fragile X syndrome (FRAX)

Males with FRAX typically suffer autistic spectrum disorder, ADHD and social anxiety; women tend to suffer social anxiety and depressive disorders (Dykens, 2000). Munir *et al.* (2000) described attentional problems in boys with FRAX. Hall *et al.* (2008) compared boys and girls with FRAX; finding boys had more self-injurious behaviour (SIB) (58% vs. 17%) and autistic spectrum disorders (50% vs. 20%).

Williams syndrome (WS)

Children and adolescents with WS demonstrate anxiety, hyperactivity, insomnia and hyperacusis (Einfeld *et al.*, 2001). Dykens (2003) found high rates of generalised anxiety (60%) and specific phobias (80%). Leyfer *et al.* (2006) reported 80% of children with WS had at least one DSM-IV disorder, primarily ADHD (65%) and phobias (54%).

Velo-cardio-facial syndrome (VCFS)

Children with VCFS have high rates of ADHD and anxiety and mood disorders; adults frequently develop psychotic disorders, particularly schizophrenia (Murphy, 2005). Antshel *et al.* (2006) reported ADHD, major depression and simple phobia. Shprintzen (2008) concluded that individuals with VCFS were 25 times more likely to manifest severe psychiatric illnesses than the general population.

Smith-Magenis syndrome (SMS)

Finucane *et al.* (2001) found nearly universal SIB in individuals with SMS. Edelman *et al.* (2007) found SIB, aggression and hyperactivity in a meta-analysis of 105 individuals with SMS.

Other aetiologies of ID currently under investigation to characterise possible behavioural phenotypes include fetal alcohol syndrome, Angelman syndrome and Rett syndrome amongst others (RCP, 2001).

Treatment of psychiatric and behavioural disorders

The lack of systematic studies of psychiatric diagnosis in ID is eclipsed by a greater dearth of treatment studies. Individuals with ID are routinely excluded from psychiatric treatment research (Dykens, 2007). Although psychotropic medications are widely utilised in individuals with ID, few large treatment trials are adequately scientifically sound to guide the field (Deb *et al.*, 2007). An exception may be risperidone, for which there does appear sufficient evidence to support its use in individuals with autistic disorders, both for disruptive and self-injurious behaviour, as well as repetitive, stereotyped core features (RUPP, 2005). However, in a recent controlled study, Tyrer *et al.* (2008) found no advantage for risperidone or haloperidol over placebo in the treatment of adults with ID and aggressive behaviour. An additional complication is the long-standing practice in ID psychiatry of treating symptoms in people with ID (e.g. aggression and self-injury), rather than disorders (Tsiouris *et al.*, 2003). In the absence of evidence-based information, a consensus-based approach has been offered (Rush and Frances, 2000).

Choice of psychotropic medication must take into account co-morbid medical conditions, be part of multidisciplinary treatment and be based on accurate psychiatric diagnosis and informed consent. Care must be taken to monitor for drug side effects using standardised instruments, seeking to use the lowest dose, with systematic reviews in place, and avoidance of frequent drug and dose changes (Kalachnik *et al.*, 1998). Reviews of psychopharmacological treatments in people with ID include Deb *et al.* (2007, 2008); King (2007); Reiss and Aman (1998); Rush and Frances (2000) and Sohanpal *et al.* (2007)

Behavioural, psychosocial and psychotherapeutic treatments are equally valid. Treatment must be individualised, and modified to address developmental level. Behavioural interventions have been successfully utilised for co-morbid depression, psychosis and anxiety/phobic disorders, although most reports are of uncontrolled studies (Benson and Havercamp, 2007). Psychosocial treatments have not yet become specialised for application to individuals with ID (Dagnan, 2007). Psychodynamic psychotherapy has been utilised in many treatment settings, including trauma/abuse, loss/bereavement, anger/aggression and sexual offending (Parkes and Hollins, 2007). Several small but methodologically sound studies support its utility. Reviews of non-pharmacological treatments of people with ID include Benson and Havercamp (2007) and Dagnan (2007).

Conclusion

Mental illness is common in people with ID. Prevalence rates in population studies range from 10% to 39%, for both children and adults, making mental illness 3–5 times more common than in those without ID. A large population study using the DC-LD more than doubled the reported prevalence of co-morbid mental illness (35%), compared to the ICD-10 and DSM-IV (Cooper *et al.*, 2007b). In institutional settings, rates are higher, ranging from 30% to 50%, and in referred populations may reach 70–90%.

Several specific psychiatric disorders are more common in people with ID. These include ADHD (15–60%); mood disorders (3.8–9%); psychotic disorders (1.3–4.4%); and anxiety disorders (2.8–27%). Less prevalent may be substance misuse and classic eating disorders. The overlap of OCD with autistic spectrum disorders complicates the understanding of the presentation of both disorders. Dementia appears more prevalent in ID than in the general population, even when individuals with DS are excluded. Personality and behavioural disorders are prevalent but more difficult to assess in people with ID. Newer diagnostic systems will hopefully address these methodological problems. Future study of behavioural phenotypes may lead the field back to an aetiologically orientated approach to psychiatric diagnosis, with less emphasis on stratification approaches based on severity of ID.

The paucity of psychiatric diagnostic research is eclipsed by even fewer methodologically sound treatment studies. Currently, the best guide for choosing psychopharmacological and/or psychosocial treatments is establishment of an accurate psychiatric diagnosis. It is hoped the advent of new diagnostic systems in ID psychiatry in the UK and USA will improve diagnostic accuracy, such that treatment studies will follow.

References

Alexander, R. and Cooray, S. (2003). Diagnosis of personality disorders in learning disability. *Br J Psychiatry*, 44(Suppl), S28–31.

Ali, Z. (2001). Pica in people with intellectual disability: a literature review of aetiology, epidemiology and complications. *J Intellect Dev Disabil*, 26, 205–15.

American Psychiatric Association (APA) (1994). *Diagnostic and Statistical Manual of Mental Disorders: Fourth Edition.* Washington DC: American Psychiatric Association.

Antshel, K. M., Fremont, W., Roizen, N. J. *et al.* (2006). ADHD, major depressive disorder, and simple phobia are prevalent psychiatric conditions in youth with velocardiofacial syndromes. *J Am Acad Child Adolesc Psychiatry*, 45, 596–603.

Bailey, N. M. and Andrews, T. M. (2003). *Diagnostic Criteria for Psychiatric Disorders for Use with Adults with Learning Disability/Mental Retardation* (DC-LD) and the diagnosis of anxiety disorders: a review. *J Intellect Disabil Res*, 47(Suppl), 50–61.

Benson, B. and Havercamp, S. (2007). Behavioural approaches to treatment: principles and practices. In *Psychiatric and Behavioural Disorders in Intellectual and Developmental Disabilities*, 2nd edn., ed. N. Bouras and G. Holt. Cambridge: Cambridge University Press, pp. 283–309.

Bodfish, J. W., Crawford, T. W., Powell, S. B. *et al.* (1995). Compulsions in adults with mental retardation: prevalence, phenomenology, and comorbidity with stereotypy and self-injury. *Am J Ment Retard*, 100(2), 183–92.

Borthwick-Duffy S. A. and Eyman, R. K. (1990). Who are the dually diagnosed? *Am J Ment Retard*, 94, 586–95.

Bouras, N., Cowley, A., Holt, G., Newton, J. T. and Sturmey, P. (2003). Referral trends of people with intellectual disability and psychiatric disorder. *J Intellect Disabil Res*, 47, 439–46.

Burgard, J. F., Donohue, B., Azrin, N. H. and Teichner, G. (2000). Prevalence and treatment of substance abuse in the mentally retarded population: an empirical review. *J Psychoactive Drugs*, 32(3), 293–8.

Clarke, D. (2007). Schizophrenia spectrum disorders in people with intellectual disabilities. In *Psychiatric and Behavioural Disorders in Intellectual and Developmental Disabilities*, 2nd edn., ed. N. Bouras and G. Holt. Cambridge: Cambridge University Press, pp. 131–42.

Clarke, D. J., Boer, H., Whittington J. *et al.* (2002). Prader-Willi syndrome, compulsion and ritualistic behavior: the first population-based survey. *Br J Psychiatry*, 180, 358–62.

Cooper, S. A. (1997). High prevalence of dementia amongst people with learning disabilities not attributed to Down syndrome. *Psychol Med*, 27, 609–16.

Cooper, S. A., Melville, C. A. and Einfeld, S. L. (2003). Psychiatric diagnosis, intellectual disabilities, and Diagnostic Criteria for Psychiatric Disorders for Use with Adults with Learning Disability/Mental Retardation (DC-LD). *J Intellect Disabil Res*, 47, 3–15.

Cooper S. A., Smiley, E., Morrison, J., Williamson, A. and Allan, L. (2007a). An epidemiological investigation of affective disorders with a population-based cohort of 1023 adults with intellectual disabilities. *Psychol Med*, 37(6), 873–82.

Cooper, S. A., Smiley, E., Morrison, J., Williamson, A. and Allan, L. (2007b). Mental ill-health in adults with intellectual disabilities: prevalence and associated factors. *Br J Psychiatry*, 190, 27–35.

Cowley, A., Holt, G., Bouras, N. *et al.* (2004). Descriptive psychopathology in people with mental retardation. *J Nerv Ment Dis*, 192, 232–7.

Craddock, N. and Owen, M. (1994). Is there an inverse relationship between Down's syndrome and bipolar affective disorder? Literature review and genetic implications. *J Intellect Disabil Res*, 38, 613–20.

Crews, W. D., Bonaventura, S. and Rowe, F. (1994). Dual diagnosis: prevalence of psychiatric disorders in a large state residential facility for individuals with mental retardation. *Am J Ment Retard*, 98, 724–31.

Dagnan, D. (2007). Psychosocial interventions for people with intellectual disabilities. In *Psychiatric and Behavioural Disorders in Intellectual and Developmental Disabilities*, 2nd edn., ed. N. Bouras and G. Holt. Cambridge: Cambridge University Press, pp. 330–8.

Deb, S., Sohanpal, S. K., Soni, L., Lenotre, L. and Unwin, G. (2007). The effectiveness of antipsychotic medication in the management of behaviour problems in adults with intellectual disabilities. *J Intellect Disabil Res*, 51, 766–77.

Deb, S., Chaplin, R., Sohanpal, S. *et al.* (2008). The effectiveness of mood stabilizers and antiepileptic medication for the management of behaviour problems in adults with intellectual disability: a systemic review. *J Intellect Disabil Res*, 52, 107–13.

Dykens, E. (2000). Psychopathology in children with intellectual disability. *J Child Psychol Psychiatry*, 41, 407–17.

Dykens, E. (2003). Anxiety, fears, and phobias in persons with Williams syndrome. *Dev Neuropsychol*, 23(1 and 2), 291–316.

Dykens, E. (2007). Psychiatric and behavioral disorders in persons with Down syndrome. *Ment Retard Dev Disabil Res Rev*, 13, 272–8.

Eaton, L. F. and Menolascino, F. J. (1982). Psychiatric disorders in the mentally retarded: types, problems, and challenges. *Am J Psychiatry*, 139, 1297–303.

Edelman, E. A., Girirajan, S., Finucane, B. *et al.* (2007). Gender, genotype, and phenotype differences in Smith-Magenis syndromes: a meta-analysis of 105 cases. *Clin Genet*, 71, 540–50.

Einfeld, S. L., Tonge, B. J. and Rees, V. W. (2001). Longitudinal course of behavioral and emotional problems in Williams syndrome. *Am J Ment Retard*, 106, 73–81.

Finucane, B., Dirrigl, K. H. and Simon, E. W. (2001). Characterization of self-injurious behaviors in children and adults with Smith-Magenis syndrome. *Am J Ment Retard*, 106, 52–8.

Fletcher, R., Loschen, E., Stavakake, C. and First, M. (2007). *Diagnostic Manual-Intellectual Disability: A Clinical Guide for Diagnosis of Mental Disorders in Persons with Intellectual Disability.* Kingston: NADD Press.

Fletcher, R. J., Havercamp, S. M., Ruedrich, S. L. *et al.* (2009). Clinical usefulness of the Diagnostic Manual-Intellectual Disability for Mental Disorders in persons with intellectual disability: results from a brief field survey. *J Clin Psychiatry*, June 2, e1–8; doi: 10.4088/JCP.08m04429.

Fox, R. A. and Wade, E. J. (1998). Attention deficit hyperactivity disorder among adults with severe and profound mental retardation. *Res Dev Disabil*, 19, 275–80.

Gravestock, S. (2003). Diagnosis and classification of eating disorders in adults with intellectual disability: The Diagnostic Criteria for Psychiatric Disorders for Use with Adults with Learning Disability/Mental Retardation (DC-LD) approach. *J Intellect Disabil Res*, 47, 72–83.

Hall, S. S., Lightbody, A. A. and Reiss, A. L. (2008). Compulsive, self-injurious and autistic behavior in children and adolescents with fragile X syndrome. *Am J Ment Retard*, 113, 44–53.

Harris, J. C. (2006). *Intellectual Disability: Understanding Its Development, Causes, Classification, Evaluation, and Treatment.* New York: Oxford University Press.

Hassiotis, A., Strydom, A., Hall, I. *et al.* (2008). Psychiatric morbidity and social functioning among adults with borderline intelligence living in private households. *J Intellect Disabil Res*, 52(2), 95–106.

Hastings, R. P., Beck, A., Daley, D. and Hill, C. (2005). Symptoms of ADHD and their correlates in children with intellectual disabilities. *Res Dev Disabil*, 26, 456–68.

Hemmings, C. P., Gravestock, S., Pickard, M. and Bouras N. (2006). Psychiatric symptoms and problem behaviours in people with intellectual disabilities. *J Intellect Disabil Res*, 50, 269–76.

Hiraiwa, R., Maegaki, Y., Oka, A. and Ohno, K. (2007). Behavioral and psychiatric disorders in Prader-Willi syndrome: a population study in Japan. *Brain Dev*, 29, 535–42.

Hodapp, R. M. and Dykens, E. M. (2007). Behavioural phenotypes: growing understandings of psychiatric disorders in individuals with intellectual disabilities. In *Psychiatric and Behavioural Disorders in Intellectual and Developmental Disabilities*, 2nd edn., ed. N. Bouras and G. Holt. Cambridge: Cambridge University Press, pp. 202–14.

Holland, A. J., Hon, J., Huppert, F. A., Stevens, F. and Watson, P. (1998). Population-based study of the prevalence and presentation of dementia in adults with Down syndrome. *Br J Psychiatry*, 172, 494–8.

Kalachnik, J. E., Leventhal, B. L., James, D. H. *et al.* (1998). Guidelines for the use of psychotropic medication. In *Psychotropic Medications and Developmental Disabilities: The International Consensus Handbook*, ed. S. Reiss and M. G. Aman. Columbus: Nisonger Press, pp. 45–72.

King, B. (2007). Psychopharmacology in intellectual disabilities. In *Psychiatric and Behavioural Disorders in Intellectual and Developmental Disabilities*, 2nd edn., ed. N. Bouras and G. Holt. Cambridge: Cambridge University Press, pp. 310–29.

King, B. H., DeAntonio C., McCracken, J. T., Forness, S. R. and Ackerland V. (1994). Psychiatric consultation in severe and profound mental retardation. *Am J Psychiatry*, 151, 1802–8.

Kishore, M. T., Nizamie, A., Nizamie, S. H. and Jahan, M. (2004). Psychiatric diagnosis in persons with intellectual disability in India. *J Intellect Disabil Res*, 48, 19–24.

Leyfer, O. T., Woodruff-Borden, J., Klein-Tasman, B. P., Fricke, J. S. and Mervis, C. B. (2006). Prevalence of psychiatric disorders in 4 to 16 year-olds with William's syndrome. *Am J Med Genet B: Neuropsychiatr Genet*, 141B, 615–22.

Lindsay, W. R. (2007). Personality disorder. In *Psychiatric and Behavioural Disorders in Intellectual and Developmental Disabilities*, 2nd edn., ed. N. Bouras and G. Holt. Cambridge: Cambridge University Press, pp. 143–53.

Lund, J. (1985). The prevalence of psychiatric morbidity in mentally retarded adults. *Acta Psychiatr Scand*, 72, 563–70.

Mantry, D., Cooper, S. A., Smiley, E. *et al.* (2008). The prevalence and incidence of mental ill-health in adults with Down syndrome. *J Intellect Disabil Res*, 52(2), 141–55.

Masi, G., Mucci, M., Favilla, L. and Poli, P. (1999). Dysthymic disorder in adolescents with intellectual disability. *J Intellect Disabil Res*, 43, 80–7.

McGillicuddy, N. B. (2006). A review of substance use research among those with mental retardation. *Ment Retard Dev Disabil Res Rev*, 12(1), 41–7.

Melville, C. A. (2003). A critique of the The Diagnostic Criteria for Psychiatric Disorder for Use with Adults with Learning Disabilities/Mental Retardation [DC-LD] chapter on non-affective psychotic disorders. *J Intellect Disabil Res*, 47, 16–25.

Morgan, V. A., Leonard, H., Bourke, J. and Jablensky, A. (2008). Intellectual disability co-occurring with schizophrenia and other psychiatric illness: a population-based study. *Br J Psychiatry*, 193, 364–72.

Munir, F., Cornish, K. M. and Wilding, J. (2000). A neuropsychological profile of attention deficits in young males with fragile X syndrome. *Neuropsychologia*, 30, 1261–70.

Murphy, K. C. (2005). Annotation: velo-cardio-facial syndrome. *J Child Psychol Psychiatry*, 46(6), 563–71.

O'Hara, J. (2007). Inter-disciplinary multi-modal assessment for mental health problems in people with intellectual disabilities. In *Psychiatric and Behavioural Disorders in Intellectual and Developmental Disabilities*, 2nd edn., ed. N. Bouras and G. Holt. Cambridge: Cambridge University Press, pp. 42–61.

Parkes, G. and Hollins, S. (2007). Psychodynamic approaches to people with intellectual disabilities: individuals, groups/systems, and families. In *Psychiatric and Behavioural Disorders in Intellectual and Developmental Disabilities*, 2nd edn., ed. N. Bouras and G. Holt. Cambridge: Cambridge University Press, pp. 339–50.

Pary, R. J. and DesNoyers-Hurley, A. (2002). Down syndrome and autistic disorder. *Ment Health Aspects Dev Disabil*, 5, 64–5.

Reiss, S. and Aman, M. G. (eds.) (1998). *Psychotropic Medications and Developmental Disabilities: The International Consensus Handbook*. Columbus: Nisonger Press.

Reiss, S., Levitan, G. W. and Szyzko, J. (1982). Emotional disturbance and mental retardation: diagnostic overshadowing. *Am J Ment Defic*, 86, 567–74.

Richards, M., Maughan, B., Hardy, R. *et al.* (2001). Long-term affective disorder in people with mild learning disability. *Br J Psychiatry*, 179, 523–7.

Research Units in Pediatric Psychopharmacology (RUPP) Autism Network (2005). Risperidone treatment of autistic disorder: longer-term benefits and blinded discontinuation after 6 months. *Am J Psychiatry* 162, 1361–9.

Royal College of Psychiatrists (RCP) (2001). *OP48. DC-LD: Diagnostic Criteria for Psychiatric Disorders for Use with Adults with Learning Disabilities/Mental Retardation*. London: Gaskell.

Rush, A. J. and Frances, A. (2000). Treatment of psychiatric and behavioral problems in mental retardation: expert consensus guideline series. *Am J Ment Retard*, 105, 159–226.

Rutter, M., Tizard, J., Yule, W., Graham, P. and Whitmore, K. (1976). Research report: Isle of Wight studies 1964–1974. *Psychol Med*, 6, 313–32.

Schroeder, S. R, Bouras N., Ellis, C. R. *et al.* (1998). Past research on psychopharmacology of people with mental retardation and developmental disabilities. In *Psychotropic Medications and Developmental Disabilities: The International Consensus Handbook*, ed. S. Reiss and M. G. Aman. Columbus: Nisonger Press, pp. 19–29.

Seager, M. C. and O'Brien, G. (2003). Attention deficit hyperactivity disorder: review of ADHD in learning disability: The Diagnostic Criteria for Psychiatric Disorder for use with Adults with Learning Disabilities/Mental Retardation [DC-LD] criteria for diagnosis. *J Intellect Disabil Res*, 47(Suppl 1), 26–31.

Sequeira, H., Howlin, P. and Hollins, S. (2003). Psychological disturbance associated with sexual abuse in people with learning disabilities: case control study. *Br J Psychiatry*, 183, 451–6.

Shprintzen, R. J. (2008). Velo-cardio-facial syndrome: 30 years of study. *Dev Disabil Res Rev*, 14, 3–10.

Sohanpal, S. K., Deb, S., Thomas, C. *et al.* (2007). The effectiveness of antidepressant medication for the management of behaviour problems in adults with intellectual disability: a systemic review. *J Intellect Disabil Res*, 51, 750–65.

Stavrakaki, C. and Lunsky, Y. (2007). Depression, anxiety and adjustment disorders in people with intellectual disabilities. In *Psychiatric and Behavioural Disorders in Intellectual and Developmental Disabilities*, 2nd edn., ed. N. Bouras and G. Holt. Cambridge: Cambridge University Press, pp. 113–30.

Stavrakaki, C. and Mintsioulis, G. (1997). Implications of a clinical study of anxiety disorders in persons with mental retardation. *Psychiatr Ann*, 27, 182–9.

Stromme, P. and Diseth, T. H. (2000). Prevalence of psychiatric diagnoses in children with mental retardation: data from a population-based study. *Dev Med Child Neurol*, 42, 266–70.

Strydom, A., Livingston, G., King, M. and Hassiotis, A. (2007). Prevalence of dementia in intellectual disability using different diagnostic criteria. *Br J Psychiatry*, 191, 150–7.

Sturmey, P. (2007). Diagnosis of mental disorders in people with intellectual disabilities. In *Psychiatric and Behavioural Disorders in Intellectual and Developmental Disabilities*, 2nd edn., ed. N. Bouras and G. Holt. Cambridge: Cambridge University Press, pp. 3–23.

Taggart, L., McLaughlin, D., Quinn, B. and Milligan, V. (2006). An exploration of substance misuse in people with intellectual disabilities. *J Intellect Disabil Res*, 50(Pt 8), 588–97.

Tonge, B. (2007). The psychopathology of children with intellectual disabilities. In *Psychiatric and Behavioural Disorders in Intellectual and Developmental Disabilities*, 2nd edn., ed. N. Bouras and G. Holt. Cambridge: Cambridge University Press, pp. 93–112.

Tsakanikos, E., Bouras, N., Costello, H. and Holt, G. (2007). Multiple exposure to life events and clinical psychopathology in adults with intellectual disability. *Soc Psychiatry Psychiatr Epidemiol*, 42(1), 24–8.

Tsiouris, J. A., Cohen, I. L., Patti, P. J. and Korosh W. M. (2003). Treatment of previously undiagnosed psychiatric disorders in persons with developmental disabilities decreased or eliminated self-injurious behavior. *J Clin Psychiatry*, 64, 1081–90.

Tyrer, P., Oliver-Africano, P. C., Ahmed, Z. *et al.* (2008). Risperidone, haloperidol, and placebo in the treatment of aggressive challenging behaviour in patients with intellectual disability: a randomized controlled trial. *Lancet*, 371, 57–63.

US Public Health Service (2001). *Closing the Gap: A National Blueprint for Improving the Health of Individuals with Mental Retardation. Report of the Surgeon General's Conference on Health Disparities and Mental Retardation.* Washington DC: US Public Health Service.

White, P., Chant, D., Edwards, N., Townsend, C. and Waghorn, G. (2005). Prevalence of intellectual disability and comorbid mental illness in an Australian community sample. *Aust NZ J Psychiatry*, 39, 395–400.

World Health Organization (WHO) (1992). *The ICD-10 Classification of Mental and Behavioural Disorders.* Geneva: World Health Organization.

Zigman, W. B., Schupf, N., Devenny, D. A. *et al.* (2004). Incidence and prevalence of dementia in elderly adults with mental retardation without Down syndrome. *Am J Ment Retard*, 109(2), 126–41.

17 Neurodevelopmental disorders

Seth A. Mensah and William I. Fraser

Introduction

Neurodevelopmental disorders encompass two broad groups of disorders with their onset before childhood development is completed; those that are defined behaviourally and those with known genetic aetiologies. Neurodevelopmental disorders are now accepted to arise from endogenous (i.e. genetic) and exogenous disturbances in brain development, often beginning in the earliest stages of embryonic development (Tager-Flusberg, 1999).

Defining the phenotype of a disorder remains central to addressing issues of intervention or remediation because, to date, pharmacological treatments have been of limited value for most neurodevelopmental disorders, and the hopes for genetic therapies still lie ahead. Instead, most efforts at intervention are directed toward educational, cognitive and behavioural change (Tager-Flusberg, 1999).

The focus of this chapter is on autistic spectrum disorder (ASD) and attention deficit hyperactivity disorder (ADHD), which are frequently associated with intellectual disability (ID).

Method

An advanced OVID search which provided a merged access to the MEDLINE, CINAHL, EMBASE, Evidence Based medicine reviews including the entire Cochrane library, and PsycINFO databases was conducted. Psychiatric, ID and autism journals were also hand searched. The NICE (National Institute for Health and Clinical Excellence) (UK) clinical guideline on the diagnosis and management of ADHD was also reviewed (NICE, 2008).

The search period was from 1966 to the present using the MeSH terms: neurodevelopmental disorder(s), intellectual disabilities/learning disabilities, mental retardation, pervasive developmental disorder, autism, Asperger syndrome, attention deficit hyperactivity disorder, hyperkinetic disorder, ADHD.

The initial search was conducted in April 2008 and was updated in August 2008. The abstracts of all articles identified were screened and only those that provided direct research findings and evidence on epidemiology, aetiology, diagnostic tools and treatment were accepted and inspected in more detail.

Intellectual Disability and Ill Health: A Review of the Evidence, ed. Jean O'Hara, Jane McCarthy and Nick Bouras. Published by Cambridge University Press. © Cambridge University Press 2010.

Table 17.1. Search results

	Autistic spectrum disorders	Attention deficit hyperactivity disorder
Before evidence-based screening	46 496	31 098
After evidence-based screening	256	235

Results

Results were combined which generated 46 496 articles for 'autism' and 31 098 articles for 'ADHD'. There were no limitations placed on the search and there were no language restrictions although we were unable to further analyse results for which there were no abstracts in English. After screening, the final number of abstracts for 'autism' was 256 and that for 'ADHD' was 235 (please refer to Table 17.1). Evidence accepted included high-quality population-based and institutional-based studies with or without comparison control groups, reviews and book chapters.

Discussion

Epidemiology

Autistic spectrum disorder

Autism has been defined as a condition involving: (1) problems of social communication, (2) inflexible language and behaviour and (3) repetitive sensorimotor movements (WHO, 1992). Some investigators have emphasised that there is a continuum in this disorder, and the phrase autistic spectrum disorder (ASD) has become acceptable and useful terminology.

There has been a notable increase in the prevalence of ASD in recent years. The prevalence rate for studies between 1966 and 1991 was 4.4 cases per 10 000, while that for the period 1992–2001 was 12.7 per 10 000 (Fombonne, 2003a). However, a recent study has reported a prevalence rate of 26.1 per 10 000 (Fombonne et al., 2001). Reasons for this apparent increase include changes in diagnostic practice, increased recognition of the disorder, earlier diagnosis, issues of study design and case ascertainment and the problem of '*diagnostic substitution*' (Croen et al., 2002).

Autistic spectrum disorders are more common in males, with an accepted male:female ratio of 4:1 established in both clinical and epidemiological samples (Ehlers and Gillberg 1993; Fombonne, 2003a, 2003b), but the cause of the observed sex difference remains unclear. The evidence for race and immigration status as potential risk factors for ASD remains controversial (Cuccaro et al., 2007; Ghanizadeh, 2008; Gillberg and Gillberg 1996). The available evidence for reports of clusters of cases or 'outbreaks' of ASD is weak (Autism and Developmental Disabilities Monitoring Network (USA), 2007). Early apparent onset of ASD has not been consistently shown to be associated with greater severity of symptoms (Volkmar et al., 2004; Wing and Potter, 2002).

Attention deficit hyperactivity disorder

Attention deficit hyperactivity disorder (ADHD) is the most prevalent childhood mental disorder and is characterised by three core behavioural symptoms of inattention, hyperactivity and impulsivity. Children with ADHD show considerable variation in the severity of their symptoms, degree of impairment and presence of co-morbid disorders.

Prevalence rates in the general population, using stringent criteria for ADHD, of between 3% and 6% (Goldman *et al.*, 1998), and up to 12% (Brown *et al.*, 2001) have been reported in recent studies. Attention deficit hyperactivity disorder is thought to be more prevalent among the people with ID with estimates ranging from 9% to 60% with greater variability as severity of ID increases (La Malfa *et al.*, 2008). Most estimates of the male:female ratio range between 3:1 and 4:1 (James and Taylor, 1990) in clinical samples and 2:1 (Spira and Fischel, 2005) in community-based samples. Attention deficit hyperactivity disorder is more common in urban settings than in rural areas.

Aetiology

Autistic spectrum disorder

The current evidence suggests that ASD represents a heterogeneous group of disorders with a complex multifactorial aetiology. The notion that ASD might be caused by measles, mumps and Rubella (MMR) immunisation, either directly through exposure to some pathogenic agent (such as the measles virus) or some vaccine preservative (such as mercury), is not supported by the available evidence (Geier and Geier, 2007; Honda *et al.*, 2005). (Please refer to Chapter 5 on Immune system diseases.)

There has been a recent development of psychological models of ASD which centre on the constructs of '*theory of mind*' skills (the '*theory of mind*' model), a cognitive drive for central coherence (the '*weak central coherence*' model) and a group of neuropsychological skills clustered together by the term '*executive functions*' (the '*executive dysfunction*' model). For more detailed information on these models, see Baron-Cohen (1995), Happé and Frith (1996), Klin *et al.* (2000) and Ozonoff (1997). The '*theory of mind*' model lacks specificity to ASD (Klin *et al.*, 2000; Ozonoff and Miller, 1995). Other hypotheses (deficits in joint attentional skills, preferential orientation to social stimuli, drive or motivation for social engagement, central deficits in imitation) have been proposed but the evidence to support them is very weak (Happé and Frith, 1996; Klin *et al.*, 2003; Mundy and Neal, 2001).

Significant changes in white matter volume in relation to grey matter volume, and dysfunction of the limbic system particularly amygdala and hippocampus, have been proposed as causal models for ASD (Casanova, 2007; Dager *et al.*, 2007; Mostofsky *et al.*, 2007). Recent MRI, post-mortem and additional studies have confirmed the observation first made by Kanner (1943) of enlarged head circumference possibly the result of excess levels of neuropeptides and neurotrophins, glial overproduction and dysregulation of synaptic and dendritic pruning (Courchesne, 2002; Courchesne *et al.*, 2003; Nelson *et al.*, 2001), and with the tendency towards size normalisation after this early overgrowth. This increase in size appears to be a shift of the entire brain and head size distribution rather than merely an excess of megalencephaly (Courchesne *et al.*, 2003).

The implication of the consistent finding of high peripheral 5-hydroxytryptamine (5-HT, serotonin) in about a third of children with ASD remains unclear, and the examination of other neurotransmitter systems have not yet generated consistent results (Veenstra-VanderWeele *et al.*, 2002).

Epidemiological, twin, adoption and family data provide evidence to support the view that ASD arises on the basis of a complex genetic predisposition, involving interactions between a number of susceptibility loci (Yang and Gill, 2007). Recent genetic research has shown promise and focused on 5-HT receptor genes, allelic variation in the promoter of the 5-HT transporter gene, Hox genes, forkhead domain (*FOXP2*) genes which are also associated with neurodevelopmental verbal dyspraxia, paired box 3 (*PAX3*) gene, *EN2* (engrailed 2) gene, tuberous sclerosis type 2 gene, adenosine deaminase, the GABAA receptor gene cluster, maternally derived X chromosome and *MECP2* gene, but all have so far produced inconsistent results. Recurrent or *de novo copy number variation* is reported to occur in 10–20% of people with ASD (Gupta and State 2007; Szatmari *et al.*, 2007; Swackhammer and Tatum, 2007). Zhao *et al.* (2007) have reported that there are two types of genetically determined dominant transmission: (1) in sporadic ASD in low-risk families, but with high penetrance in males, and (2) in high-risk families, mainly in females who are unaffected but carry the causative mutation.

Many different chromosomes have been associated with ASD. Regions suggestive of linkage have been identified on chromosomes 1, 2, 3, 4, 5, 6, 7, 9, 10, 13, 14, 16, 17, 19, 21, 22 and X, and unravelling this remains a challenge (Gupta and State, 2007; Vorsanova *et al.*, 2007).

Some investigators have suggested that ASD is associated with elevated fetal testosterone levels but the evidence for this remains unconvincing (Baron-Cohen, 1999; Bohm *et al.*, 2007).

Attention deficit hyperactivity disorder

The exact cause of ADHD is unknown, and multiple pathways may lead to its phenotypic expression. Cerebral lesions, predominantly of the frontal lobe and dysfunction of striatal connections, have been linked with symptoms of hyperkinesia, impulsivity, distractibility and inattention (Biederman and Faraone, 2002; Zametkin and Rapoport, 1987a, 1987b).

Attention deficit hyperactivity disorder is a highly heritable disorder and genetic factors account for an estimated 80% of the aetiology of ADHD (Biederman and Faraone, 2002; Smalley, 1997). Studies of familial transmission of ADHD ascertained through girls suggest that the genetic contributions to ADHD are similar in both boys and girls (Faraone *et al.*, 2000). First-degree relatives of individuals with ADHD have a five- to sixfold higher risk of being affected than the general population (Biederman *et al.*, 1990). Twin studies have shown 79% concordance in monozygotic twins compared with 32% in same-gender dizygotic twins (Khan and Faraone, 2006; Smalley, 1997) but adoption studies support the role of both genetic and environmental factors in the aetiology of ADHD. There is currently a lack of evidence to support individual chromosomal involvement in ADHD.

A recent review of molecular genetic studies supported the involvement of the dopamine receptor and dopamine transporter genes (e.g. *DAT1*) in the genesis of ADHD. Genetic studies emphasise the role of dopaminergic genes in both clinical phenotypes and observed drug effects (Khan and Faraone, 2006). The gene–environment interaction is now accepted as an important mechanism in the aetiology and development of ADHD, with some genes (e.g. *DAT1*) thought to affect individual sensitivity to environmental aetiological factors (Swanson *et al.*, 2007; Thapar *et al.*, 2007).

Environmental factors that have been found to be associated with ADHD have been classified as prenatal, perinatal and postnatal in origin (Millichap, 2008; St Sauver *et al.*, 2004) but the evidence to fully support these remains controversial. It is thought that these factors increase dopamine receptor availability and cause deficient dopaminergic neurotransmission and the subsequent development of ADHD.

Maternal smoking has attracted the greatest attention in the recent literature and has consistently showed a significant environmentally mediated association (Linnet *et al.*, 2003; Thapar *et al.*, 2003).

Diagnosis and diagnostic tools

Autistic spectrum disorder

Both the ICD-10 (WHO, 1992) and DSM-IV (APA, 1994) systems of classification adopt the classic triad of impairments in reciprocal social interaction and communication, and a restricted stereotyped and repetitive repertoire of interests and activities, plus an age of onset before three years as core criteria for diagnosis. The lack of a clear description of the boundaries, and the broadening conceptualisation of ASD have made the categorical diagnosis of people whose symptoms fall outside the boundaries of definite ASD more challenging, even while it has become easier within the boundaries (Willemsen-Swinkels and Buitelaar, 2002).

Various standardised instruments including the Autism Diagnostic Interview-Revised (ADI-R) have been developed and validated for use in clinical practice and research (Lord and Corsello, 2005; Mahoney et al., 1998; Volkmar et al., 1994, 2004). The current evidence suggests that there is the need for other instruments that can provide more continuous measures of the broader phenotype of ASD (Lord and Corsello 2005; Mahoney et al., 1998; Volkmar et al., 1994). Measurements of severity that take into account chronological age, language level and cognitive skills are still yet to be developed (Volkmar et al., 2004). There is enough evidence now to suggest that ASD can be reliably diagnosed in children as young as two years old although there is more variability in children with early diagnoses of atypical ASD (Moore and Goodson, 2003).

The IQ distribution of ASD has also shifted, from the earlier studies in which up to 70% of children were classed as having ID, to the current estimates in which fewer than 50% have non-verbal IQs of less than 70 (Chakrabarti and Fombonne, 2001).

Attention deficit hyperactivity disorder

The DSM-IV and ICD-10 have almost identical criteria for the identification of inattention, hyperactivity and impulsivity of ADHD. Diagnosis of ADHD in people with ID remains a challenge especially in those with severe and profound disabilities.

Standardised instruments including the Conners' Parent and Teacher Rating Scales-Revised have been developed and validated for use in clinical practice for the assessment and monitoring of treatment, and for research in ADHD. These have shown consistency in discriminating between individuals with and without ADHD (Atkins et al., 1985; Brown et al., 2001; Collett et al., 2003; Conners, 1997).

Attention deficit hyperactivity disorder does not resolve once the child enters puberty for as many as 65% of cases, the diagnosis may persist into adolescence and adulthood (Biederman et al., 1996; Ingram et al., 1999).

Treatment and management

Autistic spectrum disorder

Applied behaviour analysis (ABA) is the most commonly studied treatment for ASD, however, it is now generally accepted that no single approach is the best for all individuals or even across time for the same individual (Matson and Minshawi, 2006; Smith and Antolovich, 2000).

Treatment and research in treatment interventions, which have been inspired by psychological models, have tended to focus on the interplay between different treatments such as the use of social stories and written cues, individualised behaviour treatment (IBT), early individualised behavioural intervention (EIBI), modifications or expansions of behavioural treatments such as incidental teaching or pivotal responsive intervention and the TEACCH (treatment and education of children and adults with communication handicaps). This has also included interventions emphasising social skills training in children and adults. Randomised control trials using the ABA, EIBI, IBT and TEACCH have all consistently shown greater gains in children with ASD and in parent training groups but evidence for longer-term overall cost-effectiveness is yet to be addressed (Drew *et al.*, 2002; Howlin, 1998).

Pharmacological interventions in children and adults with ASD have the benefit of symptom reduction and help in profiting from behavioural and educational interventions even though empirical placebo-controlled research is lacking. Trials have been of small numbers who have often not been well characterised resulting unsurprisingly in studies not being able to be replicated.

Atypical neuroleptics have reported beneficial effects and advantages of these agents include decreased risk of extrapyramidal side effects and tardive dyskinesia but they do cause sedation and weight gain (Campbell *et al.*, 1997). Risperidone is the most extensively studied and has shown significant benefits in individuals with ASD (Jesner *et al.*, 2007; Scott and Dhillon, 2007). A recent MEDLINE database analysis of aripiprazole, olanzapine, quetiapine and ziprasidone concluded that these drugs have some efficacy in improving certain behavioural symptoms, especially aggressiveness, hyperactivity and self-injurious behaviour in ASD (Stachnik and Nunn-Thompson, 2007).

Inhibitors of 5-HT reuptake have not been extensively studied in ASD but are commonly used for the repetitive behaviours, stereotyped mannerisms and difficulties with anxiety and dealing with change (Martin *et al.*, 1999).

Other pharmacological agents, such as mood stabilisers (anticonvulsants), memantine, naltrexone and the gut hormone secretin, and non-pharmacological agents, such as music therapy, acupuncture, use of robots and massage, have shown small but inconclusive beneficial effects (Hughes, 2008; Oswald and Sonenklar, 2007; Unis *et al.*, 2002). Early intervention is helpful but there is a dearth of evidence to suggest that long-term outcome is significantly improved by any particular intervention (Eikeseth *et al.*, 2007; Howlin, 1997; McEachin *et al.*, 1993; Remington *et al.*, 2007).

Attention deficit hyperactivity disorder

A combination of medication, psychological and behavioural management approaches is supported by current evidence as the best means of ensuring long-term improvement in the disorder. Psychosocial treatments encompass a broad set of interventions, including behaviour therapy, academic interventions, family therapy and care coordination.

The current evidence base demonstrates the efficacy of stimulant medications in helping to manage the symptoms of ADHD (King *et al.*, 2006). The stimulant drugs, methylphenidate, dexamphetamine and pemoline, and the non-stimulant drug, atomoxetine, do address the behavioural symptoms of the disorder (McMaster University Evidence-Based Practice Center, 1999; Miller *et al.*, 1998). The most extensive randomised controlled trial to date is the National Institute of Mental Health Collaborative Multisite Multimodal Treatment Study of Children With Attention-Deficit/Hyperactivity Disorder (MTA) which showed improvements over time with medication management, and combined intervention of medication and intensive behavioural management (Jensen *et al.*, 2001; The MTA Cooperative Group, 1999; Swanson *et al.*, 2001). It is still debatable whether these results can be generalised to children in the UK or elsewhere.

Conclusion

Amidst the wealth of current evidence on children with neurodevelopmental disorders, clinicians cannot lose sight of the child in the family. There is enough evidence currently to support epidemiological and aetiological factors thus far identified in neurodevelopmental disorders but the areas of diagnosis and management are still awash with controversies and inconclusive data.

There is the need for future research to focus on:

- Improving integrated diagnostic methods in the early detection, from birth to two years, of neurodevelopmental disorders.
- Developing diagnostic systems aimed at the detection of the impact of ASD and ADHD in ID with the view to clarifying diagnosis of these disorders across all individuals with ID.
- Disentangling diagnostic criteria of co-morbid ADHD particularly in people with severe and profound ID.
- Developing new chemical systems and therapeutic approaches targeted specifically at individualised neurobiological and genetic architecture.
- Collaborative, multi-centre, randomised trials and well-powered longitudinal follow-up studies on the pharmacological management of co-morbid ADHD and ASD in people with ID.
- Translating the findings from research into best clinical practice in order to improve overall long-term outcome and quality of life.

Future research into treatment interventions for ASD and ADHD in people with ID must reflect particularly the most recent advances in the knowledge of the genetics of neurodevelopmental disorders.

References

American Psychiatric Association (APA) (1994). *Diagnostic and Statistical Manual of Mental Disorders: Fourth Edition.* Washington DC: American Psychiatric Association.

Atkins, M., Pelham, W. and Licht, M. (1985). A comparison of objective classroom measures and teacher ratings of attention deficit disorder. *J Abnorm Child Psychol*, 13, 155–67.

Autism and Developmental Disabilities Monitoring Network Surveillance Year 2000 Principal Investigators; Centers for Disease Control and Prevention. (2007). Prevalence of autism spectrum disorders: Autism and Developmental Disabilities Monitoring Network, six sites, United States, 2000. *MMWR Surveill Summ*, 56, 1–11.

Baron-Cohen, S. (1995). *Mind Blindness.* Cambridge, Massachusetts: MIT Press.

Baron-Cohen, S. (1999). The extreme-male-brain theory of autism. In *Neurodevelopmental Disorders*, ed., H. Tager-Flusberg. Cambridge, Massachusetts: MIT Press, pp. 401–30.

Biederman, J. and Faraone S. (2002). Current concepts on the neurobiology of attention-deficit/hyperactivity disorder. *J Atten Disord*, 6(Suppl 1), s7–16.

Biederman, J., Faraone, S., Keenan, K., Knee, D. and Tsuang, M. (1990). Family-genetic and psychosocial risk factors in DSM-III attention deficit disorder. *J Am Acad Child Adolesc Psychiatry*, 29(4), 526–33.

Biederman, J., Faraone, S., Milberger, S. *et al.* (1996). A prospective 4-year follow-up study of attention-deficit hyperactivity and related disorders. *Arch Gen Psychiatry*, 53, 437–46.

Bohm, H., McComish, J. and Stewart, M. (2007). On a possible early identification procedure for babies at high risk for autistic spectrum disorder. *Med Hypotheses*, 69, 47–51.

Brown, R., Freeman, W., Perrin, J. *et al.* (2001). Prevalence and assessment of attention-deficit/hyperactivity disorder in primary care settings. *Pediatrics*, 107(3), 1–11.

Campbell, M., Armenteros, J., Malone, R. *et al.* (1997). Neuroleptic-related dyskinesias in autistic children: a prospective, longitudinal study. *J Am Acad Child Adolesc Psychiatry*, 36, 835–43.

Casanova, M. F. (2007). The neuropathology of autism. *Brain Pathol*, 17, 422–33.

Chakrabarti, S. and Fombonne, E. (2001). Pervasive developmental disorders in preschool children. *JAMA*, 285, 3093–9.

Collett, B. R., Ohan, J. L. and Myers, K. M. (2003). Ten-year review of rating scales. V: scales assessing attention-deficit/hyperactivity disorder. *J Am Acad Child Adolesc Psychiatry*, 42, 1015–37.

Conners, C. (1997). *Conners' Rating Scales-Revised: Instruments for Use with Children and Adolescents.* New York, NY: Multi-Health Systems, Inc.

Courchesne, E. (2002). Abnormal early brain development in autism. *Mol Psychiatry*, 7, S21–3.

Courchesne, E., Carper, R. and Akshoomoff, N. (2003). Evidence of brain overgrowth in the first year of life in autism. *JAMA*, 290, 337–44.

Croen, L. A., Grether, J. K., Hoogstrate, J. and Selvin, S. (2002). The changing prevalence of autism in California. *J Autism Dev Disord*, 32, 207–15.

Cuccaro, M. L., Brinkley, J., Abramson, R. K. *et al.* (2007). Autism in African American families: clinical–phenotypic findings. *Am J Med Genet B Neuropsychiatr Genet*, 144, 1022–6.

Dager, S., Wang, L., Friedman, S. *et al.* (2007). Shape mapping of the hippocampus in young children with autism spectrum disorder. *Am J Neuroradiol*, 28, 672–7.

Drew, A., Baird, G., Baron-Cohen, S. *et al.* (2002). A pilot randomised control trial of a parent training intervention for pre-school children with autism. Preliminary findings and methodological challenges. *Eur Child Adolesc Psychiatry*, 11, 266–72.

Ehlers, S. and Gillberg, C. (1993). The epidemiology of Asperger syndrome. A total population study. *J Child Psychol Psychiatry*, 34, 1327–50.

Eikeseth, S., Smith, T., Jahr, E. and Eldevik, S. (2007). Outcome for children with autism who began intensive behavioral treatment between ages 4 and 7: a comparison controlled study. *Behav Modif*, 31, 264–78.

Faraone, S., Biederman, J., Mick E. *et al.* (2000). Family study of girls with attention deficit hyperactivity disorder. *Am J Psychiatry*, 157(7), 1077–83.

Fombonne, E. (2003a). The prevalence of autism. *JAMA*, 289, 87–9.

Fombonne, E. (2003b). Epidemiological surveys of autism and other pervasive developmental disorders: an update. *J Autism Dev Disord*, 33, 365–82.

Fombonne, E., Simmons, H., Ford, T. *et al.* (2001). Prevalence of pervasive developmental disorders in the British nationwide survey of child mental health. *J Am Acad Child Adolesc Psychiatry*, 40, 820–7.

Geier D. and Geier M. (2007). A prospective study of mercury toxicity biomarkers in autistic spectrum disorders. *J Toxicol Environ Health A*, 70, 1723–30.

Ghanizadeh, A. (2008). A preliminary study on screening prevalence of pervasive developmental disorder in school children in Iran. *J Autism Dev Disord*, 38:759–63.

Gillberg, I. and Gillberg, C. (1996). Autism in immigrants: a population-based study from Swedish rural and urban areas. *J Intellect Disabil Res*, 40, 24–31.

Goldman, L., Genel, L., Bezman, R. *et al.* (1998). Diagnosis and treatment of attention deficit hyperactivity disorder. *JAMA*, 279, 1100–17.

Gupta, A. and State, M. (2007). Recent advances in the genetics of autism. *Biol Psychiatry*, 61(4), 429–37.

Happé, F. G. and Frith, U. (1996). The neuropsychology of autism. *Brain*, 119, 1377–400.

Honda, H., Shimizu, Y. and Rutter, M. (2005). No effect of MMR withdrawal on the incidence of autism: a total population study. *J Child Psychol and Psychiatry*, 46(6), 572–9.

Howlin, P. (1997). Prognosis in autism: do specialist treatments affect long-term outcome? *Eur Child Adolesc Psychiatry*, 6, 55–72.

Howlin, P. (1998). Practitioner review: psychological and educational treatments for autism. *J Child Psychol Psychiatry*, 39, 307–22.

Hughes, J. (2008). A review of recent reports on autism: 1000 studies published in 2007. *Epilepsy Behav* 13, 425–37.

Ingram, S., Hechtman, L. and Morgenstern, G. (1999). Outcome issues in ADHD: adolescent and adult long-term outcome. *Ment Retard Dev Disabil Res Rev*, 5, 243–50.

James, A. and Taylor, E. (1990). Sex differences in the hyperkinetic syndrome of childhood. *J Child Psychol Psychiatry*, 31, 437–46.

Jensen, P., Hinshaw, S., Swanson, J. *et al.* (2001). Findings from the NIMH Multimodal Treatment Study of ADHD (MTA): implications and applications for primary care providers. *J Dev Behav Pediatr*, 22, 60–73.

Jesner, O., Aref-Adib, M. and Coren, E. (2007). Risperidone for autism spectrum disorder. *Cochrane Database Syst Rev*, (1), CD005040.

Kanner, L. (1943). Autistic disturbances of affective contact. *Nerv Child*, 2, 217–50.

Khan, S. and Faraone, S. (2006). The genetics of ADHD: a literature review of 2005. *Curr Psychiatry Rep*, 8(5), 393–7.

King, S., Griffin, S., Hodges, Z. *et al.* (2006). A systematic review and economic model of the effectiveness and cost-effectiveness of methylphenidate, dexamfetamine and atomoxetine for the treatment of attention deficit hyperactivity disorder in children and adolescents. *Health Technol Assess*, 10(23): iii–iv, xiii–146.

Klin, A., Schultz, R. and Cohen, D. J. (2000). Theory of mind in action: developmental perspectives on social neuroscience. *Understanding Other Minds: Perspectives from Developmental Neuroscience*,

2nd edn., ed. S. Baron-Cohen, R. Tager-Flusberg and D. Cohen. Oxford: Oxford University Press, pp. 357–88.

Klin, A., Jones, W., Schultz, R. and Volkmar, F. (2003). The enactive mind – from actions to cognition: lessons from autism. *Philos Trans R Soc Lond B Bio Sci*, 358, 345–60.

La Malfa, G., Lassi, S., Bertelli, M., Pallanti, S. and Albertini, G. (2008). Detecting attention-deficit/hyperactivity disorder (ADHD) in adults with intellectual disability: the use of Conners' Adult ADHD Rating Scales (CAARS). *Res Dev Disabil*, 29(2), 158–64.

Linnet, K. M., Dalsgaard, S., Obel, C. *et al.* (2003). Maternal lifestyle factors in pregnancy risk of attention deficit hyperactivity disorder and associated behaviors: review of the current evidence. *Am J Psychiatry*, 160(6), 1028–40.

Lord, C. and Corsello, C. (2005). Diagnostic instruments in autistic spectrum disorders. In *Handbook of Autism and Pervasive Developmental Disorders*, 3rd edn., ed. F. Volkmar, R. Paul, A. Klin and D. Cohen. Hoboken, NJ: John Wiley & Sons Inc., pp. 730–71.

Mahoney, W. J., Szatmari, P., MacLean, J. E. *et al.* (1998). Reliability and accuracy of differentiating pervasive developmental disorder subtypes. *J Am Acad Child Adolesc Psychiatry*, 37, 278–85.

Martin, A., Scahill, L., Klin, A. and Volkmar, F. R. (1999). Higher-functioning pervasive developmental disorders: rates and patterns of psychotropic drug use. *J Am Acad Child Adolesc Psychiatry*, 38, 923–31.

Matson, J. and Minshawi, N. (2006). *Early Intervention for Autism Spectrum Disorders: A Critical Analysis*. Oxford, England: Elsevier Science, Inc.

McEachin, J., Smith, T. and Lovaas, O. (1993). Long-term outcome for children with autism who received early intensive behavioral treatment. *Am J Ment Retard*, 97, 359–72.

McMaster University Evidence-Based Practice Center (1999). *Treatment of Attention-Deficit Hyperactivity Disorder*. Rockville, MD: Agency for Health Care

Policy and Research. Evidence Report/Technology Assessment no. 11, AHCPR Publication no. 99-E018.

Miller, A., Lee, S., Raina, P. *et al.* (1998). *A Review of Therapies for Attention-Deficit/Hyperactivity Disorder*. Ottawa, Canada: Canadian Coordinating Office for Health Technology Assessment.

Millichap, J. (2008). Etiologic classification of attention-deficit/hyperactivity disorder. *Pediatrics*, 121(2), e358–65.

Moore, V. and Goodson, S. (2003). How well does early diagnosis of autism stand the test of time? Follow-up study of children assessed for autism at age 2 and development of an early diagnostic service. *Autism*, 7, 47–63.

Mostofsky, S. H., Burgess, M. P. and Gidley Larson, J. C. (2007). Increased motor cortex white matter volume predicts motor impairment in autism. *Brain*, 130, 2117–22.

The MTA Cooperative Group (1999). Multimodal Treatment Study of Children With ADHD. A 14-month randomized clinical trial of treatment strategies for attention-deficit/hyperactivity disorder. *Arch Gen Psychiatry*, 56, 1073–86.

Mundy, P. and Neal, A. R. (2001). Neural plasticity, joint attention, and a transactional social-orienting model of autism. In *International Review of Research in Mental Retardation*, Vol. 23: *Autism*, ed. L. M. Glidden. San Diego, California: Academic Press, 23, pp. 139–68.

Nelson, K. B., Grether, J. K., Croen, L. A. *et al.* (2001). Neuropeptides and neurotrophins in neonatal blood of children with autism or mental retardation. *Ann Neurol*, 49, 597–606.

NICE (2008). *Guideline on the Diagnosis and Management of ADHD in Children*. London: National Institute of Health and Clinical Excellence, CG 72.

Oswald, D. and Sonenklar, N. A. (2007). Medication use among children with autism spectrum disorders. *J Child Adolesc Psychopharmacol*, 17, 348–55.

Ozonoff, S. (1997). Components of executive function deficits in autism and other Disorders. In: *Autism as an Executive*

Disorder, ed. J. Russel. Oxford: Oxford University Press, pp. 179–211.

Ozonoff, S. and Miller, J. N. (1995). Teaching theory of mind: a new approach to social skills training for individuals with autism. *J Autism Dev Disord*, 25, 415–33.

Remington, B., Hastings, R. P., Kovshoff, H. *et al.* (2007). Early intensive behavioural intervention: outcomes for children with autism and their parents after two years. *Am J Ment Retard*, 112(6), 418–38.

Scott, L. and Dhillon, S. (2007). Risperidone: a review of its use in the treatment of irritability associated with autistic disorder in children and adolescents. *Paediatr Drugs*, 9, 343–54.

Smalley, S. (1997). Genetic influences in childhood-onset psychiatric disorders: autism and attention deficit/hyperactivity disorder. *Am J Hum Genet*, 60(6), 1276–82.

Smith, T. and Antolovich, M. (2000). Parental perceptions of supplemental interventions received by young children with autism in intensive behaviour analytic treatment. *Behav Intervent*, 15, 83–97.

Spira, E. and Fischel, J. (2005). The impact of preschool inattention, hyperactivity, and impulsivity on social and academic development: a review. *J Child Psychol Psychiatry*, 46(7), 755–73.

St Sauver, J., Barbaresi, W., Katusic, S. *et al.* (2004). Early life risk factors for attention-deficit/hyperactivity disorder: a population-based cohort study. *Mayo Clin Proc*, 79(9), 1124–31.

Stachnik, J. and Nunn-Thompson, C. (2007). Use of atypical antipsychotics in the treatment of autistic disorder. *Ann Pharmacother*, 41, 626–34.

Swackhammer, R. and Tatum, O. (2007). Survey of candidate genes for autism susceptibility. *J Assoc Genet Technol*, 33, 8–16.

Swanson, J., Kraemer, H., Hinshaw, S. *et al.* (2001). Clinical relevance of the primary findings of the MTA: success rates based on severity of ADHD and ODD symptoms at the end of treatment. *J Am Acad Child Adolesc Psychiatry*, 40(2), 168–79.

Swanson, J., Kinsbourne, M., Nigg, J. *et al.* (2007). Etiologic subtypes of attention-deficit/hyperactivity disorder: brain imaging, molecular genetic and environmental factors and the dopamine hypothesis. *Neuropsychol Rev*, 17(1), 39–59.

Szatmari, P., Paterson, A., Zwaigenbaum, L. *et al.* (2007). For the Autism Genome Project Consortium. Mapping autism risk loci using genetic linkage and chromosomal rearrangements. *Nat Genet*, 39, 319–28.

Tager-Flusberg, H. (1999). Research on neurodevelopmental disorders. In: *Neurodevelopmental Disorders from a Cognitive Neuroscience Perspective*, ed. H. Tager-Flusberg. Cambridge, MA: The MIT Press, pp. 3–21.

Thapar, A., Fowler, T., Rice, F. *et al.* (2003). Maternal smoking during pregnancy and attention deficit hyperactivity disorder symptoms in offspring. *Am J Psychiatry*, 160(11), 1985–9.

Thapar, A., Langley, K., Asherson, P. and Gill, M. (2007). Gene-environment interplay in attention-deficit hyperactivity disorder and the importance of a developmental perspective. *Br J Psychiatry*, 190, 1–3.

Unis, A. S., Munson, J. A., Rogers, S. J. *et al.* (2002). A randomized, double-blind, placebo controlled trial of porcine versus synthetic secretin for reducing symptoms of autism. *J Am Acad Child Adolesc Psychiatry*, 41, 1315–21.

Veenstra-VanderWeele, J., Kim, S. J., Lord, C. *et al.* (2002). Transmission disequilibrium studies of the serotonin 5-HT2A receptor gene (HTR2A) in autism. *Am J Med Genet*, 114, 277–83.

Volkmar, F., Lord, C., Bailey, A., Schultz, R. and Klin, A. (2004). Autism and pervasive developmental disorders. *J Child Psychol Psychiatry*, 45(1), 135–70.

Volkmar, F. R., Klin, A., Siegal, B. *et al.* (1994). Field trial for autistic disorder in DSM-IV. *Am J Psychiatry*, 151, 1361–7.

Vorsanova, S., Yurov, I., Demidova, I. *et al.* (2007). Variability in the heterochromatin regions of the chromosomes and chromosomal anomalies in children with autism: identification of genetic markers of autistic spectrum disorders. *Neurosc Behav Physiol*, 37, 553–8.

Willemsen-Swinkels, S. H. and Buitelaar, J. K. (2002). The autistic spectrum: subgroups, boundaries, and treatment. *Psychiatr Clin North Am*, 25, 811–36.

Wing, L. and Potter, D. (2002). The epidemiology of autistic spectrum disorders; is the prevalence rising? *Ment Retard Dev Disabil Res Rev*, 8, 151–61.

World Health Organization (WHO) (1992). *International Statistical Classification of Diseases and Related Health Problems*, 10th Revision Geneva: World Health Organization.

Yang, M. and Gill, M. (2007). A review of gene linkage, association and expression studies in autism and an assessment of convergent evidence. *Int J Dev Neurosci*, 25, 69–85.

Zametkin, A. and Rapoport, J. (1987a). Neurobiology of ADHD. *J Am Acad Child Adolesc Psychiatry*, 26(5), 676–86.

Zametkin, A. and Rapoport, J. (1987b). Quantitative brain magnetic resonance imaging in attention-deficit hyperactivity disorder. *Arch Gen Psychiatry*, 53(7), 607–16.

Zhao, X., Leotta, A., Kustanovich, V. *et al.* (2007). A unified genetic theory for sporadic and inherited autism. *Proc Nat Acad Sci USA*, 104, 128321–6.

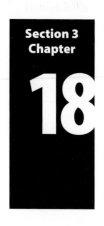

18 Diseases of the nervous system I: epilepsy, hydrocephalus and nervous system malformations

Basil Cardoza and Mike Kerr

Introduction

Epilepsy

The association between intellectual disability (ID) and epilepsy is well known. Studies have shown higher prevalence rates both in institutions and in the community and commented on the profound effect it has on individuals and their families. Nervous system malformations (including brain malformation) and hydrocephalus are often associated with ID. Many people with ID, especially of a more severe degree, also have neurological impairments. Epilepsy will be discussed in the first section of this chapter, followed by hydrocephalus and nervous system malformations.

Hydrocephalus and nervous system malformations

Over the past few years, increased availability of neuroimaging such as MRI has led to more discoveries of developmental brain disorders with co-morbid epilepsy and ID (Barkovich *et al.*, 2001). Malformations of cortical development (MCD) describes a broad range of conditions of developmental origin. They are important causes of chronic epilepsy and encompass many varied developmental disorders, with diverse clinical manifestations including focal cortical dysplasia, periventricular heterotopia, polymicrogyria, band heterotopia and lissencephaly, dysembryoplastic neuroepithelial tumours and microdysgenesis (Sisodiya, 2004). Brodtkorb *et al.* (1992) suggest that MCD may be seen in 14% of individuals with ID and epilepsy.

Method

Electronic databases, MEDLINE OVID (1950 to September 2008), EMBASE (1980 to September 2008) and PsycINFO (1806 to September 2008) were searched, along with selective hand searches. All abstracts were screened, relevant abstracts read and potentially relevant articles were inspected in more detail. Other well-known publications outside this search, from the Cochrane collaboration and published textbooks, were also included in this review. There were no exclusion criteria and no restriction as to language or origin of study.

Table 18.1. Search results

	Total	Relevant
Epilepsy		
EMBASE	483	81
MEDLINE	276	61
PsycINFO	125	55
Hydrocephalus and nervous system malformations		
EMBASE	51	7
MEDLINE	48	8
PsycINFO	65	12

The following search terms were included: learning disability, developmental disability, mental retardation, mental handicap, intellectual disability, intellectual handicap, intellectual impairment.

These search terms were used for epilepsy: epilepsy, focal epilepsy, generalised epilepsy, intractable epilepsy, seizure, convulsion, temporal lobe epilepsy, absence, complex partial epilepsy. (Please refer to Table 18.1.)

These search terms were used for hydrocephalus and nervous system malformations: hydrocephalus, communicating hydrocephalus, normotensive hydrocephalus, nervous system malformations, neural tube deficits, malformations of cortical development, central nervous system malformations. (Please refer to Table 18.1.)

Papers were selected depending on the subject matter and relevance to the topic studied, looking specifically at the association between ID and epilepsy or ID and hydrocephalus/nervous system malformations. Papers on learning difficulties such as dyslexia were not included in the study.

Results

The number of references identified is shown in Table 18.1.

Discussion

Epilepsy

Aetiology

Many epilepsy syndromes are benign and are not associated with ID, but others are severe and are frequently associated with significant disability. These syndromes are also termed epileptic encephalopathies and any intellectual impairment is considered to be related to a combination of the underlying disorder, the frequency of seizures and abnormal inter-ictal epileptiform EEG activity.

A potential and important cause of ID is the aetiology of the epilepsy syndrome itself, although an individual epilepsy syndrome may have many causes. This may occur as part of a chromosomal disorder (e.g. Down syndrome, Ring chromosome 20), a genetic syndrome (e.g. Prader-Willi, Rett syndrome) or as a consequence of early brain injury. A significant number of epilepsy syndromes are cryptogenic or idiopathic, without an identified aetiology.

Epilepsy syndromes

Lennox-Gastaut syndrome, with a peak age of onset between two and six years, is one of the more common epilepsy syndromes and is characterised by severe ID, multiple seizure types (tonic, atypical absence, atonic and tonic–clonic) and characteristic EEG changes (paroxysms of slow, spike and slow-wave activity, frequency of 1–2 Hz) (Crumrine, 2002; Niedermeyer, 2002).

Landau-Kleffner syndrome or 'acquired aphasia of childhood with epilepsy' presents with verbal agnosia and expressive aphasia and the majority of individuals develop multiple seizures. Global intellectual impairment may be seen if the syndrome is diagnosed late or response to treatment is poor (Robinson *et al.*, 2001).

Infantile spasms are sudden brief seizures, usually seen as part of West syndrome and of the infants who survive, more than 75% have ID (Appleton, 2001).

Epileptic encephalopathies with burst-suppression on the EEG (including Ohtahara syndrome) present in the first few weeks or months of life with multiple seizure types and have a poor prognosis; leaving survivors with refractory epilepsy and severe ID (Yamatogi and Ohtahara, 2002).

Migrating partial seizures in infancy are rare and seizures originate from different parts of the cortex. The long-term prognosis is poor and includes severe ID and death (Coppola *et al.*, 1995).

Severe myoclonic epilepsy in infancy often presents with drug-resistant tonic–clonic and clonic seizures and most children develop severe ID (Kanazawa, 2001).

Chromosomal and genetic syndromes

The more common chromosomal and genetic disorders associated with ID and epilepsy are Down syndrome (Stafstrom and Konkol, 1994), Fragile X syndrome, Ring chromosome 20, Ring chromosome 14 and Wolf-Hirschhorn syndrome (Singh *et al.*, 2002).

In Down syndrome (Trisomy 21), epilepsy is seen in 5–10% of individuals and infantile spasms in 1–13% (Stafstrom and Konkol, 1994). An evaluation of 62 individuals with Fragile X syndrome showed 23% had a history of seizures, all controlled with antiepileptic drugs (Wisniewski *et al.*, 1991).

Ring chromosome 20 (r20) syndrome is a rare disorder characterised by mild to moderate ID, behavioural disorders, epilepsy and various dysmorphic features (Alpman *et al.*, 2005). Wolf-Hirschhorn syndrome (4p 16.3 deletion) comprises of moderate to severe ID, epilepsy and dysmorphic facial features (Battaglia *et al.*, 1999).

Angelman syndrome presents in the first year of life with developmental delay, is usually caused by deletion on chromosome 15q 11–13 (maternal arm) and 90% of children will develop seizures. However, Prader-Willi syndrome, caused by a similar deletion on paternal chromosome 15, is not usually associated with epilepsy.

X-linked myoclonic epilepsy with generalised spasticity and ID (XMESID) is a rare X-linked myoclonic epilepsy seen in males (Scheffer *et al.*, 2002).

Rett syndrome is almost exclusively seen in girls and is usually caused by a mutation in the *MeCP2* gene (methyl-CpG binding protein 2) at Xq 28. Severe ID is common and multiple seizure types are seen in the vast majority of individuals (Steffenburg *et al.*, 2001).

Treatment-resistant epilepsy with mild to severe ID are characteristic features of most neurocutaneous syndromes such as tuberous sclerosis (Appleton and Fryer, 1995), Sturge-Weber syndrome (Kramer *et al.*, 2000) and Neurofibromatosis type 1 (Suenobu *et al.*, 2008).

Facioscapulohumeral muscular dystrophy results from deletion of tandem repeats on chromosome 4q35, presenting with sensorineural hearing loss, ID and epilepsy (Hobson-Webb and Caress, 2006).

Pallister-Killian syndrome is a rare sporadic genetic disorder characterised by dysmorphic features, ID and epilepsy. It is caused by a mosaic supernumerary isochromosome 12p (Sanchez-Carpintero et al., 2005).

Miscellaneous syndromes

Kabuki syndrome is a dysmorphogenic syndrome of unknown aetiology, reported in over 300 people with mild to moderate ID. Neurological anomalies are frequently reported, including epilepsy in 8% (Powell et al., 2003).

In a study of seven children with central nervous system (CNS) folate deficiency (CFD), five met the criteria for autistic spectrum disorder (ASD) (Moretti et al., 2008). The study concludes that autistic features are salient in CFD and suggests that a subset of children with developmental regression, ID, seizures, dyskinesia and ASD may have CNS folate abnormalities.

Epidemiology

There seems to be an over-representation of epilepsy in people with ID. Prevalence rates in the community have ranged from 6% in children with mild ID (Ross and Peckham, 1983 (cited in Krishnamoorthy, 2003, pp. 17–18)) to 24% in severe ID (Steffenburg et al., 1995) and 50% in profound ID (Corbett, 1998 (cited in Krishnamoorthy, 2003, pp. 17–18)). A global estimate is that between 15% (mild ID) and 30% (severe ID) of children have co-morbid epilepsy (Sillanpää, 1996).

The prevalence of epilepsy in a study of 1595 adults with an ID by Morgan et al. (2003) was found to be 16.1%. A study of 318 adults with ID from 40 general practices found 18% to have epilepsy, of which 26% were seizure free and 34% had extremely poorly controlled seizures, supporting the high occurrence and chronicity of epilepsy in this population (Matthews et al., 2008). A population-based prevalence study using the Leicester Learning Disability Register, identified from structured home interviews with carers, gave a prevalence of 26%, with 68% experiencing seizures despite antiepileptic medication (McGrother et al., 2006). Lund (1985) in a study of 302 individuals with ID found 18.2% to have had epilepsy sometime in their lives and 8.35% to have active epilepsy. There was a strong correlation between the level of disability and prevalence of epilepsy.

A study comparing 25 patients with ID and 263 patients without ID found that a higher proportion of the group with ID had epilepsy as well as psychogenic non-epileptic seizures (PNES) and a higher proportion were taking antiepileptic drugs at the time of diagnosis of PNES (Duncan and Oto, 2008)

In a study of 201 adults with Down syndrome, of whom 15.9% had epilepsy, a bimodal age distribution for seizure onset in childhood and later in middle-age was found (Prasher, 1995). A study of a sample of 108 people with tuberous sclerosis found 44.5% had ID and that all individuals with ID had a history of seizures that usually commenced before 12 months of age, often presenting as infantile spasms (Joinson et al., 2003). In a study of 66 participants with microcephaly (2–19 years old), overall prevalence of epilepsy was 40.9%. There was a significantly higher prevalence of epilepsy in males, mostly generalised tonic-clonic seizures. Intellectual disability was diagnosed in 93.9% and profound ID was evident in 43.9% of participants (Abdel-Salam et al., 2000).

A Canadian study found that children with epilepsy often grew into adults with significant social problems including decreased employment (Camfield and Camfield, 2007).

The educational and social progress of a child with epilepsy depends not only on seizure control, but also on cognitive and behavioural factors. The Lennox-Gastaut syndrome often has a poor prognosis in this regard (Besag, 2006).

Psychiatric co-morbidity

The Camberwell study, which compared children with and without ID, with and without epilepsy, found no significant difference in the frequency of behavioural disturbance (Corbett, 1981 (cited in Krishnamoorthy, 2003, pp. 18–19)). Caplan et al. (1991) reported hyperactivity, antisocial behaviour and schizophrenia-like psychosis in children with ID, especially in association with temporal lobe epilepsy.

Deb et al. (1987) and Espie et al. (1989) comparing adults with ID, with and without epilepsy, also found no differences in the rates of maladaptive behaviour. Deb and Hunter (1991a,b,c) in a comparison of 150 individuals with ID and epilepsy and the same number without epilepsy found that over 50% exhibited severe maladaptive behaviour. Although the behaviours were slightly more severe in the population with epilepsy, the results were not statistically significant.

Data collected retrospectively on the rate and type of psychiatric illness and behavioural problems in 143 adults with ID and epilepsy showed 55% to have behavioural problems, 19% to have physical aggression, 17% to have verbal aggression and temper tantrums and 13% to have self-injurious behaviour. A psychiatric diagnosis was seen in 12.6% (Deb and Joyce, 1999). In a study on epilepsy and psychopathology in 186 people with ID, one-third of participants met criteria for possible psychiatric disorder or possibly affective/neurotic disorder (Espie et al., 2003). A retrospective study of 175 individuals with epilepsy and ID found that depression and psychoses were more common in those with no seizures in the preceding three months compared to patients who had at least one seizure in the same period (Ring et al., 2007). Rates of psychosis were higher in those with milder disability, whereas depression rates were higher in those with severe disability.

Seizure types

In a study on the characteristics of epilepsy in a population of 143 adults with ID, generalised tonic–clonic seizure was the most common seizure type (Deb and Joyce, 1999).

A Swedish study examining co-morbidity pattern, seizure characteristics and aetiology in a group of 90 children with ASD, active epilepsy and ID found that partial seizures tended to be more common and generalised seizures less common in the group with ASD compared with the group without ASD. Seizure onset was later in the group with ASD (Steffenburg et al., 2003).

Outcome measures

The measurement of outcomes in people with ID and epilepsy has been limited and is currently based on seizure frequency, severity and quality-of-life measures, but these have not been validated in people with ID (Kerr and Espie, 1997).

The Epilepsy and Learning Disabilities Quality of Life scale (ELDQOL), a 70-item questionnaire covering items related to seizures, antiepileptic drug side effects, mood, cognition and social functioning, was found to have a high reliability and validity, making it a promising instrument for assessing quality of life in children and young adults with epilepsy and ID (Buck *et al.*, 2007).

Treatment

Pharmacological

Epilepsy and its treatment can have a profound effect on individuals with ID. This impact on physical health, psychological health and mortality has, in turn, a further impact on the families and carers for these individuals (Kerr and Bowley, 2001). A major systematic review on pharmacological interventions for epilepsy in people with ID, assessing data from randomised controlled trials, confirmed that in the majority of cases where antiepileptic drugs were trialled moderate reduction in seizure frequency and occasional seizure freedom were obtained. Antiepileptic drugs proven effective in the general population were also effective in refractory epilepsy in people with ID. Side effects seem to be the same as in the general population and behavioural side effects leading to discontinuation of treatment were rare (Beavis *et al.*, 2007a).

Implementing NICE (National Institute for Health and Clinical Excellence) guidelines showed improvements to individuals' seizure assessments and epilepsy management, in a review of 23 British patients, in an outpatient service for people with ID, which in turn led to identifiable improvement in documentation and patient care (Whitten and Griffiths, 2007).

A study investigating the prevalence and psychopathological features of psychiatric side effects in 118 patients with ID, in therapy with levetiracetam, found that 15% experienced psychiatric side effects (1.75% developed an affective disorder, 7.6% aggressive behaviour, 1.7% emotional lability and 1.7% personality changes such as agitation, anger and hostile behaviour) (Mula *et al.*, 2004). A retrospective, open, observational study to assess antiepileptic efficacy and tolerability of gabapentin (used as add-on therapy) on 29 patients with ID and severe treatment-resistant epilepsy found that 10.3% had a reduction of seizure frequency by 50% or more and side effects occurred in 37.9%, somnolence and ataxia being most common (Huber and Tomka-Hoffmeister, 2003). Skin drug reactions to antiepileptic drugs were significantly less often seen in patients with ID than in others (7% vs. 16%) and more common in females than males in a study of 663 patients with the three most common drugs implicated being carbamazepine, phenytoin and lamotrigine (Alvestad *et al.*, 2007).

A comparison of the long-term drug retention rates at two years of newly licensed antiepileptic drugs in a residential community of adults with chronic epilepsy and ID showed figures of 85% (oxcarbazepine), 57% (lamotrigine), 56% (levetiracetam), 45% (topiramate), 24% (tiagabine) and 15% (gabapentin). Topiramate had the highest rate of adverse events at the maximum tried dose (60%), whereas levetiracetam had the lowest (16%) (Simister *et al.*, 2007).

An audit to ascertain outcomes for people who had taken or were still taking three antiepileptic drugs, lamotrigine, levetiracetam and topiramate, found that one-third of people with ID derived substantial benefit, although the rate of seizure freedom was lower than in the population without ID (Chappell and Crawford, 2005). The findings of another audit on 37 patients with ID and refractory epilepsy suggest that the outcome for the majority of patients may be better than has been previously reported, with 10 patients becoming seizure free, 76% experiencing an improvement in seizure frequency, 65% being regarded as being more aware and interactive with their surroundings and 49% reported to be more assertive (Scheepers *et al.*, 2004).

A retrospective study evaluating the effects of levetiracetam in routine therapy in 46 patients with ID and therapy-resistant epilepsy found that 41.3% had a 50% reduction in seizure frequency (Huber *et al.*, 2004). Response rates were higher in focal and multifocal epilepsy as compared to symptomatic generalised epilepsy/Lennox-Gastaut syndrome. A prospective, uncontrolled, open study exploring the efficacy of sulthiame on 52 patients with refractory epilepsy and ID showed promising results with 22 patients achieving seizure freedom in the short term (Koepp *et al.*, 2002).

A study on the outcome at adulthood, of the continuous spike-waves during slow sleep (CSWS) and Landau-Kleffner syndromes in seven young adults, confirmed that the epilepsy associated with these syndromes has a good prognosis, with only one patient having active epilepsy (Praline *et al.*, 2003).

An examination of a community model of epilepsy care for people with ID revealed that 22.7% of individuals with ID and epilepsy had been free of seizures for over one year and 95.1% were taking antiepileptic drugs (Reuber *et al.*, 2008).

A study on seizure outcome after resective surgery in patients with low IQ in Sweden (data from the Swedish National Epilepsy Surgery Register), on 72 patients with an IQ less than 70, found seizure freedom as follows: 22% (IQ less than 50) and 37% (IQ 50 to 69) (Flink and Rydenhag, 2008).

Non-pharmacological

A systematic review of non-pharmacological interventions for epilepsy in people with ID found no randomised controlled studies in this population, highlighting the need for well-designed randomised controlled trials in this area (Beavis *et al.*, 2007b). Interventions studied in populations without ID include relaxation, behaviour therapy, hypnosis, acupuncture, biofeedback, seizure alert dogs and aromatherapy, with varying results.

Hydrocephalus and nervous system malformations

Aetiology

Focal cortical dysplasia is one of the most common MCD found either in imaging studies or in surgical specimens and is invariably associated with refractory epilepsy (Taylor *et al.*,1971).

Periventricular nodular heterotopia (PNH) is a rare neuronal migration disorder occurring predominantly in females and associated with near average intelligence. Periventricular nodular heterotopia with ID has been reported in 15 male patients with several syndromes and various congenital abnormalities such as craniosynostosis, frontonasal malformation and agenesis of the corpus callosum (Balci *et al.*, 2007).

Two families with an autosomal dominant syndrome of abnormalities of the hands and feet, short palpebral fissures, microcephaly and ID have been reported. The phenotype is similar to that observed in 13q22-qter deletion patients without any chromosomal abnormalities detected (Brunner and Winter, 1991).

Heterozygous, *de novo*, loss-of-function mutations in *SOX2* have been shown to cause bilateral anophthalmia along with ID, seizures, brain malformation, specific motor abnormalities, male genital tract malformations, mild facial dysmorphism, and postnatal growth failure (Ragge *et al.*, 2005).

The rates of ASD, ID and brain abnormalities were examined in 20 participants diagnosed as falling within the oculoauriculovertebral spectrum (OAV). Two individuals met diagnostic criteria for ASD, one for autistic-like condition and five for autistic traits. Four had mild ID, three had severe, two had profound, and two borderline intellectual functioning, suggesting that at least a subgroup of ASD may be associated with errors in early embryonic brain development (Johansson *et al.*, 2007).

The case of a 12-year-old Turkish boy with an IQ of 46 and a normal karyotype (46, XY) has been reported with subcortical/subependymal heterotopia associated with corpus callosum dysgenesis, craniofacial dysmorphism, severe eye abnormalities, growth retardation and ID. It is hypothesised that this phenotype could be a new syndrome (Caksen *et al.*, 2003).

Epidemiology, co-morbidity and treatment

A population-based study of 114 children, 70 with infantile hydrocephalus and 44 with hydrocephalus associated with myelomeningocoele (MMC), showed that ID was present in 47% of children with infantile hydrocephalus, compared with 16% of those with MMC (Persson *et al.*, 2006). A similar Swedish study of 103 children with hydrocephalus showed that one-third of the children had an average IQ, 30% had a low average IQ of 70–84 and 37% had ID with an IQ of less than 70 (Lindquist *et al.*, 2005).

In a study of 107 children with hydrocephalus born in western Sweden, the majority of children were found to have behavioural problems (39–67%) and 13% had ASD (Lindquist *et al.*, 2006).

Thirty adolescents with spina bifida and hydrocephalus were matched for age and IQ with 30 controls of different aetiology (Hurley *et al.*, 1983). The index group differed from the controls in having a greater difference between verbal and performance IQ and better complex motor skills. Eleven adults (mean age 18.4 years) shunted for congenital hydrocephalus related to spina bifida and eight adults (mean age 17.7 years) shunted for hydrocephalus related to aqueductal stenosis were administered an extensive neuropsychological battery (Hommet *et al.*, 1999). Results showed no discrepancies between Wechsler performance IQ or verbal IQ in either group. Those individuals with spina bifida appeared more cognitively impaired than those with aqueductal stenosis, who performed normally on the Wechsler Adult Intelligence Scale-Revised.

Conclusion

Epilepsy

A wide range of aetiologies have been described for people with ID co-morbid with epilepsy, including some rare genetic syndromes. Individuals with epilepsy and ID seem to have increased rates of mental ill health and behavioural disorder. However, it is not clear whether this increased burden is attributable to epilepsy.

Antiepileptic drug therapy seems to be the main mode of treatment, similar to the general population, with the same range of drugs used, although there is evidence of increased prevalence of treatment-resistant epilepsy. Almost all studies on non-pharmacological methods of management have been conducted in populations without ID. Although some of these results look promising, they are not of proven value and further research in this area is clearly required.

Hydrocephalus and nervous system malformations

Malformations of cortical development, which may affect large areas of the cortex, are common causes of ID and are usually associated with epilepsy. The presence of ID is suggestive of more damage than can be seen on neuroimaging and is considered to be a poor prognostic factor. There are very few studies on the outcome of intellectual functioning in individuals with nervous system malformations following surgical treatment and more studies are required in this area.

References

Abdel-Salam, G. M., Halasz, A. A. and Czeizel, A. E. (2000). Association of epilepsy with different groups of microcephaly. *Dev Med Child Neurol*, 42(11), 760–7.

Alpman, A., Serdaroglu, G., Cogulu, O. *et al.* (2005). Ring chromosome 20 syndrome with intractable epilepsy. *Dev Med Child Neurol*, 47(5), 343–6.

Alvestad, S., Lydersen, S. and Brodtkorb, E. (2007). Rash from antiepileptic drugs: influence by gender, age, and learning disability. *Epilepsia*, 48(7), 1360–5.

Appleton, R. E. (2001). West syndrome: long term prognosis and social aspects. *Brain Dev*, 23, 688–91.

Appleton, R. E. and Fryer, A. E. (1995). Neurological manifestations of tuberous sclerosis complex. *CNS Drugs*, 3, 174–85.

Balci, S., Unal, A., Engiz, O. *et al.* (2007). Bilateral periventricular nodular heterotopia, severe learning disability, and epilepsy in a male patient with 46,XY, der (19)t(X;19)(q11.1–11.2;p13.3). *Dev Med Child Neurol*, 49(3), 219–24.

Barkovich, A. J., Kuzniecky, R. I., Jackson, G. D., Guerrini, R. and Dobyns, W. B. (2001). Classification system for malformations of cortical development: update 2001. *Neurology*, 57, 2168–78.

Battaglia, A., Carey, J. C., Cederholm, P. *et al.* (1999). Natural history of Wolf-Hirschhorn syndrome: experience with 15 cases. *Pediatrics*, 103, 830–6.

Beavis, J., Kerr, M. and Marson, A. G. (2007a). Pharmacological interventions for epilepsy in people with intellectual disabilities. *Cochrane Database Syst Rev*, Issue 3. Art.No.:CD005399. DOI:10.1002/14651858.CD005399.pub2

Beavis, J., Kerr, M. and Marson, A. G. (2007b). Non-pharmacological interventions for epilepsy in people with intellectual disabilities. *Cochrane Database Syst Rev*, Issue 4.Art.No.:CD005502. DOI:10.1002/14651858.CD005502.pub2

Besag, F. M. C. (2006). Cognitive and behavioural outcomes of epileptic syndromes: implications for education and clinical practice. *Epilepsia*, 47(2), 119–25.

Brodtkorb, E., Nilsen, G., Smevik, O. and Rinck, P. A. (1992). Epilepsy and anomalies of neuronal migration: MRI and clinical aspects. *Acta Neurol Scand*, 86, 24–32.

Brunner, H. G. and Winter, R. M. (1991). Autosomal dominant inheritance of abnormalities of the hands and feet with short palpebral fissures, variable microcephaly with learning disability, and oesophageal/duodenal atresia. *J Med Genet*, 28(6), 389–94.

Buck, D., Smith, M., Appleton, R., Baker, G. A. and Jacoby, A. (2007). The development and validation of the Epilepsy and Learning Disabilities Quality of life (ELDQOL) scale. *Epilepsy Behav*, 10(1), 38–43.

Caksen H., Tuncer O., Atasl B. *et al.* (2003). A Turkish case of subcortical/subependymal heterotopia associated with corpus callosum dysgenesis, craniofacial dysmorphism, severe eye abnormalities, and growth-mental retardation. *Genet Couns*, 14(3), 343–8.

Camfield, C. S. and Camfield, P. R. (2007). Long term social outcomes for children with epilepsy. *Epilepsia*, 48(9), 3–5.

Caplan, R., Shields, W. R., Mori, L. and Yudovin, S. (1991). Middle childhood onset of interictal psychosis. *J Am Acad Child Adolesc Psychiatry*, 30, 893–6.

Chappell, B. and Crawford, P. (2005). An audit of lamotrigine, levetiracetam and topiramate usage for epilepsy in a district general hospital. *Seizure*, 14(6), 422–8.

Coppola, G., Plouin, P., Chiron, C., Robain, O. and Dulac, O. (1995). Migrating partial seizures in infancy: a malignant disorder with developmental arrest. *Epilepsia*, 36, 1017–24.

Crumrine, P. K. (2002). Lennox-Gastaut syndrome. *J Child Neurol*, 17(Suppl 1), 70–5.

Deb, S. and Hunter, D. (1991a). Psychopathology of people with mental handicap and epilepsy. I: Maladaptive behaviour. *Br J Psychiatry*, 159, 822–6.

Deb, S. and Hunter, D. (1991b). Psychopathology of people with mental handicap and epilepsy. II: Psychiatric illness. *Br J Psychiatry*, 159, 826–30.

Deb, S. and Hunter, D. (1991c). Psychopathology of people with Mental handicap and Epilepsy. III: Personality disorder. *Br J Psychiatry*, 159, 830–4.

Deb, S. and Joyce, J. (1999). Characteristics of epilepsy in a population based cohort of adults with learning disability. *Ir J Psychol Med*, 16(1), 5–9.

Deb, S., Cowie, V. A. and Richens, A. (1987). Folate metabolism and problem behaviour in mentally handicapped epileptics. *J Ment Defic Res*, 31, 163–8.

Duncan, R. and Oto, M. (2008). Psychogenic nonepileptic seizures in patients with learning disability: comparision with patients with no learning disability. *Epilepsy Behav*, 12(1), 183–6.

Espie, C. A., Pashley, E. S., Bonham, K. G., Sourindham, I. and O'Donovan, M. (1989). The mentally handicapped person with epilepsy: a comparative study investigating psychosocial functioning. *J Ment Defic Res*, 33, 123–35.

Espie, C. A., Watkins, J., Curtice, L. *et al.* (2003). Psychopathology in people with epilepsy and intellectual disability: an investigation of potential explanatory variables. *J Neurol Neurosurg Psychiatry*, 74(11), 1485–92.

Flink, R. and Rydenhag, B. (2008). Seizure outcome after resective epilepsy surgery in patients with low IQ. *Brain*, 131(Pt 2), 535–42.

Hobson-Webb, L. D. and Caress, J. B. (2006). Facioscapulohumeral muscular dystrophy can be a cause of isolated childhood cognitive dysfunction. *J Child Neurol*, 21(3), 252–3.

Hommet, C., Billard, C., Barthez, M. A. *et al.* (1999). Neuropsychological and adaptive functioning in adolescents and young adults shunted for congenital hydrocephalus. *J Child Neurol*, 14(3), 144–50.

Huber, B. and Tomka-Hoffmeister, M. (2003). Limited efficacy of gabapentin in severe therapy-resistant epilepsies of learning disabled patients. *Seizure*, 12(8), 602–3.

Huber, B., Bommel, W., Hauser, I. *et al.* (2004). Efficacy and tolerability of levetiracetam in patients with therapy-resistant epilepsy and learning disabilities. *Seizure*, 13(3), 168–75.

Hurley, A. D., Laatsch, L. K. and Dorman, C. (1983). Comparison of spina bifida, hydrocephalic patients and matched controls on neuropsychological tests. *Z Kinderchir*, 38(Suppl 2), 116–18.

Johansson, M., Billstedt, E., Danielsson, S. *et al.* (2007). Autism spectrum disorder and underlying brain mechanism in the oculoauriculovertebral spectrum. *Dev Med Child Neurol*, 49(4), 280–8.

Joinson, C., O'Callaghan, F. J., Osborne, J. P. *et al.* (2003). Learning disability and epilepsy in an epidemiological sample of individuals with tuberous sclerosis complex. *Psychol Med*, 33(2), 335–44.

Kanazawa, O. (2001). Refractory grand mal seizures with onset during infancy including severe myoclonic epilepsy in infancy. *Brain Dev*, 23, 749–56.

Kerr, M. and Bowley, C. (2001). Evidence-based prescribing in those with learning disability and epilepsy. *Epilepsia*, 42(Suppl1), 44–5.

Kerr, M. P. and Espie, C. A. (1997). Learning disability and epilepsy. 1, towards common outcome measures. *Seizure*, 6(5), 331–6.

Koepp, M. J., Patsalos, P. N. and Sander, J. W. A. S. (2002). Sulthiame in adults with refractory epilepsy and learning disability: an open trial. *Epilepsy Res*, 50(3), 277–82.

Kramer, U., Kahana, E., Shorer, Z. and Ben-Zeer, B. (2000). Outcome of infants with unilateral Sturge-Weber syndrome and early onset seizures. *Dev Med Child Neurol*, 42, 756–9.

Krishnamoorthy, E. S. (2003). Neuropsychiatric epidemiology at the interface between learning disability and epilepsy. In *Learning Disability and Epilepsy: An Integrative Approach*, ed. M. Trimble. Guildford, UK: Claruis Press Ltd, pp. 17–25.

Lindquist, B., Carlsson G., Persson, E.-K. and Uvebrant, P. (2005). Learning disabilities in a population-based group of children with hydrocephalus. *Acta Paediat*, 94(7), 878–83.

Lindquist, B., Carlsson, G., Persson, E.-K. and Uvebrant, P. (2006). Behavioural problems and autism in children with hydrocephalus: a population based study. *Eur Child Adolesc Psychiatry*, 15(4), 214–19.

Lund, J. (1985). Epilepsy and psychiatric disorder in the mentally retarded adult. *Acta Psychiatr Scand*, 71, 557–62.

Matthews, T., Weston, N., Baxter, H., Felce, D. and Kerr, M. (2008). A general practice-based prevalence study of epilepsy among adults with intellectual disabilities, and of its association with psychiatric disorder, behaviour disturbance and carer stress. *J Intellect Disabil Res*, 52(Pt 2), 163–73.

McGrother, C. W., Bhaumik, S., Thorp, C. F. *et al.* (2006). Epilepsy in adults with intellectual disabilities: prevalence, associations and service implications. *Seizure*, 15(6), 376–86.

Moretti, P., Peters, S. U., Del Gaudio, D. *et al.* (2008). Brief report: autistic symptoms, developmental regression, mental retardation, epilepsy, and dyskinesias in CNS folate deficiency. *J Autism Dev Disord*, 38(6), 1170–7.

Morgan, C. L., Baxter, H. and Kerr, M. P. (2003). Prevalence of epilepsy and associated health service utilization and mortality among patients with intellectual disability. *Am J Ment Retard*, 108(5), 293–300.

Mula, M., Trimble, M. R. and Sander, J. W. A. S. (2004). Psychiatric adverse events in patients with epilepsy and learning disabilities taking levetiracetam. *Seizure*, 13(1), 55–7.

Niedermeyer, E. (2002). Lennox-Gastaut syndrome. Clinical description and diagnosis. *Adv Exp Med Biol*, 497, 61–75.

Persson, E.-K., Hagberg, G. and Uvebrant, P. (2006). Disabilities in children with hydrocephalus–a population based study of children aged between four and twelve years. *Neuropediatrics*, 37(6), 330–6.

Powell, H. W. R., Hart, P. E. and Sisodiya, S. M. (2003). Epilepsy and perisylvian polymicrogyria in a patient with Kabuki syndrome. *Dev Med Child Neurol*, 45(12), 841–3.

Praline, J., Hommet, C., Barthez, M. *et al.* (2003). Outcome at adulthood of the continous spike-waves during slow sleep and Landau-Kleffner syndromes. *Epilepsia*, 44(11), 1434–40.

Prasher, V. P. (1995). Epilepsy and associated effects on adaptive behaviour in adults with Down syndrome. *Seizure*, 4(1), 53–6.

Ragge, N. K., Lorenz, B., Schneider, A. *et al.* (2005). SOX2 anophthalmia syndrome. *Am J Med Genet A*, 135(1), 1–7.

Reuber, M., Gore, J., Wolstenhome, J. *et al.* (2008). Examining a community model of epilepsy care for people with learning disabilities. *Seizure*, 17(1), 84–91.

Ring, H., Zia, A., Lindeman, S. and Himlok, K. (2007). Interactions between seizure frequency, psychopathology, and severity of intellectual disability in a population with epilepsy and a learning disability. *Epilepsy Behav*, 11(1), 92–7.

Robinson, R. O., Baird, G., Robinson, G. and Simonoff, E. (2001). Landau-Kleffner syndrome: course and correlates with outcome. *Dev Med Child Neurol*, 43, 243–7.

Sanchez-Carpintero, R., McLellan, A., Parmeggiani, L. *et al.* (2005). Pallister-Killian syndrome: an unusual cause of epileptic spasms. *Dev Med Child Neurol*, 47(11), 776–9.

Scheepers, B., Salahudeen, S. and Morelli, J. (2004). Two-year outcome audit in an adult learning disability population with refractory epilepsy. *Seizure*, 13(8), 529–33.

Scheffer, I. E., Wallace, R. H., Phillips, F. L. *et al.* (2002). X-linked myoclonic epilepsy with spasticity and intellectual disability. *Neurology*, 59(3), 348–56.

Sillanpää, M. (1996). Epilepsy in the mentally retarded. In: *Epilepsy in Children*, Ed. S. Wallace. London: Chapman and Hall, pp. 417–27.

Simister, R. J., Sander, J. W. and Koepp, M. J. (2007). Long-term retention rates of new antiepileptic drugs in adults with chronic epilepsy and learning disability. *Epilepsy Behav*, 10(2), 336–9.

Singh, R., Gardner, R. J. M., Crossland, K. M., Scheffer, I. E. and Berkovic, S. F. (2002). Chromosomal abnormalities and epilepsy: a review for clinicians and gene hunters. *Epilepsia*, 43, 127–40.

Sisodiya, S. M. (2004). Malformations of cortical development: burdens and insights from important causes of human epilepsy. *Lancet Neurol*, 3(1), 29–38.

Stafstrom, C. E. and Konkol, R. J. (1994). Infantile spasms in children with Down syndrome. *Dev Med Child Neurol*, 36, 576–85.

Steffenburg, S., Steffenburg, U. and Gillberg, C. (2003). Autism spectrum disorders in children with active epilepsy and learning disability: co-morbidity, pre- and perinatal background, and seizure characteristics. *Dev Med Child Neurol*, 45(11), 724–30.

Steffenburg, U., Hagberg, G. and Kyllerman, M. (1995). Active epilepsy in mentally retarded children. II. Etiology and reduced pre- and perinatal optimality. *Acta Paediatr Scand*, 84, 1153–9.

Steffenburg, U., Hagberg, G. and Hagberg, B. (2001). Epilepsy in a representative series of Rett syndrome. *Acta Paediatr*, 90(1), 34–9.

Suenobu, S.-I., Akiyoshi, K., Maeda, T., Korematsu, S. and Izumi, T. (2008). Clinical presentation of patients with neurofibromatosis type 1 in infancy and childhood: genetic traits and gender effects. *J Child Neurol*, 23(11), 1282–7.

Taylor, D. C., Falconer, M. A., Bruton, C. J. and Corsellis, J. A. (1971). Focal dysplasia of the cerebral cortex in epilepsy. *J Neurol Neurosurg Psychiatry*, 34, 369–87.

Whitten, E. and Griffiths, A. (2007). Implementing epilepsy guidelines within a learning disability service. *Seizure*, 16(6), 471–8.

Wisniewski, K. E., Segan, S. M., Miezejeski, C. M., Sersen, E. A. and Rudelli, R. D. (1991). The Fra(X) syndrome: neurological, electrophysiological, and neuropathological abnormalities. *Am J Med Genet*, 38(2–3), 476–80.

Yamatogi, Y. and Ohtahara, S. (2002). Early infantile epileptic encephalopathy with suppression bursts, Ohtahara syndrome; its overview referring to our 16 cases. *Brain Dev*, 24, 13–23.

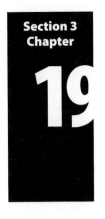

Diseases of the nervous system II: neurodegenerative diseases including dementias

Muthukumar Kannabiran and Shoumitro Deb

Introduction

Neurodegenerative diseases (ND) are hereditary and sporadic conditions, characterised by progressive nervous system dysfunction (MeSH, 2009). They include Alzheimer's disease (AD) and other dementias, and conditions such as Huntington's disease, multiple sclerosis and motor neurone disease. It is now well known that a high proportion of people with Down syndrome (DS) develop AD at an early age (McCarron *et al.* (2005); also see Deb (2003) for a review). This chapter will review dementia in people with intellectual disability (ID) without DS, before discussing AD in people with DS in detail.

Method

We used a broad search strategy using the National Library for Health (NLH) Advanced Search (AMED, BNI, EMBASE, HMIC, MEDLINE, PsycINFO, CINAHL and HEALTH BUSINESS ELITE) and Google Scholar. All relevant abstracts were read and relevant articles were inspected in more detail. Intellectual disability journals were hand searched for relevant papers. The following search terms were used: dementia, neurodegenerative, learning AND disability, intellectual AND disability, developmental AND disability, and mental AND retardation. The MeSH terms used were mental retardation and neurodegenerative disease. The first search was made in October 2008 and updated in December 2008.

Results

The results of the search are shown in Table 19.1.

Discussion

Neurodegenerative disorders

The bulk of the studies identified by the search were on dementia and a small number of papers were on Fragile X-associated tremor/ataxia syndrome (FXTAS). The latter is a multi-system neurological disorder characterised by progressive cerebellar ataxia, parkinsonism, dementia and autonomic dysfunction, reported in individuals with the Fragile X premutation expansion (of 55–200 CGG repeats in the *FMR1* gene) (Baba and Uitti, 2005). Jacquemont

Intellectual Disability and Ill Health: A Review of the Evidence, ed. Jean O'Hara, Jane McCarthy and Nick Bouras. Published by Cambridge University Press. © Cambridge University Press 2010.

Table 19.1. Search results

Search terms	Number of references/hits
1. (dementia OR neurodegenerative)	270 470
2. (intellectual OR learning OR developmental AND disability)	72 704
3. 1 AND 2	1 691

et al. (2004) report that mild dementia may be present in 20% of males with FXTAS, with other authors reporting dementia (Karmon and Gadoth, 2008) and multiple sclerosis (Greco *et al.*, 2008) in women with the *FMR1* premutation.

Dementia in persons with ID without DS

A number of studies of dementia in people with ID (who do not have DS) have been undertaken. Cooper (1997) reports an increased prevalence of dementia (21.6%) in a study of 134 adults with ID aged 65 years and above. In a cross-sectional study involving adults with ID (without DS), aged ≥ 60 years, AD was the most common subtype (prevalence of 8.6%), followed by Lewy body, fronto-temporal and vascular dementias (Strydom *et al.*, 2007). Strydom *et al.* (2009) found increased prevalence (18.3%) of dementia in 284 adults over 65 years of age with ID (without DS), with the prevalence not differing with the severity of ID. The study confirmed a downward shift in age-associated risk, with an earlier age of dementia onset in this population compared with the general population. In contrast, Zigman *et al.* (2004) reported rates of dementia in adults with ID (without DS) equivalent to or lower than the expected rates from the general population (AD prevalence of 2.7% in those over 65 years of age; 4.1% in the over 75 age group). Patel *et al.* (1993) found a prevalence of dementia of 11.4% among 105 adults aged 50 years and over who had ID. Between 31% and 78% of adults with ID but not DS show AD neuropathology, whereas almost all people with DS aged over 50 are known to develop AD neuropathology (Deb, 2003).

Alzheimer's disease and Down syndrome

Coppus *et al.* (2006) studied 506 people with DS, aged 45 years or older. The overall prevalence of dementia was 16.8%, the prevalence doubling every 5 years up to 60 years and decreasing slightly in individuals who were 60 years and older (attributed to increased mortality up to age 60).

Aetiopathology and risk factors for AD in DS

Extracellular neuritic amyloid plaques and intracellular neurofibrillary tangles (phosphorylated tau protein) are the hallmarks of AD neuropathology. The deposition of β amyloid is related to mutations in presenilin 1 (*PS 1*) and presenilin 2 (*PS 2*) genes and to over expression of the amyloid precursor protein (*APP*) gene, located on the long arm of chromosome 21. Mutations in these three genes are shown to be associated with early-onset familiar type of AD (Schupf, 2002). In a study of 105 adults with DS, Margallo-Lana *et al.* (2004) found a 13-year difference in the age of onset of dementia associated with the number of APP repeats and concluded that APP is an important locus in predicting age of onset of dementia in people with DS. Individuals with increased plasma levels of amyloid peptide β 42 were twice

> **Box 19.1** Risk factors for AD in people with DS
>
> AD in DS is more commonly seen with
>
> - increasing age
> - higher pre-morbid level of functioning (cognitive reserve)
> - menopause and early onset of menopause
> - higher frequencies of APOE ε4 allele
>
> Zigman and Lott, 2007; Bush and Beail, 2004.

as likely to develop AD and participants with AD had higher levels of plasma amyloid peptide β 42 (Schupf *et al.*, 2007).

Three alleles (ε2, ε3 and ε4) encode for the Apolipoprotein E (*APOE*) gene (located on chromosome 19) which is involved in cholesterol transport and lipid metabolism (Dupuy *et al.*, 2001). Apolipoprotein E ε4 is considered to increase the risk of early-onset AD. Coppus *et al.* (2008) found APOE ε4 was associated with increased long-term ($\geq$ 3 years) incidence of dementia in 425 people with DS. In a longitudinal study of 252 individuals, Prasher *et al.* (2008c) reported that participants with APOE ε4 had significantly increased risk of developing AD (hazard ratio (HR) = 1.8; 1.12–2.79), with an earlier age of onset and more rapid progression to death. Deb *et al.* (2000) in their meta-analysis found an association between APOE ε4 and an increased rate of dementia in people with DS but they did not find any such association with presenilin 1 or 2 polymorphism (Deb *et al.*, 1998).

Oxidative stress (OS) is the imbalance between the production and removal of reactive oxygen species (ROS), and has been postulated to be the 'bridge' between DS and AD (Zana *et al.*, 2007). Oxidative stress is thought to precede the development of the characteristic pathology in AD (Moreira *et al.*, 2006) and amyloid deposition and tau hyperphosphorylation are considered to be compensatory cellular responses to OS.

Compared with a control group, individuals with DS (n = 19) showed a tendency towards higher serum cytokine concentrations, with a significantly higher level of macrophage inflammatory protein-1α (MIP-1α) (Carta *et al.*, 2002). The authors suggest involvement of MIP-1α in pathogenesis of AD in DS, as MIP-1α level was directly proportional to age. Given the role of APOE in cholesterol transport, in a study of 179 people with DS, Prasher *et al.* (2008a) found no significant association between total serum cholesterol and AD, though cholesterol levels were significantly increased in individuals with APOE ε4.

A number of risk factors for developing AD have been identified in persons with DS (please refer to Box 19.1). In a comparison of two groups of individuals with DS, with and without symptoms of AD, the level of cognitive functioning correlated with environmental factors (Temple *et al.*, 2001). Individuals with higher levels of cognitive functioning were found to be less likely to develop dementia. Interestingly, no significant difference was found in season of birth for individuals with DS and dementia, compared with those without dementia (Prasher *et al.*, 2008a).

Clinical presentation

Prasher (1995a) described mental deterioration, slowing, confusion, reduced speech and deterioration in gait and personality change as the common early symptoms of dementia among adults with DS. Evenhuis (1990) on the other hand described apathy and withdrawal

---

Box 19.2 Symptoms in early stage AD in DS

- Forgetfulness – impairment of recent memory (with relatively intact distant memory)
- Confusion
- Slowness in activities and speech*
- Speech and language problems – speech initiation*, lack of expression*, flattening of tone, repetitive questioning (when not present previously)
- Difficulty following more than one instruction at a time
- Sleep disturbance – early morning wakening, wandering at night
- Loss of skills – requiring more prompting and help
- Loss of interest in activities* and slowness of movement*
- Social withdrawal*
- Balance problems – unsteady gait, fear of kerbs
- Emergence of emotional and behaviour problems – crying spells, shouting and screaming
- Visual hallucinations and illusions
- 'Covering up for the loss of memory'
- Personality change – aggressive, behaviourally disturbed, change from previous personality

* Frontal lobe symptoms.
Deb *et al.*, 2007a.

---

symptoms as the most common early features of dementia among those with both moderate as well as severe ID. The late features of dementia among adults with ID include severe intellectual deterioration, marked change in personality and mood, loss of sphincter control, onset of epileptic seizures, loss of mobility with increased muscle tone and eventual complete loss of all self-help skills (Prasher, 1995b).

Deb *et al.* (2007a) found that there were many similarities in the clinical presentation of dementia in adults with DS and the general population. Forgetfulness and confusion were common, and presented early in dementia among adults with DS. However, many 'frontal lobe' related symptoms that are usually manifested later in the process of dementia among the general population were seen at an early stage of dementia among adults with DS (please refer to Box 19.2).

Studies have examined the nature and course of cognitive impairment in this population. Krinsky-McHale *et al.* (2002) compared changes in memory in early-stage AD in 14 adults with DS to the changes in those with normal ageing, using a modified version of the Selective Reminding Test (SRT). Participants with early-stage AD had deficits in their ability to code and retrieve information from long-term memory compared with controls, with these deficits preceding other symptoms of dementia by one to three years. However, considerable debate exists regarding the overlap of age-related cognitive decline and dementia in the general population as well as in people with ID. Studies that have mapped out cognitive decline among adults with ID, with and without DS, using prospective designs show a trend of relatively greater decline in verbal abilities compared with performance abilities, than has been shown in the general population (Carr, 2005; Devenny *et al.*, 2000). However, the exact features associated with normal ageing and their overlap with dementia symptoms have never been properly studied among people with ID.

With progressive dyspraxia being recognised as an early symptom of AD in people with DS (Dalton and Fedor, 1998), older persons with DS show significant deterioration in

> **Box 19.3** Schema for diagnosis of dementia in people with ID
>
> - History from the person and from an informant
> - Examination or check for
>   - Sensory impairments such as hearing and vision
>   - Medical conditions, particularly hypothyroidism and epilepsy
>   - 'functional' psychiatric disorders such as depression
>   - associated drug treatment
> - Laboratory investigations
> - Blood tests for differential diagnosis and cause of dementia (full blood count, vitamin B12 etc.)
> - Neuroimaging (structural to exclude space-occupying lesion; functional, particularly SPECT (Deb *et al.*, 1992) to help with the differential diagnosis)
> - Baseline and longitudinal use of neuropsychological tests and observer-rated questionnaires
>
> Modified from Deb, 2003.

dyspraxia scores, thought to be suggestive of preclinical signs of AD. Kittler *et al.* (2006) suggested that increase in verbal intrusion errors during a working memory task in adults with DS may signal future cognitive decline. Dalton *et al.* (1999) reported that deterioration of memory and learning (at a mean age of 54.2 years) may precede impairment in praxis (mean age 56.9 years) in adults with DS ($\geq$ 50 years).

Diagnosis

The diagnosis of dementia in people with ID in general and DS in particular remains difficult, particularly in the early stage of the disease. The components of the diagnostic process include history-taking, examination, investigations and specialised testing (please refer to Box 19.3). Cognitive abilities in most people with ID are at a below average level even before they develop dementia. Therefore, the screening instruments commonly used in the general population such as the Mini Mental State Examination (MMSE) (Folstein *et al.*, 1975) cannot be used in this population because of possible floor effect. For similar reasons direct neuropsychological tests cannot be administered in any meaningful way to most people with DS (Deb and Braganza, 1999). Only experienced professionals can administer neuropsychological tests, not carers (Aylward *et al.*, 1997). Some of the early symptoms of dementia may be subtle or may present as an exacerbation of the existing behavioural traits or manifest differently in people with DS than they do in people without ID. Only carers will notice these early and sometimes unusual changes in the person's behaviour and only by asking carers can we ensure that such symptoms are included in any case-detection instrument. Therefore the use of a combination of informant-rated scales and neuropsychological tests adapted for use in people with ID, particularly in a prospective way, is the best way to detect dementia among people with ID. In an effort to standardise the approach to diagnosing dementia in ID, one working group proposed a test battery (Burt and Aylward, 2000).

Ball *et al.* (2004) reported that the Cambridge Examination for Mental Disorders of the Elderly (CAMDEX), modified to emphasise change in cognitive function, has good validity and reliability in diagnosing AD in people with DS. Margallo-Lana *et al.* (2007) followed

---

Box 19.4 Instruments used for screening dementia among adults with ID

Observer/informant-rated instruments

- Dementia Questionnaire for Persons with Mental Retardation (DMR) (Evenhuis, 1996)
- Dementia Scale for Down Syndrome (DSDS) (Gedye, 1995)
- Multidimensional Observation Scale for Elderly Subjects (MOSES) (Dalton and Fedor 1997; Dalton *et al.*, 2002)
- Early Signs of Dementia Checklist (Visser *et al.*, 1997)
- Adaptive Behaviour Scale (ABS) (Nihira *et al.*, 1974)
- Modified CAMDEX informant interview (Ball et al., 2004)
- Dementia Screening Questionnaire for Individuals with Intellectual Disabilities (DSQIID) (Deb *et al.*, 2007b)

Neuropsychological tests

- Modified MMSE (Folstein *et al.*, 1975)
- Modified Boston Naming Test (Kaplan *et al.*, 1978)
- McCarthy Verbal Fluency (McCarthy, 1972)
- Modified Fuld (Altman, 1977; Seltzer, 1997)
- Modified Purdue Pegboard (Tiffin and Asher, 1948)
- Brief Praxis Test (Dalton, 1992)
- Spatial Recognition Span (Moss *et al.*, 1986)
- Test for Severe Impairment (TSI) (Albert and Cohen, 1992)

Modified from Deb, 2003.

---

up 92 hospitalised persons with DS over a 15-year period, using the Prudhoe Cognitive Function Test (PCFT) and the Adaptive Behaviour Scale (ABS). They found that 21% developed dementia and the median age of onset was 55.5 (45–74) years. Instruments such as PCFT and ABS are reportedly useful in making a diagnosis of dementia in people with less severe ID, while behavioural and neurological criteria are required for diagnosis in those with more profound ID. Deb *et al.* (2007b) have recently developed the Dementia Screening Questionnaire for Individuals with Intellectual Disabilities (DSQIID), with excellent psychometric properties. To ensure face validity, the DSQIID items were collated by asking carers to describe changes in behaviour of the person with DS as they developed dementia. Box 19.4 lists dementia screening instruments for adults with ID.

Management of AD

Pharmacological and psychological approaches are used in the management of AD. The mainstays of treatment are acetylcholinesterase inhibitors (donepezil, rivastigmine and galantamine) or the NMDA antagonist memantine (Prasher, 2004). In a 24-week, double-blind, placebo-controlled trial involving 30 patients with DS and AD treated with donepezil, the treatment group had a (non-significant) reduction in deterioration in global functioning, adaptive behaviour and cognitive functions (Prasher *et al.*, 2002). The participants in this study continued on to an open-label phase to study the long-term effect of donepezil (Prasher *et al.*, 2003). After 104 weeks, the treatment group showed significant reduction in deterioration of cognitive functions and adaptive behaviour.

In an open-label trial of patients with DS and dementia comparing nine patients treated with donepezil with nine untreated, matched patients with DS and dementia, significant improvement was reported in the treatment group over a three- to five-month period

> **Box 19.5** Novel treatment strategies in AD Tanzi, 2008
>
> - M1 muscarinic agonists, M2 muscarinic antagonists and nicotinic agonists (Fisher, 2008)
> - Intranasal insulin (Reger *et al.*, 2008)
> - β-amyloid immunotherapy (Nitsch and Hock, 2008)
> - γ-secretase (Wolfe, 2008)
> - β-secretase inhibitors (Ghosh *et al.*, 2008)
> - 5-HT6 receptor antagonists (Upton *et al.*, 2008)
> - Ketone bodies (Henderson, 2008)
> - Peroxisome proliferator-activated receptor gamma (PPAR-γ) – Rosiglitazone (Landreth *et al.*, 2008)
> - Tau-based treatment strategies (Schneider and Mandelkow, 2008)

(p = 0.03) (Lott *et al.*, 2002). Prasher *et al.* (2005) compared 17 patients with DS and AD treated with rivastigmine with 13 patients treated with placebo. Both groups deteriorated over a 24-week period, but the rate of decline was less in the rivastigmine group. Meta-analyses of studies of agents with antioxidant effect in DS, including Gingko Biloba, piracetam and vitamins have pointed towards either insufficient evidence or lack of positive evidence of cognitive improvement (see review by Zana *et al.* (2007)). Box 19.5 lists new treatments for AD under investigation.

Conclusion

There have been a number of recent reports of neurodegenerative diseases in people with ID, especially with FXATS. Further studies will identify the epidemiology and clarify whether there are shared underlying pathogenic mechanisms, which may guide development of potential therapies. Much is known about dementia, especially AD and DS, in this population, however, there is scant evidence on treatment, with much of this being extrapolated from studies involving people without ID. A number of promising approaches are being explored in the management of AD and it is vital that studies include people with ID to establish a good evidence base for future treatments.

References

Albert, M. and Cohen, C. (1992). The Test for Severe Impairment: an instrument for the assessment of patients with severe cognitive dysfunction. *J Am Geriatr Soc*, 40, 449–53.

Altman, P. (1977). *Fuld Object-Memory Evaluation: Instruction Manual*. IL, USA: Stoelting, Wheat Dale.

Aylward, E. H., Burt, D. B., Thorpe, L. U., Lai, F. and Dalton, A. (1997). Diagnosis of dementia in individuals with intellectual disability. *J Intellect Disabil Res*, 41(2), 152–64.

Baba, Y. and Uitti, R. J. (2005). Fragile X-associated tremor/ataxia syndrome and movement disorders. *Curr Opin Neurol*, 18, 393–8.

Ball, S. L., Holland, A. J., Huppert, F. A. *et al.* (2004). The modified CAMDEX informant interview is a valid and reliable tool for use in the diagnosis of dementia in adults with Down's syndrome. *J Intellect Disabil Res*, 48(6), 611–20.

Burt, D. B. and Aylward, E. H. (2000). Test battery for the diagnosis of dementia in individuals with intellectual disability. *J Intellect Disabil Res*, 44(2), 175–80.

Bush, A. and Beail, N. (2004). Risk factors for dementia in people with down syndrome: issues in assessment and diagnosis. *Am J Ment Retard*, 109(2), 83–97.

Carr J. (2005). Stability and change in cognitive ability over the life span: a comparison of populations with and without Down's syndrome. *J Intellect Disabil Res*, 49(12), 915–28.

Carta, M. G., Serra, P., Giani, A. *et al.* (2002). Chemokines and pro-inflammatory cytokines in Down's syndrome: an early marker for Alzheimer-type dementia? *Psychother Psychosom*, 71, 233–6.

Cooper, S.-A. (1997). High prevalence of dementia among people with learning disabilities not attributable to Down's syndrome. *Psychol Med*, 27, 609–16.

Coppus, A., Evenhuis, H., Verberne, G. J. *et al.* (2006). Dementia and mortality in persons with Down's syndrome. *J Intellect Disabil Res*, 50(10), 768–77.

Coppus, A. M. W., Evenhuis, H. M., Verberne, G. *et al.* (2008). The impact of apolipoprotein E on dementia in persons with Down's syndrome. *Neurobiol Aging*, 29, 828–35.

Dalton, A. J. (1992). Dementia in Down syndrome: methods of evaluation. In *Alzheimer's Disease and Down Syndrome*, ed. L. Nadel and C. J. Epstein. New York, USA: Wiley Liss, pp. 51–76.

Dalton, A. J. and Fedor, B. L. (1997). The Multi-dimensional Observation Scale for Elderly Subjects applied for persons with Down syndrome. In *Proceedings of the International Congress III on the Dually Diagnosed*. Washington DC, USA: National Association for the Dually Diagnosed, pp. 173–8.

Dalton, A. J. and Fedor, B. L. (1998). Onset of dyspraxia in aging persons with Down syndrome: longitudinal studies. *J Intellect Disabil*, 23(1), 13–24.

Dalton, A. J., Mehta, P. D., Fedor, B. L. and Patti, P. J. (1999). Cognitive changes in memory precede those in praxis in aging persons with Down syndrome. *J Intellect Dev Disabil*, 24(2), 169–87.

Dalton, A. J., Fedor, B. L., Patti, P. J., Tsiouris, J. A. and Mehta, P. D. (2002). The Multidimensional Observation Scale for Elderly Subjects (MOSES): studies in adults with intellectual disability. *J Intellect Dev Disabil*, 27(4), 310–24.

Deb, S. (2003). Dementia in people who have an intellectual disability. *Rev Clin Gerontol*, 13, 137–44.

Deb, S. and Braganza, J. (1999). Comparison of rating scales for the diagnosis of dementia in adults with Down's syndrome. *J Intellect Disabil Res*, 43(5), 400–7.

Deb, S., de Silva, P., Gemmell, H. G. *et al.* (1992). Alzheimer's disease in adults with Down's syndrome: the relationship between regional cerebral blood flow deficits and dementia. *Acta Psychiatr Scand*, 86, 340–5.

Deb, S., Braganza, J., Owen, M. *et al.* (1998). No significant association between a PS-1 intronic polymorphism and dementia in Down's syndrome. *Alzheimers Rep*, 1(6), 365–8.

Deb, S., Braganza, J., Norton N. *et al.* (2000) APOE epsilon 4 influences the manifestation of Alzheimer's dementia in adults with Down's syndrome. *Br J Psychiatry*, 176, 468–72.

Deb, S., Hare, M. and Prior, L. (2007a). Symptoms of dementia among adults with Down's syndrome: a qualitative study. *J Intellect Disabil Res*, 51(9), 726–39.

Deb, S., Hare, M., Prior, L. and Bhaumik, S. (2007b). Dementia Screening Questionnaire for Individuals with Intellectual Disabilities (DSQIID). *Br J Psychiatry*, 190, 440–4.

Devenny, D. A., Krinsky-Hale, S. J., Sersen, G. and Silverman, W. P. (2000). Sequence of cognitive decline in adults with Down's syndrome. *J Intellect Disabil Res*, 44, 654–65.

Dupuy, A. M., Mas, E., Ritchie, K. *et al.* (2001). The relationship between apolipoprotein E4 and lipid metabolism is impaired in Alzheimer's disease. *Gerontology*, 47, 213–18.

Evenhuis, H. M. (1990). The natural history of dementia in Down's syndrome. *Arch Neurol*, 47(3), 263–7.

Evenhuis, H. M. (1996). Further evaluation of the Dementia Questionnaire for Persons with Mental Retardation (DMR). *J Intellect Disabil Res*, 40, 369–73.

Fisher, A. (2008). Cholinergic treatments with emphasis on M1 muscarinic agonists as potential disease-modifying agents for Alzheimer's disease. *Neurotherapeutics*, 5, 433–42.

Folstein, M. F., Folstein, S. E. and McHugh, P. R. (1975). 'Mini Mental State'. A practical method for grading the cognitive state of patients for the clinician. *J Psychiatr Res*, 12, 189–98.

Gedye, A. (1995). *Dementia Scale for Down Syndrome Manual*. Vancouver, British Columbia: Gedye Research and Consulting.

Ghosh, A. K., Gemma, S. and Tang, J. (2008). B-Secretase as a therapeutic target for Alzheimer's disease. *Neurotherapeutics*, 5, 399–408.

Greco, C. M., Tassone, F., Garcia-Arocena, D. *et al.* (2008). Clinical and neuropathological findings in a woman with the FMR1 premutation and multiple sclerosis. *Arch Neurol*, 65(8), 1114–16.

Henderson, S. T. (2008). Ketone bodies as a therapeutic for Alzheimer's disease. *Neurotherapeutics*, 5, 470–90.

Jacquemont, S., Farzin, F., Hall, D. *et al.* (2004). Aging in individuals with the FMR1 mutation. *Am J Ment Retard*, 109, 154–64.

Kaplan, E., Goodglass, H. and Weubtraub, S. (1978). *The Boston Naming Test*. Philadelphia, PA, USA: Lea and Febiger.

Karmon, Y. and Gadoth, N. (2008). Fragile X tremor/ataxia syndrome (FXTAS) with dementia in a female harbouring FMR1 premutation. *J Neurol, Neurosurg Psychiatry*, 79, 738–9.

Kittler, P., Krinsky-McHale, S. J. and Devenny, D. A. (2006). Verbal intrusions precede memory decline in adults with Down syndrome. *J Intellect Disabil Res*, 50(1), 1–10.

Krinsky-McHale, S. J., Devenny, D. A. and Silverman, W. P. (2002). Changes in explicit memory associated with early dementia in adults with Down's syndrome. *J Intellect Disabil Res*, 46(3), 198–208.

Landreth, G., Jiang, Q., Mandrekar, S. and Heneka, M. (2008). PPARγ agonists as therapeutics for the treatment of Alzheimer's disease. *Neurotherapeutics*, 5, 481–9.

Lott, I. T., Osann, K., Doran, E. and Nelson, L. (2002). Down syndrome and Alzheimer disease. *Arch Neurol*, 59, 1133–6.

Margallo-Lana, M., Morris, C. M., Gibson, A. M. *et al.* (2004). Influence of the amyloid precursor protein locus on dementia in Down syndrome. *Neurology*, 63, 1996–8.

Margallo-Lana, M. L., Moore, P. B., Kay, D. W. K. *et al.* (2007). Fifteen-year follow-up of 92 hospitalized adults with Down's syndrome: incidence of cognitive decline, its relationship to age and neuropathology. *J Intellect Disabil Res*, 51(6), 463–77.

McCarron, M., Gill, M., McCallion, P. and Begley, C. (2005). Health co-morbidities in ageing persons with Down syndrome and Alzheimer's dementia. *J Intellect Disabil Res*, 49, 560–6.

McCarthy, D. (1972). *Manual for the McCarthy Scales of Children's Ability*. San Antonio, TX, USA: The Psychological Corporation.

MeSH (2009). National Library of Medicine – Medical Subject Headings Available from: www.nlm.nih.gov/mesh/MBrowser.html.

Moreira, P. I., Honda, K., Zhu, X. *et al.* (2006). Brain and brawn: parallels in oxidative strength. *Neurology*, 66(Suppl 1), S97–101.

Moss, M. B., Albert, M. S., Butters, N. and Payne, M. (1986). Differential patterns of memory loss among patients with Alzheimer's disease, Huntington's disease, and alcoholic Korsakoff's syndrome. *Arch Neurol*, 43, 239–46.

Nihira, K., Foster, R., Shellhass, M. and Leland, H. (1974). *AAMD Adaptive Behavior Scale*. Washington DC, USA: American Association on Mental Retardation.

Nitsch, R. M. and Hock, C. (2008). Targeting β-amyloid pathology in Alzheimer's disease with Aβ immunotherapy. *Neurotherapeutics*, 5, 415–20.

Patel, P., Goldberg, D. and Moss, S. (1993). Psychiatric morbidity in older people with moderate and severe learning disability (mental retardation). Part II: The prevalence study. *Br J Psychiatry*, 163, 481–91.

Prasher, V. P. (1995a). Age-specific prevalence, thyroid dysfunction and depressive symptomatology in adults with Down's syndrome and dementia. *Int J Geriatr Psychiatry*, 10, 25–31.

Prasher, V. P. (1995b). End-stage dementia in adults with Down's syndrome. *Int J Geriatr Psychiatry*, 10, 1067–9.

Prasher, V. P. (2004). Review of donepezil, rivastigmine, galantamine and memantine for the treatment of dementia in Alzheimer's disease in adults with Down syndrome: implications for the intellectual disability population. *Int J Geriatr Psychiatry*, 19, 509–15.

Prasher, V. P., Huxley, A. and Haque, M. S.; Down syndrome Ageing Study Group.

(2002). A 24-week, double-blind, placebo-controlled trial of donepezil in patients with Down syndrome and Alzheimer's disease-pilot study. *Int J Geriatr Psychiatry*, 17, 270–8.

Prasher, V. P., Adams, C. and Holder, R. (2003). Long term safety and efficacy of donepezil in the treatment of dementia in Alzheimer's disease in adults with Down syndrome: open label study. *Int J Geriatr Psychiatry*, 18, 549–51.

Prasher, V. P., Fung, N. and Adams, C. (2005). Rivastigmine in the treatment of dementia in Alzheimer's disease in adults with Down syndrome. *Int J Geriatr Psychiatry*, 20, 496–7.

Prasher, V. P., Airuehia, E., Patel, A. and Haque, M. S. (2008a). Total serum cholesterol levels and Alzheimer's dementia in patients with Down syndrome. *Int J Geriatr Psychiatry*, 23, 937–42.

Prasher, V. P., Kapadia, H. M. and Haque, M. S. (2008b). Season of birth: dementia in Alzheimer's disease in adults with Down syndrome. *Int J Geriatr Psychiatry*, 23, 441–2.

Prasher, V. P., Sajith, S. G., Rees, S. D. *et al.* (2008c). Significant effect of APOE Epsilon 4 genotype on the risk of dementia in Alzheimer's disease and mortality in persons with Down syndrome. *Int J Geriatr Psychiatry*, 23, 1134–40.

Reger, M. A., Watson, G. S., Green, P. S. *et al.* (2008). Intranasal insulin improves cognition and modulates β-amyloid in early AD. *Neurology*, 70, 440–8.

Schneider, A. and Mandelkow, E. (2008). Tau-based treatment strategies in neurodegenerative diseases. *Neurotherapeutics*, 5(3), 443–57.

Schupf, N. (2002). Genetic and host factors for dementia in Down's syndrome. *Br J Psychiatry*, 180, 405–10.

Schupf, N., Patel, B., Pang, D. *et al.* (2007). Elevated plasma amyloid b-peptide Ab42, incident dementia and mortality in Down syndrome. *Arch Neurol*, 64(7), 1007–13.

Seltzer, G. B. (1997). *Modified Fuld Object Memory Evaluation*. Madison, WI, USA:

Waisman Center, University of Wisconsin Madison.

Strydom, A., Livingston, M. K. and Hassiotis, A. (2007). Prevalence of dementia in intellectual disability using different diagnostic criteria. *Br J Psychiatry*, 191, 150–7.

Strydom, A., Hassiotis, A., King, M. and Livingston, G. (2009). The relationship of dementia prevalence in older adults with intellectual disability (ID) to age and severity of ID. *Psychol Med*, 39, 13–21.

Tanzi, R. E. (2008). Novel therapeutics for Alzheimer's disease. *Neurotherapeutics*, 5, 377–80.

Temple, V., Jozsvai, E., Konstantareas, M. M. and Hewitt, T.-A. (2001). Alzheimer's dementia in Down's syndrome: the relevance of cognitive ability. *J Intellect Disabil Res*, 45(1), 47–55.

Tiffin, J. and Asher, E. J. (1948). The Purdue pegboard: norms and studies of reliability and validity. *J Appl Psychol*, 32, 234–47.

Upton, N., Chuang, T. T., Hunter, A. J. and Virley, D. J. (2008). 5-HT6 receptor antagonists as novel cognitive enhancing agents for Alzheimer's disease. *Neurotherapeutics*, 5, 458–69.

Visser, F. E., Aldenkamp, A. P., van Huffelen, A. C. *et al.* (1997). Prospective study of the prevalence of Alzheimer-type dementia in institutionalised individuals with Down syndrome. *Am J Ment Retard*, 101, 404–12.

Wolfe, M. S. (2008). Inhibition and modulation of γ-secretase for Alzheimer's disease. *Neurotherapeutics*, 5, 391–8.

Zana, M., Janka, Z. and Kálmán, J. (2007). Oxidative stress: a bridge between Down's syndrome and Alzheimer's disease. *Neurobiol Aging*, 28, 648–76.

Zigman, W. B. and Lott, I. R. (2007). Alzheimer's disease in Down syndrome: neurobiology and Risk. *Ment Retard Dev Disabil*, 13, 237–46.

Zigman, W. B., Schupf, N., Devenny, D. A. *et al.* (2004). Incidence and prevalence of dementia in elderly adults with mental retardation without Down syndrome. *Am J Ment Retard*, 109(2), 126–41.

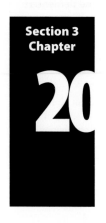

20 Diseases of the nervous system III: cerebral palsy, movement disorders and pain perception

Henry Kwok and Wai-Him Cheung

Introduction

Diseases of the nervous system are often encountered in people with intellectual disability (ID). This is logical and understandable because intelligence is a function of the human brain. Lin *et al.* (2006) found in Taiwan that neurological disorder was the most common illness (12.6%) reported by carers of people with ID (n = 1007) in the previous seven months. This chapter focuses on cerebral palsy (CP), movement disorders and altered pain perception.

Method

Searches in Ovid MEDLINE (R) without Revisions (1950–2008), EMBASE and PsycINFO were made to find all studies on the association between intellectual disabilities (or learning disabilities or mental retardation or mental deficiency) and cerebral palsy, movement disorders and pain.

Results

The results of the searches are shown in Table 20.1

The number of references was 277, 223 and 130 respectively for cerebral palsy, movement disorders and pain. All potentially relevant articles were inspected but more emphasis was put on studies published in the recent years.

Discussion

Cerebral palsy

Cerebral palsy (CP) is a group of non-progressive neurological conditions resulting from brain injury that occurs before cerebral development is complete. It is characterised by impaired body movement and muscle coordination. Pathologically, there is denervation of target neuron centres within the neuraxis. Although compensatory reinnervation occurs by acquiring synaptic sprouts from neurons in the neighbourhood, such reorganisations are often maladaptive and result in incomplete recovery with compromised functioning (Krishnan, 2006). The presentation can be global mental and physical dysfunction or isolated

Intellectual Disability and Ill Health: A Review of the Evidence, ed. Jean O'Hara, Jane McCarthy and Nick Bouras. Published by Cambridge University Press. © Cambridge University Press 2010.

Table 20.1. Search results

	Number of references
Cerebral palsy	277
Movement disorders	223
Pain	130

disturbances in gait, cognition or sensation (Krigger, 2006). Spasticity is common and may result in contractures or joint dislocation.

Epidemiology

Cerebral palsy is not an uncommon condition, with mean prevalence rates of 2.0–2.5 for every 1000 children (Fehlings *et al.*, 2007). The variation in the reported rates among countries may be due to a genuine difference but the study design may also be responsible. In a recent study on the population born between 1990 and 1997 in southern Sweden, the prevalence rate of CP was found to be 2.4/1000 (95% CI 2.1–2.6) in children of 4–11 years of age. This figure excluded postnatally acquired CP and those children who were born aboard (Westbom *et al.*, 2007). Another cohort study in Saudi Arabia covered 99 788 live births at a hospital from 1984 to 2003 (Al-Asmari *et al.*, 2006). Based on medical information collected from medical files, 412 positive cases of children with CP between 1 and 10 years old were identified. This gave a rate of 4.1 per 1000.

Therefore, continued monitoring of the prevalence using a reliable and valid surveillance system is necessary to provide accurate information for planning of services and collaboration of health care for this group of children and adults. One such network is the Surveillance of Cerebral Palsy in Europe (SCPE) aimed at developing a central database across Europe (McManus *et al.*, 2006).

Aetiology and risk factors

Cerebral palsy can be caused by a wide variety of cerebral insults occurring prenatal, perinatal and postnatal. However, the cause remains unknown in 50% of cases (Jan, 2006). Birth asphyxia is an important perinatal cause and neonates who develop severe hypoxic ischaemic encephalopathy have a high risk of neurological sequelae that leads to CP (Premila and Arulkumaran, 2008). The most important neonatal risk factors are prematurity, low birth weight, intrauterine infections and twinning or multiple gestations (Odding *et al.*, 2006; Yan *et al.*, 2006).

Extreme prematurity confers about a 100-fold increase in the risk of CP relative to birth at term gestation (O'Shea, 2008). In a French study that assessed 5-year-old children who were born very preterm (22–32 weeks of gestation) in 1997, CP was diagnosed in 159 (9%) of 1817 surviving children (Larroque *et al.*, 2008). On the other hand, a meta-analysis has found chorioamnionitis to be associated with an increased incidence of CP (Wu and Colford, 2000). One of the human pathogens that can target and damage the fetal brain is lymphocytic choriomeningitis virus (LCMV). A study of 20 children with serologically confirmed infection with this virus all had structural brain anomalies with profound ID, epilepsy and CP (Bonthius *et al.*, 2007).

Types

Cerebral palsy is usually classified according to the clinical presentation. There are four main categories: spastic, dyskinetic (athetoid), ataxic and mixed depending on the type of motor disturbance. The first three categories are in turn due to involvement of the pyramidal tracts, extrapyramidal tracts and the cerebellum respectively. Spastic CP is the commonest type while ataxic CP is the rarest form (Krigger, 2006). Data from Europe for the cohort of people with CP born from 1980 to 1996 (n = 9128) found that 53.9% had bilateral spastic CP, 31.0% had unilateral spastic CP, 6.6% had dyskinetic CP and 4.1% ataxic CP (McManus et al., 2006).

Associated disabilities and impairments

There is a wide continuum of co-morbidity associated with CP. In a review of the literature from 1965 to 2004 by Odding et al. (2006), 25–80% of people with CP had additional impairments. As hemiplegic CP is a less severe condition than quadriplegic CP, it has been demonstrated that the former is also associated with a significantly lower prevalence of cognitive impairments and sensory deficits (Lagunju and Adedokun, 2008). A recent study was carried out in Norway on all children with CP born in 1996–8. A total of 374 children were identified. Intellectual disability was present in 31%, active epilepsy in 28%, severely impaired speech in 28%, severely impaired vision in 5% and severely impaired hearing in 4% of the children (Andersen et al., 2008).

Recent evidence suggests that walking ability could be an indicator of the total disability load in children with CP. In a study that investigated walking ability in 9012 patients gathered from 14 European centres, it was found to be related significantly not only to the type of CP but also to IQ level, active epilepsy and severe visual and hearing impairment. Logistic regression revealed that intellectual capacity was the variable most associated with walking ability in all types of CP. The presence of severe intellectual impairment increased the risk of being unable to walk 56 times in unilateral spastic CP and 9 times in bilateral spastic CP (Beckung et al., 2008).

Management

The goal of management of CP is not to cure but to increase functionality and sustain health in terms of locomotion, cognitive development, social interaction and independence. A multidisciplinary team approach focusing on early intervention and total patient development will bring about the best clinical outcome within the limits of their deficits (Krigger, 2006). Providing family support and improving caregivers' skills are also important elements of the management plan (Raina et al., 2005).

There have been considerable advances in the pharmacological management of spasticity. Early medical intervention may prevent contractures and reduce the need for future orthopaedic operations (Aker and Anderson, 2007). Although the usefulness of botulinum toxin (Botox) is now well recognised, it is recommended that it should always be adjunctive to a programme of physical intervention (Ward, 2008). This toxin is derived from the bacterium clostridium botulinum and it blocks the release of acetylcholine. Truong and Bhidayasiri (2008) commented that its effectiveness in the treatment of sialorrhoea is also established. However, some individuals show no further response after the initial few injections and it has been suggested that the formation of neutralising antibodies against botulinum toxin can be a reason for this phenomenon (Berweck et al., 2007).

Movement disorders

Movement disorders are neurological conditions that affect the speed, fluency, quality and ease of movement of a person. Almost any disease of the nervous system can produce a disorder of movement. They include parkinsonism, dyskinesia, dystonia, tics, chorea and myoclonus. Although clinical features may overlap, recent technological advances in neuro-imaging, genetic studies and neurochemistry have enabled more precise delineation of one motor disorder from another.

Parkinsonism

Parkinsonism refers to a clinical condition that consists of tremor, rigidity and bradykine-sia in the absence of Parkinson's disease. Loss of dopaminergic input to the striatum causes the rigidity and bradykinesia. Thalamic, cerebellar and basal ganglia abnormalities are the probable cause of thalamocortical oscillations underlying the resting tremor (Obeso *et al.*, 1997). Stone *et al.* (1989) found that the prevalence of parkinsonism was 3% in a large sam-ple of people with developmental disability (n = 1227), which was higher than that in general population, and increased with age and male gender.

The majority of parkinsonism observed in people with ID is drug-induced. The com-monest causative agent is a conventional antipsychotic while tetrabenazine, tricyclic antide-pressants and selective 5-hydroxytryptamine (5-HT, serotonin) reuptake inhibitors have also been reported to be associated with this problem (Leo, 1996). Clinical presentations closely resemble Parkinson's disease, although symmetric involvement at onset and the presence of akathisia or dyskinesia help to distinguish the former from the latter. Drug-induced parkin-sonism may continue up to one year after the drug is withdrawn (Kaufman, 2007).

In adults with Down syndrome who develop Alzheimer's disease, 20% were reported to show flexed posture, bradykinesia, masked face and cogwheel rigidity of parkinsonism in their late stage (Lai and Williams, 1989).

Dyskinesia

Dyskinesia is a generic neurological term for 'any type of hyperkinetic movement disorders except tremor' (Marsden *et al.*, 1975).

Guanidinoacetate methyltransferase (GAMT) deficiency is an autosomal recessive disor-der of creatine synthesis. Affected individuals usually present with ID, severe developmental delay, epileptic seizures and movement disorders. Clinical features consist of dyskinetic or dystonic involuntary movements, pyramidal signs and myoclonic jerks. Neuroimaging tech-niques have revealed marked myelination delay (Schulze *et al.*, 1997; Stockler *et al.*, 1996a). Oral substitution of creatine and dietary restriction of arginine may improve the movement disorder but the degree of ID remains unchanged (Stockler *et al.*, 1996b).

Tardive dyskinesia (TD) refers to dyskinesias that develop during the course of long-term exposure to dopamine-blocking agents. People with ID are vulnerable to developing this con-dition (Brasic *et al.*, 2004) and reducing antipsychotic medication in this population was also found to be associated with increased dyskinesia (Ahmed *et al.*, 2000). The involuntary move-ments are usually complex, repetitive and coordinated. They often involve the oral/perioral musculature but sometimes the trunk and limbs may also be affected. The underlying cause is thought to be due to the supersensitivity of dopamine receptors after a period of chronic blockade. Unless carers have received specific training, TD movements may easily be missed in the early stage. Prevention of this condition is important and Taylor (2002) has suggested the use of a screening tool by community nurses to identify an individual's risk of developing TD before commencing antipsychotic medication in people with ID.

Dystonia

Dystonia is a syndrome of sustained muscle contractions, frequently causing twisting and repetitive movements or abnormal postures (Fahn *et al.*, 1987). Dystonia is worse with emotion or stress, improves with relaxation and disappears in sleep.

Lesch-Nyhan syndrome is an X-linked disorder with ID and progressive motor deterioration leading to spasticity, choreoathetosis and dystonia. Affected individuals have deficiency of hypoxanthine-guanine phosphoribosyltransferase. Both self-injurious and violent behaviour are common. Premature death in early adulthood due to respiratory or renal failure is the usual result.

Tics

Tics are involuntary muscle contractions that are sudden, repetitive, stereotypic and rapid in nature. They are often preceded by a premonitory urge and they can be motor or vocal. The prevalence is highly variable and the onset is typically during childhood. The intensity of tics may wax and wane over weeks, months or years. Tourette's syndrome is characterised by multiple motor and vocal tics. A review of the literature by Robertson (2003) has indicated that this syndrome occurs in around 1% of mainstream school children and is even more common in students with special educational needs. Research has suggested that this syndrome is inherited as a highly penetrant, sex-influenced, autosomal dominant trait (Pauls and Leckman, 1986).

Altered pain perception

Pain is defined as an unpleasant sensory and emotional experience associated with actual or potential tissue damage (International Association for the Study of Pain). The subjective experience and the way pain is expressed do not correspond to the magnitude of the stimulus in a simple manner. In people with ID, such a subjective experiential state is further complicated by their impairments in cognitive function, communication skills and motor activities.

Defrin *et al.* (2006) investigated whether level of cognitive impairment affects acute pain behaviour and how it is manifested. In their study, 121 individuals with cognitive impairment (divided into groups of mild, moderate, severe and profound) were compared with 38 controls without cognitive impairment before and during acute pain produced by influenza vaccination. Their behaviours were coded using the Facial Action Coding System (FACS; scores facial reactions to pain) and the Non-communication Children's Pain Checklist (scores both facial and general body reactions). The results showed that both scores of individuals with mild to moderate cognitive impairment increased significantly during vaccination ($p < 0.001$). In contrast, individuals with severe to profound cognitive impairment exhibited high rates of freezing reaction on the face and therefore the FACS scores were not elevated.

In an earlier, similar study, Hennequin *et al.* (2000) compared the latency of cold stimuli on the wrist and the temple between individuals with Down syndrome (n = 26) and a control group with no disability (n = 75). It was found that the group with Down syndrome had significantly longer median detection latencies than the control group and more difficulties in localising the cold stimulus.

The issue of altered pain sensation has also been investigated using the animal model and the histological approach. Price *et al.* (2007) have demonstrated decreased responses to ongoing nociceptive stimuli in mice lacking the Fragile X mental retardation protein. The authors commented that this observation supported the hypothesis that self-injurious behaviour (SIB) in individuals with Fragile X syndrome could be related to deficits in nociceptive sensitisation. On the other hand, microscopic examination of skin biopsy samples from adults with ID with chronic SIB revealed morphological abnormalities in the epidermal nerve fibres with increased substance P fibre density two to three times that of a control group of people without ID and with no SIB (Symons *et al.*, 2008b).

Evidence from research is accumulating to improve our assessment, treatment and understanding of pain in people with ID (Symons *et al.*, 2008a).

Conclusion

Cerebral palsy has been the focus of research for many decades but other movement disorders and altered pain perception in people with ID are receiving increasing attention. These areas of research are important for clinical practice and they also have major implications on the quality of life and psychosocial functioning of this population.

Evidence has clearly shown that CP is associated with a wide range of health problems. Early identification of these co-morbidities and early intervention will often improve individuals' capabilities. Similarly, people with ID are more likely to have medical conditions that are painful, or require painful treatment, such as physiotherapy or surgery (Breau *et al.*, 2007). A better understanding of their pain perception will assist healthcare professionals to develop more effective programmes or strategies to reduce the intrusion of pain in their lives. More research is needed to determine the additional impact of CP, movement disorder and pain on the mental health of people with ID.

References

Ahmed, Z., Fraser, W., Kerr, M. P. *et al.* (2000). Reducing antipsychotic medication in people with a learning disability. *Br J Psychiatry*, 176, 42–6.

Aker, J. and Anderson, D. J. (2007). Perioperative care of patients with cerebral palsy. *AANA J*, 75(1), 65–73.

Al-Asmari, A., Al Moutaery, K., Akhdar, F. and Al Jadid, M. (2006). Cerebral palsy: incidence and clinical features in Saudi Arabia. *Disabil Rehabil*, 28(22), 1373–7.

Andersen, G. L., Irgens, L. M., Haagaas, I. *et al.* (2008). Cerebral palsy in Norway: prevalence, subtypes and severity. *Eur J Paediatr Neurol*, 12(1), 4–13.

Beckung, E., Hagberg, G., Uldall, P. and Cans, C. (2008). Probability of walking in children with cerebral palsy in Europe. *Paediatrics*, 121(1), e187–92.

Berweck, S., Schroeder, A. S., Lee, S. H., Bigalke, H. and Heinen, F. (2007). Secondary non-response due to antibody formation in a child after three injections of botulinum toxin B into the salivary glands. *Dev Med Child Neurol*, 49(1), 62–4.

Bonthius, D. J., Wright, R., Tseng, B. *et al.* (2007). Congenital lymphocytic choriomeningitis virus infection: spectrum of disease. *Ann Neurol*, 62(4), 347–55.

Brasic, J. R., Barnett, J. Y., Kowalik, S., Tsaltas, M. O. and Ahmad, R. (2004). Neurobehavioural assessment of children and adolescents attending a developmental disabilities clinic. *Psychol Rep*, 95(3 Pt 2), 1079–86.

Breau, L. M., Camfield, C. S., McGrath, P. J. and Finley, G. A. (2007). Pain's impact on adaptive functioning. *J Intellect Disab Res*, 51(Pt 2), 125–34.

Defrin, R., Lotan, M. and Pick, C. G. (2006). The evaluation of acute pain in individuals with cognitive impairment: a differential effect of the level of impairment. *Pain*, 124(3), 312–20.

Fahn, S., Marsden, C. D. and Calne, D. B. (1987). Classification and investigation of dystonia. In *Movement Disorders*, Vol. 2, (ed. S. Fahn and C. D. Marsden). London: Butterworths, pp. 332–58.

Fehlings, D., Hunt, C. and Rosenbaum, P. (2007). Cerebral Palsy. In *A Comprehensive Guide to Intellectual and Developmental Disabilities*, ed. I. Brown and M. Percy. Baltimore MD, USA: Paul H. Brookes Publishing, pp. 279–85.

Hennequin, M., Morin, C. and Feine, J. S. (2000). Pain expression and stimulus localisation in individuals with Down's syndrome. *Lancet*, 356(9245), 1882–7.

International Association for the Study of Pain (http://www.iasp-pain.org).

Jan, M. M. (2006). Cerebral palsy: comprehensive review and update. *Ann Saudi Med*, 26(2), 123–32.

Kaufman, D. M. (2007). Involuntary movement disorders. In *Clinical Neurology for Psychiatrists*, 6th edn. Philadelphia: W. B. Saunders, pp. 401–64.

Krigger, K. W. (2006). Cerebral palsy: an overview. *Am Fam Physician*, 73(1), 91–100.

Krishnan, R. V. (2006). Relearning toward motor recovery in stroke, spinal cord injury, and cerebral palsy: a cognitive neural systems perspective. *Int J Neurosci*, 116(2), 127–40.

Lagunju, I. A. and Adedokun, B. O. (2008). A comparison of quadriplegic and hemiplegic cerebral palsy. *J Paediatr Neurol*, 6(1), 25–30.

Lai, F. and Williams, R. S. (1989). A prospective study of Alzheimer disease in Down syndrome. *Arch Neurol*, 46(8), 849–53.

Larroque, B., Ancel, P. Y., Marret, S. *et al.*, EPIPAGE Study Group. (2008). Neurodevelopmental disabilities and special care of 5-year-old children born before 33 weeks of gestation (the EPIPAGE study): a longitudinal cohort study. *Lancet*, 371(9615), 813–20.

Leo, R. J. (1996). Movement disorders associated with the serotonin selective reuptake inhibitors. *J Clin Psychiatry*, 57(10), 449–54.

Lin, J. D., Yen, C. F., Loh, C. H. *et al.* (2006). A cross-sectional study of the characteristics and determinants of emergency care utilisation among people with intellectual disabilities in Taiwan. *Res Dev Disabil*, 27(6), 657–67.

Marsden, C. D., Tarsy, D. and Baldessarini, R. J. (1975). Spontaneous and drug-induced movement disorders in psychotic patients. In *Psychiatric Aspects of Neurological Disease*, ed. D. F. Benson and D. Blumer. New York: Grune and Stratton, pp. 219–66.

McManus, V., Guillem, P., Surman, G. and Cans, C. (2006). SCPE work, standardisation and definition – an overview of the activities of SCPE: a collaboration of European CP registers. *Zhongguo Dang Dai Er Ke Za Zhi*, 8(4), 261–5.

Obeso, J. A., Guridi, J., Obeso, J. A. and DeLong, M. (1997). Surgery for Parkinson's disease. *J Neurol Neurosurg Psychiatry*, 62(1), 2–8.

Odding, E., Roebroeck, M. E. and Stam, H. J. (2006). The epidemiology of cerebral palsy: incidence, impairments and risk factors. *Disabil Rehabil*, 28(4), 183–91.

O'Shea, M. (2008). Cerebral palsy. *Semin Perinatol*, 32(1), 35–41.

Pauls, D. L. and Leckman, J. F. (1986). The inheritance of Gilles de la Tourette's syndrome and associated behaviours. Evidence for autosomal dominant transmission. *N Engl J Med*, 315, 993–7.

Premila, S. and Arulkumaran, S. (2008). Intrapartum fetal surveillance. *Obstet, Gynaecol Reprod Med*, 18(1), 12–17.

Price, T. J., Rashid, M. H., Millecamps, M. *et al.* (2007). Decreased nociceptive sensitization in mice lacking the fragile X mental retardation protein: role of mGluR $1/5$ and mTOR. *J Neurosci*, 27(51), 13958–67.

Raina, P., O'Donnell, M., Rosenbaum, P. *et al.* (2005). The health and well-being of caregivers of children with cerebral palsy. *Paediatrics*, 115(6), e626–36.

Robertson, M. M. (2003). Diagnosing Tourette syndrome: is it a common disorder? *J Psychosom Res*, 55(1), 3–6.

Schulze, A., Hess, T., Wevers, R. *et al.* (1997). Creatine deficiency syndrome caused by guanidinoacetate methyltransferase deficiency: diagnostic tools for a new inborn error of metabolism. *J Paediatr*, 131(4), 626–31.

Stockler, S., Hanefeld, F. and Frahm, J. (1996a). Creatine replacement therapy in guanidinoacetate methyltransferase deficiency, a novel inborn error of metabolism. *Lancet*, 348(9030), 789–90.

Stockler, S., Isbrandt, D., Hanefeld, F., Schmidt, B. and von Figura, K. (1996b). Guanidinoacetate methyltransferase deficiency: the first inborn error of creatine metabolism in man. *Am J Hum Genet*, 58(5), 914–22.

Stone, R. K., May, J. E., Alvarez, W. F. and Ellman, G. (1989). Prevalence of dyskinesia and related movement disorders in a developmentally disabled population. *J Ment Defic Res*, 33(Pt 1), 41–53.

Symons, F. J., Shinde, S. K. and Gilles, E. (2008a). Perspectives on pain and intellectual disability. *J Intellect Disabil Res*, 52, 275–86.

Symons, F. J., Wendelschafer-Crabb, G., Kennedy, W. *et al.* (2008b). Evidence of altered epidermal nerve fiber morphology in adults with self-injurious behaviour and neurodevelopmental disorders. *Pain*, 134(1–2), 232–7.

Taylor, J. (2002). Development of a screening tool to assess risk of tardive dyskinesia. *Br J Nurs*, 11(6), 374–8.

Truong, D. D. and Bhidayasiri, R. (2008). Evidence for the effectiveness of botulinum toxin for sialorrhoea. *J Neural Transm*, 115(4), 631–5.

Ward, A. B. (2008). Spasticity treatment with botulinum toxins. *J Neural Transm*, 115(4), 607–16.

Westbom, L., Hagglund, G. and Nordmark, E. (2007). Cerebral palsy in a total population of 4–11 year olds in southern Sweden. Prevalence and distribution according to different CP classification systems. *BMC Paediatr*, 7, 41.

Wu, Y. W. and Colford, J. M. Jr. (2000). Chorioamnionitis as a risk factor for cerebral palsy: a meta-analysis. *JAMA*, 284(11), 1417–24.

Yan, H., Zhang, H. J., Qin, R. *et al.* (2006). Characteristics of 40 twins with cerebral palsy. *Chin J Clin Rehabil*, 10(8), 44–6.

Index

Note: page numbers in *italics* refer to figures, tables and boxes.